COMPLICATIONS OF MYOCARDIAL INFARCTION

Clinical Diagnostic Imaging Atlas

DVD Table of Contents

Complications of
Myocardial Infarction

CLINICAL DIAGNOSTIC IMAGING ATLAS

Complications of Myocardial Infarction

CLINICAL DIAGNOSTIC IMAGING ATLAS

Stuart J. Hutchison
MD, FRCPC, FACC, FAHA, FASE, FSCMR, FSCCT

Clinical Associate Professor of Medicine
University of Calgary
Foothills Medical Center
Stephenson Cardiac Magnetic
Resonance Imaging Center
Libin Cardiovascular Institute of Alberta
Calgary, Canada

SAUNDERS

ELSEVIER

Original artwork and animations by
Gail Rudakewich, Myra Rudakewich, and **Stuart J. Hutchison**

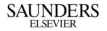

SAUNDERS
ELSEVIER

1600 John F. Kennedy Blvd.
Ste 1800
Philadelphia, PA 19103-2899

COMPLICATIONS OF MYOCARDIAL INFARCTION: ISB3N: 978-1-4160-5272-2
CLINICAL DIAGNOSTIC IMAGING ATLAS

Notice

Knowledge and best practice in this field are constantly changing. As new research and experience broaden our knowledge, changes in practice, treatment, and drug therapy may become necessary or appropriate. Readers are advised to check the most current information provided (i) on procedures featured or (ii) by the manufacturer of each product to be administered, to verify the recommended dose or formula, the method and duration of administration, and contraindications. It is the responsibility of the practitioner, relying on his or her experience and knowledge of the patient, to make diagnoses, to determine dosages and the best treatment for each individual patient, and to take all appropriate safety precautions. To the fullest extent of the law, neither the Publisher nor the Author assumes any liability for any injury and/or damage to persons or property arising out of or related to any use of the material contained in this book.

The Publisher

Library of Congress Cataloging-in-Publication Data
Hutchison, Stuart J.
    Complications of myocardial infarction : clinical diagnostic imaging atlas with DVD / Stuart J. Hutchison.—
1st ed.
        p. ; cm.—(Cardiovascular emergencies : atlas and multimedia series)
    Includes bibliographical references.
    ISBN 978-1-4160-5272-2
    1. Myocardial infarction—Complications—Atlases.   2. Cardiovascular system—Imaging—Atlases.
I. Title.   II. Series.
    [DNLM: 1. Myocardial Infarction—complications—Atlases.   2. Myocardial Infarction—diagnosis—
Atlases.   3. Diagnostic Techniques, Cardiovascular—Atlases. WG 17 H978c 2009]
    RC685.I6H88 2009
    616.1′2075—dc22   2008018561

Executive Publisher: Natasha Andjelkovic
Publishing Services Manager: Frank Polizzano
Project Manager: Rachel Miller
Design Direction: Lou Forgione
Illustration Direction: Ceil Nuyianes
Multimedia Producer: Bruce Robison

Printed in China.

Last digit is the print number: 9   8   7   6   5   4   3   2   1

To Noel Keith and Cindy Hutchison, for the immeasurable gifts of love and time.

To Keith Radley Hutchison (1957–1997)
and Richard Ross Hutchison (1936–2005)—*memor esto.*

To my father, J. Lawrence Hutchison, surely one of the most natural physicians I have ever known. Gracious and studious, open-minded and strictly honest, progressive and tenacious when someone needed him to be, he taught a great many by example. In an era when medicine lost its way, he practiced it as it was always meant to be—a calling.

Foreword

I am very pleased and honored to introduce the book titled *Complications of Myocardial Infarction: Clinical Diagnostic Imaging Atlas* written by Dr. Stuart Hutchison. Dr. Hutchison is the sole author of this outstanding book, which deals with the complications of acute myocardial infarction. This text-atlas describes not only the myriad potential complications of acute myocardial infarction but also their pathophysiology, epidemiology, diagnosis, and management. It also describes the process of remodeling, diagnosis of the ischemic-infarcted myocardium, and the potential therapies for prevention of remodeling. Thus, although the focus of this work is on the application of the latest imaging modalities for timely and accurate diagnosis, it also provides up-to-date information for various aspects of prevention and therapy of the complications of acute myocardial infarction. This book documents all the imaging modalities available today to illustrate all the aspects of the complications of acute myocardial infarction.

I have been involved in the studies of acute coronary syndromes for over three decades and have never encountered a book as clinically useful as this one. Sincerest congratulations to Dr. Hutchison on such an outstanding book.

Kanu Chatterjee, MB, FRCP, FACC, FCCP, MACP
Ernest Gallo Distinguished Professor of Medicine
Chatterjee Center for Cardiac Research
University of California, San Francisco
San Francisco, California

Preface

The principal responsibility and the purpose of coronary care is to minimize the complications of myocardial infarction and thereby the loss of patients' lives and their burden of symptoms. The coronary care unit (CCU) is an endlessly challenging, inevitably purposeful, always humbling, and definitely satisfying venue for practicing medicine, for teaching from within, and for continuing to learn both about the nature of disease and about the relevance of medical technology and therapeutics.

Patients don't die of myocardial infarctions—they die of complications of infarction. The large majority of cases of myocardial infarction evolve well, without complication, and remain low-risk throughout. A minority of patients, though, develop complications and become at risk of death, thereby representing the most significant CCU cases—the ones faced with the highest risk, and the ones wherein prompt recognition of complications and their adept management do save lives—the rationale, and raison d'être, of the CCU. The complicated cases of infarction become the focus, justification, and purpose of CCU professionals. Although the algorithmic management of coronary syndromes has hugely advanced the management of patients with coronary syndromes, the management of patients with complications of myocardial infarctions remains individualized, discretionary, and both taxing and validating of clinical skill and dedication, in success and defeat. The ablest of clinical teams relentlessly focus on anticipating complications of infarction.

Some complications of infarction, such as most degrees of heart failure, are managed solely within the realm of the CCU, but others require timely mobilization of the cardiac surgery, cardiac anesthesia, and critical care services. Interservice cooperation and coordination are often best exemplified by the management of such emergent cases.

My sustained interest in the complicated cases of myocardial infarction is based on their indisputable and dominant relevance to the dedication and professionalism of CCU physicians, nurses, and trainees. The highest-risk cases are simply the ones in which our impact, relevance, and contribution are the greatest. It is my hope that by review of chapters that emphasize the relation of coronary anatomy to pathology and associated pathophysiology and also the anatomic and physiologic basis of imaging, the reader will learn the background of and gain a handle on the reality of these most important of CCU cases.

In this book and its companion DVD, I have tried to present a systematic and integrated approach to the complications of infarction and to offer a complementary case-based approach with each chapter. The chapters and cases in the book present still images, and the DVD offers the respective dynamic images; thus, it is a true companion to the book's content.

Stuart J. Hutchison, MD

Acknowledgments

I would like to extend my sincere appreciation and gratitude to Inga Tomas; Simon Abrahmson, MD; Natasha Andjelkovic, PhD; Daniel Bonneau, MD; Jagdish Butany, MD; John Burgess, MD; Jason Burstein, MD; Warren Cantor, MD; Kanu Chatterjee, MB; Robert Chisholm, MD; the CCU, cardiac ward, cardiac OR, and CVICU nurses; Patrick Disney, MD; Lee Errett, MD; Neil Fam, MD; Matthias Friedrich, MD; Michael Heffernan, MD; Majo Joseph, MD; David Latter, MD; Yves Leclerc, MD; Anne Lenehan; Mat Lotfi, MD; Danny Marcuzzi, MD; David Mazer, MD; Rachel Miller; Abdulelah Mobeirek, MD; Juan Carlos Monge, MD; Ashok Mukherjee, MD; Mark Peterson, MD; Susan Pioli; Bill Parmley, MD; Geoffrey Puley, MD; Michael Regan; Gail Rudakewich; Myra Rudakewich; Nazmi Said, RVT; Jan-Peter Smedema, MD; Jim Stewart, MD; Bradley Strauss, MD; Subodh Verma, MD; Randy Watson, MD; and Andrew Yan, MD.

Stuart J. Hutchison, MD

Abbreviations

ACC/AHA, American College of Cardiology/American Heart Association
ACE, angiotensin-converting enzyme
ACE-I, angiotensin-converting enzyme inhibitor
ACS, acute coronary syndrome
AI, aortic insufficiency
ALPM, anterolateral papillary muscle
AMI, acute myocardial infarction
AS, aortic stenosis
ASA, acetylsalicylic acid
AV, atrioventricular
BBB, bundle branch block
BiPAP, bilevel positive airway pressure
BP, blood pressure
bpm, beats per minute
BSA, body surface area
CAD, coronary artery disease
CCS, Canadian Cardiovascular Society
CCU, coronary care unit
CHF, congestive heart failure
CI, cardiac index; confidence interval
CK, creatine kinase
CO, cardiac output
COPD, chronic obstructive pulmonary disease
CPR, cardiopulmonary resuscitation
CPS, cardiopericardial silhouette
CT, computed tomography
CVP, central venous pressure
DBP, diastolic blood pressure
DVT, deep venous thrombosis
ECG, electrocardiography; electrocardiogram
EDP, end-diastolic pressure
EF, ejection fraction
EMS, emergency medical services
ERNA, equilibrium radionuclide angiography
ESV, end-systolic volume
ESVI, end-systolic volume index
ET, endotracheal
GI, gastrointestinal
HR, heart rate
IABP, intra-aortic balloon counterpulsation
ICD, implantable cardioverter-defibrillator
ICU, intensive care unit
INR, international normalized ratio

IV, intravenous
IVC, inferior vena cava
IVRT, isovolumic relaxation time
JVD, jugular venous distention
JVP, jugular venous pressure
LA, left atrium; left atrial
LAD, left anterior descending coronary artery
LAO, left anterior oblique
LBBB, left bundle branch block
LCA, left coronary artery
LCx, left circumflex artery
LLSB, left lower sternal border
LMCA, left main coronary artery
LV, left ventricle; left ventricular
LVAD, left ventricular assist device
LVEDP, left ventricular end-diastolic pressure
LVEDVI, left ventricular end-diastolic volume index
LVEF, left ventricular ejection fraction
LVH, left ventricular hypertrophy
LVOT, left ventricular outflow tract
LVSP, left ventricular systolic pressure
MAP, mean arterial pressure
MDP, mean diastolic pressure
MI, myocardial infarction
MR, magnetic resonance; mitral regurgitation
MRI, magnetic resonance imaging
MUGA, multiple gated acquisition
NIDDM, non–insulin-dependent diabetes mellitus
NSAIDs, nonsteroidal anti-inflammatory drugs
NYHA, New York Heart Association
OM, obtuse marginal branch
OR, odds ratio
PA, pulmonary artery
PACs, premature atrial contractions
PAP, pulmonary artery pressure
PCI, percutaneous coronary intervention
PCWP, pulmonary capillary wedge pressure
PDA, posterior descending coronary artery
PE, pulmonary embolism
PEA, pulseless electrical activity
PEEP, positive end-expiratory pressure
PFO, patent foramen ovale
PISA, proximal isovelocity surface area
PIV, posterior descending interventricular

PMPM, posteromedial papillary muscle
PMR, papillary muscle rupture
PND, paroxysmal nocturnal dyspnea
PTCA, percutaneous transluminal coronary angioplasty
PVCs, premature ventricular contractions
PVR, pulmonary vascular resistance
RA, right atrium; right atrial
RAO, right anterior oblique
RAP, right atrial pressure
RCA, right coronary artery
RLSB, right lower sternal border
RR, respiratory rate
RV, right ventricle; right ventricular
RVEF, right ventricular ejection fraction
RVH, right ventricular hypertrophy
RVMI, right ventricular myocardial infarction
RVOT, right ventricular outflow tract
RVSP, right ventricular systolic pressure
SA, sinoatrial
SAM, systolic anterior motion
SBP, systolic blood pressure
SEM, systolic ejection murmur

SPECT, single-photon emission computed tomography
SSFP, steady-state free precession
STEMI, ST elevation myocardial infarction
SV, saphenous vein; stroke volume
SVC, superior vena cava
SVR, systemic vascular resistance
SW, stroke work
SWI, stroke work index
TEE, transesophageal echocardiography
TIMI, Thrombolysis in Acute Myocardial Infarction
TnI, troponin I
tPA, tissue-type plasminogen activator
TR, tricuspid regurgitation
TTE, transthoracic echocardiography
TVI, time-velocity integral
VD, ventricular dilation
VF, ventricular fibrillation
VSD, ventricular septal defect
VSR, ventricular septal rupture
VT, ventricular tachycardia
VTI, velocity-time integral
WMSI, wall motion score index

Contents

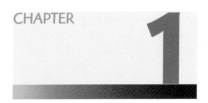

CHAPTER

1

Cardiogenic Shock

Treat the treatable. Reverse the reversible.

KEY POINTS

▶ Most cardiogenic shock is due to left ventricular pump failure, although 10% is due to mechanical complications, which are managed differently.

▶ Most cardiogenic shock develops in the hospital and is not present at admission.

▶ Recognition of cardiogenic shock remains clinically difficult and necessitates repeated bedside examination, composite assessment, and often balloon flotation pulmonary artery catheterization.

▶ Physical diagnosis findings are less sensitive in the setting of cardiogenic shock, necessitating use of noninvasive imaging and invasive assessment.

▶ Early angiography, IABP support, and revascularization (percutaneous coronary intervention and aortocoronary bypass surgery) as is appropriate for coronary anatomy and clinical context are all indicated.

DEFINITION AND ETIOLOGY OF CARDIOGENIC SHOCK

Cardiogenic shock develops in 7% to 10% of patients admitted with acute myocardial infarction and remains the principal cause of in-hospital death of patients experiencing acute infarction.[1] The mortality of cardiogenic shock depends on the patient's profile.[2] Although the mortality from cardiogenic shock is believed to be decreasing, it still is likely to exceed 80%, and other than prehospital cardiac arrest, it is the worst complication of acute infarction that may arise.

The syndrome of cardiogenic shock is one of organ dysfunction due to hypoperfusion caused by cardiac dysfunction. The heart itself is susceptible to the hypoperfusion it is causing and also to the consequences of peripheral organ failure (hypoxemia, fluid overload, metabolic depression)—thus, in cardiogenic shock, the usual occurrence of accumulating metabolic insults and of progressive deterioration.

Cardiogenic shock ensues when cardiac compensatory mechanisms fall short of achieving a cardiac output that is adequate to sustain peripheral organ function. The most obvious cardiac compensatory mechanism is that of tachycardia, which affords an expensive means to compensate for reduced forward stroke volume, as it increases myocardial oxygen demand. The presence of hypotension despite tachycardia bespeaks critically reduced stroke volume and essentially that compensatory mecha-

nisms of tachycardia, recruitment of myocardial reserve, and peripheral vasoconstriction have not been able to normalize blood pressure to its usual state (which for many patients with cardiogenic shock is actually of hypertension). The hyperadrenergic state of cardiogenic shock recruits myocardial contractility in nondiseased myocardial segments supplied by nonsignificantly diseased coronary arteries. Peripheral compensatory mechanisms to maintain blood pressure include venoconstriction to increase effective circulating blood volume, withdrawal of parasympathetic tone, and increase in neurohormonal activation (renin-angiotensin-aldosterone, vasopressin) leading to peripheral arterial vasoconstriction. Although increasing peripheral resistance increases blood pressure, it also reduces tissue perfusion. In cardiogenic shock, given the often high systemic vascular resistance that can be achieved in previously hypertensive patients, there is frankly poor correlation between blood pressure and tissue perfusion. It is unproven that overall clinical outcomes are improving among cardiogenic shock cases. Reperfusion is likely to be improving outcomes, but at the same time, the population is aging, increasing overall mortality.

Overt shock is readily recognized but less than overt shock; it remains a difficult and often belated diagnosis. There is no adequate single clinical finding, test, modality, or parameter to identify cardiogenic shock; hence, cardiogenic shock remains a clinical diagnosis based on the composite findings of bedside observations of poor tissue perfusion (agitation, diminished level of consciousness, cool extremities, oliguria), of serum lactate and mixed venous saturation, and of hemodynamic measurements of severely reduced cardiac index despite adequate or elevated filling pressures. Use of blood pressure alone to exclude the presence of shock is prone to error given the imperfect correlation of blood pressure to perfusion in cardiogenic shock, an unknown baseline state of frank hypertension in many patients, and the hyperadrenergic and hypertensive response to stress in many older and previously hypertensive patients. A systolic blood pressure less than 90 mm Hg is strongly suggestive of shock in cardiac patients. A fall of blood pressure by more than 25% to 30% is also consistent with shock, but unfortunately the baseline blood pressure level is seldom known at the time of presentation with myocardial infarction.

The large majority of cases of cardiogenic shock represent complications of myocardial infarction, but cardiogenic shock in other cases may be due to acute or chronic myopathic disease, valvular disease, pericardial disease, congenital heart disease, or to mixed cardiac diseases. By far the most common (65% to 80%) cause of postinfarction cardiogenic shock is pump failure (Fig. 1-1), but "mechanical complications" (myocardial ruptures—free wall, septal, and papillary; development of severe "ischemic" mitral regurgitation) and right ventricular infarction or failure account for up to 12% of cardiogenic shock cases.[2,3] A few cases of postinfarction cardiogenic shock result from apical infarction and dynamic left ventricular outflow tract (LVOT) obstruction. The different therapeutic options for the different causes of cardiogenic shock require that the specific causes of shock be promptly established.

Clinical factors, such as age and female gender, do correlate with risk in cardiogenic shock, but indices of left ventricular "pump" function, such as cardiac power index (mean arterial pressure × cardiac index/451) (W), are the strongest predictors of outcome of this disorder that is dominated by pump failure.[4]

There are differences in the populations of patients with ST elevation myocardial infarction (STEMI) and non-STEMI that develop cardiogenic shock. Non-STEMI patients are older, are more commonly diabetic, and generally have underlying multi-vessel disease and develop shock progressively while in the hospital rather than at admission.[5] As Table 1-1 reveals, most cardiogenic shock states occur in the hospital (after admission) rather than at admission. In the SHOCK registry, it was observed that at admission, 10% of cardiogenic shock cases had developed; by 6 hours, 47% of shock cases had developed; and by 24 hours, 75% of cardiogenic shock cases had developed, leaving only the remaining 25% to occur or to be recognized after 24 hours.[6] Similar observations were made in the GUSTO I trial.[7] Cardiogenic shock occurs earlier when it is caused by STEMI rather than by non-STEMI, when it is due to left main coronary disease or right coronary artery (RCA) disease rather than left anterior descending (LAD) coronary artery disease. Ongoing ischemia and recurrent ischemia are prominent causes of later development of cardiogenic shock. The 10-hour period for STEMI and the 3-day period for non-STEMI cases to develop shock[5] highlights the importance of repeated evaluation during the first several days in the hospital to identify the occurrence of shock before irreversible organ dysfunction has ensued.

In the majority of cases, cardiogenic shock is progressive because the hypotension and metabolic consequences of inadequate peripheral tissue perfusion (metabolic acidosis or acidemia, hypoxemia, myocardial depressant factors) are detrimental to remaining cardiac function and vascular tone, resulting in myocardial depression, bradycardia, and vasodepression. Falling arterial blood pressure, in combination with elevated filling pressures, leads to a fall in the myocardial perfusion gradient.

Coronary autoregulation, achieved by degrees of resistance of vessel vasodilation or constriction, is able to maintain coronary blood flow appropriate to myocardial demands, across a range of blood pressures (Fig. 1-2). Myocardial ischemia eliminates coronary autoregulation and renders the myocardium highly dependent on adequate aortic diastolic pressure. Progressive hypotension contributes to deterioration of myocardial function. Many other factors can contribute, such as infarct expansion or early aneurysm formation, ongoing ischemia or infarction (of the infarct "penumbra"), recurrent ischemia or infarction, ischemia at distance, ischemic mitral regurgitation, falling transmural perfusion pressure, and collateral interdependence (Fig. 1-3).

Pathologic evaluation of hearts of individuals dying of cardiogenic shock reveals little that would be unexpected, other than a high incidence of left ventricular thrombi due to local low flow aggravated by low overall cardiac output.

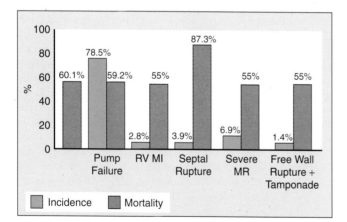

Figure 1-1. The large majority (78.5%) of SHOCK registry cases were left ventricular pump failure. Right ventricular infarction and "mechanical complications" accounted for the remainder. MI, myocardial infarction; MR, mitral regurgitation; RV, right ventricle. (From Hochman JS, Buller CE, Sleeper LA, et al: Cardiogenic shock complicating acute myocardial infarction—etiologies, management and outcome: a report from the SHOCK Trial Registry. Should we emergently revascularize Occluded Coronaries for cardiogenic shocK? J Am Coll Cardiol 2000;36[Suppl A]:1063-1070, with permission from Elsevier.)

Table 1-1. Differences in the STEMI and non-STEMI Patient Populations That Develop Cardiogenic Shock

	STEMI	Non-STEMI
Occurrence	4.2%	2.9%
Time to onset of shock	9.6 hr	76.2 hr
Average age	70 yr	73 yr
Prior MI	24%	44%
Diabetic	21%	34%
Three-vessel CAD	30%	65%
30-day mortality	63%	73%

CAD, coronary artery disease; MI, myocardial infarction; STEMI, ST elevation myocardial infarction.

From Holmes DR Jr, Berger PB, Hochman JS, et al: Cardiogenic shock in patients with acute ischemic syndromes with and without ST-segment elevation. Circulation 1999;100:2067.

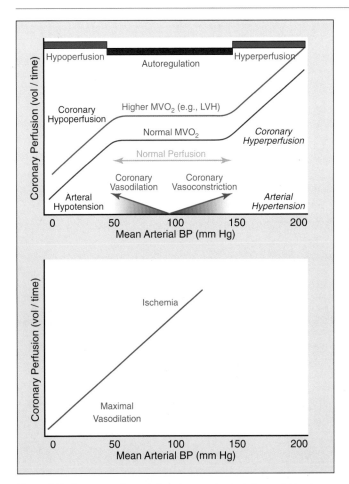

Figure 1-2. Coronary autoregulation ensures steady delivery of blood flow, appropriate to a myocardial work expenditure, across a range of blood pressures. Autoregulation is achieved by resistance vessel vasodilation to increase flow at lower perfusion pressure and vasoconstriction to reduce perfusion at higher perfusion pressure. Because the amount of vasodilation and vasoconstriction that can be effected is finite, it is possible for tissue to be hypoperfused or hyperperfused. In ischemia, there is maximal vasodilation; hence, there is a linear perfusion pressure : flow relationship and a critical reliance on driving pressure and transmural perfusion pressure. LVH, left ventricular hypertrophy.

Angiographic Disease in Cardiogenic Shock

The underlying coronary artery anatomic patterns that may be seen in cardiogenic shock cases are quite variable, other than the finding of occlusions or poor flow (TIMI 0 or I), which is seen in two thirds (67%) of both pump failure and mechanical complications cases. The mean ejection fraction of cardiogenic shock cases is 33% ± 14%,[3] indicating that an acute fall of stroke volume to less than half of normal incites shock. A slight majority of pump failure cases have three-vessel coronary artery disease (56%) or left mainstem disease (16%). LAD disease is responsible for 42% of cardiogenic shock cases, RCA disease for 30%, and left circumflex disease for only 14%. Left mainstem saphenous graft disease accounts for the remainder.

General characteristics of myocardial infarction patients who develop cardiogenic shock versus those who do not include older age, female gender, diabetes, second (or third) infarction, anterior infarction, and STEMI or Q-wave infarction (Fig. 1-4).[8]

DIAGNOSIS OF CARDIOGENIC SHOCK

Initial Assessment of Cardiogenic Shock

Initial assessment of cardiogenic shock should include the following:

- Brief history: time to onset of symptoms, chest pain, shortness of breath, previous cardiac disease and treatments, review of symptoms (fevers)
- Physical examination (Table 1-2): determination of vitals, identification of pulsus paradoxus, right- versus left-sided heart failure, murmurs or thrills, gallops, apex characteristics, peripheral perfusion, pulmonary congestion and Killip class
- Electrocardiography: rhythm, rate, ST deviation, voltage
- Chest radiography: heart size; pulmonary vasculature and edema
- O_2 saturation (oximetry, arterial blood gases)
- Chemistries, renal function, biomarkers, lactate
- Blood counts

The Challenge of Recognizing Shock

A heart rate above 100 bpm and a systolic blood pressure below 100 mm Hg (the "100 thing") are conspicuous and worrisome findings that indicate that recruiting tachycardia was not adequate to sustain blood pressure. Outcomes in such patients are nearly as poor as in those with cardiogenic shock of conventional definition.

Recognition of cardiogenic shock is critical but unfortunately often not straightforward; the systematic tendency is to underrecognize findings. At least one sixth of myocardial infarction cases with an elevated pulmonary capillary wedge pressure (PCWP) and one sixth of cases of low cardiac index (CI) are not recognized clinically. The percentages are higher in cardiogenic shock.[9]

Older acute myocardial infarction categorization schemes (Killip classification)[10] emphasized pulmonary edema findings, but it has emerged that physical diagnosis of pulmonary edema is poor in shock cases. Accordingly, the clinical category of absence of pulmonary edema does not establish a better prognosis than that of presence of pulmonary edema.[11]

Poor mentation, urine output of less than 35 mL/hr, and cool extremities are bedside signs of low output. However, use of these signs fails to recognize 15% to 25% of cases in which the cardiac index is proven to be less than 2.2 L/min/m².

Pulmonary rales, although present in most cases of shock, are absent in a significant subset, often because inspiratory effort is failing or there is underlying lung disease. Rales are absent in 15% to 25% of cases of heart failure and in an even higher percentage of cardiogenic shock cases. In the SHOCK registry, the patient subset of "isolated hypoperfusion" (identified by bedside clinical assessment and chest radiography) was composed of many cases with PCWP above 18 mm Hg; the mean PCWP of the isolated hypoperfusion subset was 22 mm Hg, and that of the pulmonary edema subset was 24 mm Hg. Furthermore, the mortality of patients without clinical pulmonary edema was not less than that of those with pulmonary edema (70% versus 60%; P = .04). It appears that among shock patients, the recognition of pulmonary edema is at its worst; 28% of proven cardiogenic shock

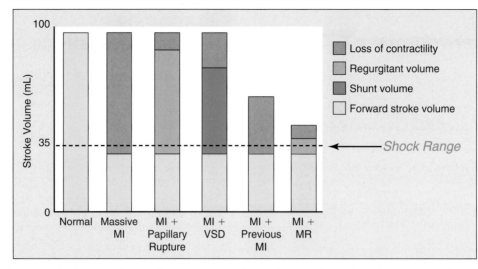

Figure 1-3. The fundamental basis of shock is tissue dysfunction due to inadequate tissue perfusion. In cardiogenic shock, the loss of forward stroke volume is critical and cannot be sufficiently compensated for by increasing heart rate. Normal stroke volume index is 45 ± 13 mL/m^2; hence, the average stroke volume for an adult man is approximately 100 mL. A critically reduced stroke volume can occur for several individual reasons or combined reasons. The loss of contractile function from a massive infarction, a small loss of contractile function (small infarction) and large regurgitant volume (severe MR), a moderate loss of contractile function (moderate-sized infarct) and a large shunt volume (VSD flow), and a reduced initial stroke volume due to prior infarction combined with an acute fall in contractile function with or without new regurgitant lesions may all result in an inadequate forward stroke volume. MI, myocardial infarction; MR, mitral regurgitation; VSD, ventricular septal defect.

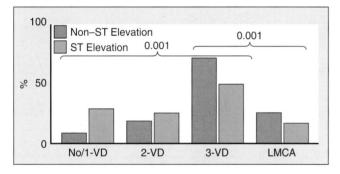

Figure 1-4. Most non–ST elevation infarctions are due to three-vessel coronary artery disease (3-VD) or left main coronary artery (LMCA) disease. (From Jacobs AK, French JK, Col J, et al: Cardiogenic shock with non–ST-segment elevation myocardial infarction: a report from the SHOCK Trial Registry. SHould we emergently revascularize Occluded coronaries for Cardiogenic shocK? J Am Coll Cardiol 2000;36[Suppl A]:1091-1096, with permission from Elsevier.)

cases did not appear to have pulmonary edema. Absence of clinically evident pulmonary edema does not exclude a diagnosis of cardiogenic shock and is not associated with a better prognosis (Fig. 1-5).

Electrocardiography and Cardiogenic Shock

Elevated heart rate (tachycardia) bespeaks inadequate stroke volume, significant hypoxia, or pain. Atrial fibrillation, the most common tachyarrhythmia, suggests elevated left atrial pressure or left atrial distention, lessens left ventricular filling, and may increase myocardial oxygen consumption if the ventricular response is tachycardic. ST deviations are significant findings. ST elevation is useful to localize the site of infarction except for the posterior territory, which is systematically underrepresented on the surface electrocardiogram. ST elevation results from acute

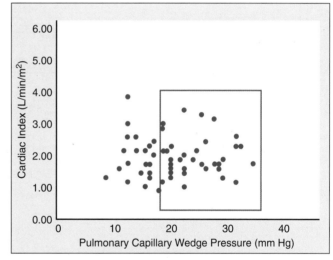

Figure 1-5. In the SHOCK registry, the clinically established category of isolated hypoperfusion cases (n = 61) according to presence or absence of rales or pulmonary congestion revealed, compared with hemodynamic parameters, how difficult it is to establish the presence of pulmonary congestion in shock cases. At least half of the isolated hypoperfusion (no pulmonary congestion) cases had frankly high pulmonary capillary wedge pressures. (From Menon V, White H, LeJemtel T, et al: The clinical profile of patients with suspected cardiogenic shock due to predominant left ventricular failure: a report from the SHOCK Trial Registry. SHould we emergently revascularize Occluded Coronaries in cardiogenic shocK? J Am Coll Cardiol 2000;36[Suppl A]:1071-1076, with permission from Elsevier.)

infarction, chronic aneurysm, pericarditis, or myopericarditis. Q waves depict infarction but may represent "electrocardiographic stunning." Myopathic disease may confer a pseudoinfarction pattern of ST deviations and Q waves, but with little evolution compared with typical infarction evolution. Bundle branch blocks are relevant: a right bundle branch block bespeaks extensive ante-

Table 1-2. Physical Signs of Cardiogenic Shock

Sign	Possible Causes
Appearance of shock	
Agitation, poor mentation	Impaired perfusion, hypoxemia, hypercarbia, acidosis
Cool	Impaired perfusion, high SVR
Clammy	Vagal state, impaired perfusion
Vital signs	
Tachypnea	Pulmonary congestion, acidosis, shock
Tachycardia	Pain, pulmonary congestion, small forward stroke volume
Hypotension	Small forward stroke volume, vasodepression—acidosis, vagal, drugs
Tachycardia and hypotension	Small forward stroke volume
Fever	Endocarditis, infarction, tachypnea
Pulsus paradoxus	Tamponade, pulmonary congestion
Venous distention	Tamponade, RV infarction, RV failure
Gallop rhythms	
S_3	Elevated filling pressures
S_4	Stiff ventricle
Rub	Pericarditis, early rupture
Murmur	
Holosystolic	MR, septal rupture, papillary rupture, TR, false aneurysm
Short systolic murmur	Papillary muscle rupture
Systolic ejection murmur	Concurrent aortic valve sclerosis or stenosis
To-and-fro	False aneurysm
Thrill	Septal rupture, papillary rupture
Apex	
Enlarged apex	Anteroapical dilation, anterolateral false aneurysm
Displaced apex	Anteroapical dilation, anteroapical displacement
Sustained apex	Dyskinetic anteroapex, pressure overload, anterolateral false aneurysm
Mesoapical impulse	Septal aneurysm
Parasternal impulse	RV enlargement, RV overload, severe MR
Rales	Pulmonary congestion
	Almost any other pulmonary disease can also generate rales.

MR, mitral regurgitation; RV, right ventricular; SVR, systemic vascular resistance; TR, tricuspid regurgitation.

rior ischemia; a left bundle branch block is unlikely to be due to acute infarction but massively attenuates its electrocardiographic representation. Similarly, a paced rhythm virtually obscures signs of infarction. Low-voltage presentation suggests massive infarction, a large pericardial effusion, or myocarditis. Increased voltages are consistent with left ventricular hypertrophy.

A slight majority of cardiogenic shock cases are due to anterior infarction (55%). Approximately 45% of cardiogenic shock cases are associated with inferior infarction and often due to the associated right ventricular infarction.

Chest Radiography and Cardiogenic Shock

A normal-sized cardiopericardial silhouette (CPS) is consistent with a previously normal heart; conversely, an enlarged CPS is consistent with prior structural heart disease. A globular or flask-like heart is consistent with a pericardial effusion or chronic myopathic disease. An abnormal cardiac contour suggests an aneurysm or false aneurysm. Cardiogenic shock with clear lung fields on the chest radiograph strongly suggests right ventricular failure or pericardial disease (tamponade). Most cases of left-sided heart failure have more pulmonary congestion than was appreciated clinically.

In addition to establishing the degree of radiographic pulmonary edema, chest radiography performed after intubation or mechanical ventilation, intra-aortic balloon counterpulsation (IABP), and line insertion provides a useful means to verify correct position and absence of complications.

The aortic contour is normal in the large majority of cardiogenic shock cases due to myocardial infarction.

Echocardiography and Cardiogenic Shock

Echocardiography is a valuable test to establish cardiac cause of shock and to exclude a surgical or "mechanical" cause. Although left ventricular failure underlies the majority of cases of cardiogenic shock, there are a significant number of cases due to other causes and complications, that can be recognized with echocardiography. Murmurs due to mitral insufficiency in particular may be short and soft in cardiogenic shock, reflecting high atrial and low ventricular pressures; they may be obscured by ventilator and IABP sounds, leaving a significant yield to echocardiography (and contrast ventriculography) among cardiogenic shock cases.

Among cardiogenic shock cases in the SHOCK registry, echocardiography was the most commonly employed test to evaluate left ventricular function (59%), contrast ventriculography was the second most common method (37%), and blood pool scanning was the least common (4%). The average ejection fraction of survivors was 33% ± 13%; of nonsurvivors, it was 27% ± 12% ($P < .001$).[2]

Cardiac cause of shock can be explained only by severe left or right ventricular systolic dysfunction, severe valve lesions, pericardial tamponade, or mechanical complications of infarction (papillary rupture, septal rupture, or free wall rupture). When transthoracic echocardiography (TTE) does not yield conclusive or confidence-achieving images, transesophageal echocardiography (TEE) should be performed. In a series of 100 consecutive shock cases of unknown cause in which echocardiography was requested to determine if shock was cardiogenic or noncardiogenic, evidence of cardiogenic shock was accepted if there was severe left or right ventricular systolic dysfunction, a severe left-sided valve lesion, pericardial tamponade, or a mechanical complication of infarction (validated with surgery, autopsy, catheterization, or other objective testing). Meticulous TTE identified cardiac cause in 58 of 59 cases, achieving 98% sensitivity and 100% specificity.[12]

TEE achieves morphologic detail superior to that of TTE for imaging of the mitral valve anatomy, including the papillary muscles, and superior pulmonary venous flow recording. TEE also facilitates assessment of false aneurysm cases that are small and posteriorly located and the echocardiographic evaluation of any case that is poorly imaged by transthoracic views.

Hemodynamics in Cardiogenic Shock

Pulmonary artery catheterization retains a role in most cardiogenic shock cases as it establishes baseline hemodynamics that are confirmatory of the diagnosis (elevated filling pressures, low output). Cardiac output calculations from pulmonary artery thermistors yield pulmonary artery flow, not systemic flow.

American College of Cardiology/American Heart Association (ACC/AHA) indications for hemodynamic (pulmonary artery) catheterization in acute infarction cases are as follows.[13]

Class I
- Severe or progressive congestive heart failure (CHF) or pulmonary edema
- Cardiogenic shock or progressive hypotension
- Suspected mechanical complications of acute infarction (i.e., ventricular septal defect, papillary muscle rupture, or pericardial tamponade)

Class IIa
- Hypotension that does not respond promptly to fluid administration in a patient without pulmonary congestion

The most useful scenarios for use of pulmonary artery catheterization are as follows:

- to exclude hypovolemia as a reversible cause of cardiogenic shock;
- to distinguish pulmonary disease from left-sided heart failure;
- to identify suspected septal rupture or severe mitral insufficiency;
- to monitor response to treatment of septal rupture or severe mitral insufficiency cases; and
- to monitor response to IABP use or inotrope or vasopressor use.

Arterial line blood pressure monitoring is additionally useful for blood gas and blood chemistry testing.

Coronary Angiography

The Killip (physical diagnosis) and Forrester (hemodynamic)[9] classifications of heart failure are commonly referred to (Tables 1-3 and 1-4). The Forrester classification is more reproducible (Fig. 1-6).

A subset of infarction patients with shock are intravascularly depleted or hypovolemic from medical or surgical comorbidities, early or excessive diuretic use, fluid restriction or nausea, vomiting, and diaphoresis and are in a low-output state because of underfilling. Preload requirements are greater in large infarctions, and normal filling pressures are commonly inadequate ("low output, low filling").

Table 1-3. Killip Classification of Heart Failure

Class	Subclass	Characteristics	Mortality (1967)
I	A	No heart failure No rales or S_3	6%
II	B	Heart failure Rales (<50% lungs), S_3, and venous hypertension	17%
III	C	Severe heart failure: frank pulmonary edema Rales (>50% lungs)	38%
IV	D	Cardiogenic shock Signs include hypotension (systolic blood pressure <90 mm Hg or less) and evidence of peripheral vasoconstriction, such as oliguria, cyanosis, and diaphoresis Heart failure, often with pulmonary edema, has also been present in the majority of these patients.	81%

From Killip T III, Kimball JT: Treatment of myocardial infarction in a coronary care unit. A two year experience with 250 patients. Am J Cardiol 1967;20:457-464, with permission from Elsevier.

Table 1-4. Forrester Classification of Heart Failure

Class		Hemodynamic Subsets			Clinical Subsets		
		PCWP	CI	Mortality	Mortality	PCWP	CI
I		<18	>2.2	3%	11%	12 ± 7	2.7 ± 0.05
II	Pulmonary congestion	>18	>2.2	9%	11%	23 ± 5	2.3 ± 0.4
III	Peripheral hypoperfusion	<18	<2.2	23%	18%	12 ± 5	1.9 ± 0.4
IV	Pulmonary congestion and peripheral hypoperfusion	>18	<2.2	51%	60%	27 ± 8	1.6 ± 0.6

CI, cardiac index; PCWP, pulmonary capillary wedge pressure.
From Forrester JS, Diamond GA, Swan HJ: Correlative classification of clinical and hemodynamic function after acute myocardial infarction. Am J Cardiol 1977;39:137-145, with permission from Elsevier.

Early coronary angiography in a STEMI or bundle branch block cohort not undergoing primary percutaneous coronary intervention is an ACC/AHA class I indication.[13] Coronary angiography in most ST depression cardiogenic shock cases identifies three-vessel or left mainstem disease.

MANAGEMENT OF CARDIOGENIC SHOCK

The management of cardiogenic shock is directed toward timely intervention (percutaneous or surgical) with appropriate supportive and stabilizing measures.

Fibrinolytics

It is unproven that fibrinolytics afford benefit in cardiogenic shock cases; at best, the effect is limited.[14] Fibrinolytic trials included few shock patients, and results were not positive. In GISSI 1, the only fibrinolytic trial that did not exclude cardiogenic shock cases, mortality among the 2.4% of patients assigned to

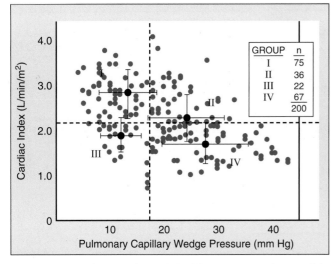

Figure 1-6. Hemodynamic subsets, derived from 200 cases of myocardial infarction. (From Forrester JS, Diamond GA, Swan HJ: Correlative classification of clinical and hemodynamic function after acute myocardial infarction. Am J Cardiol 1977;39:137-145, with permission from Elsevier.)

Killip class IV was 70% in both the streptokinase and placebo groups. The Fibrinolytic Therapy Trialists' data demonstrate mortality reduction in *hypotensive* (systolic BP < 100 mm Hg) patients (not solely cardiogenic shock): fibrinolytic 28.9% versus control 35%.[15] Observational data suggest that fibrinolytics achieve a reperfusion rate of 40% in cardiogenic shock compared with an overall reperfusion rate of about 70%. Experimental data demonstrate that there is less fibrinolytic effect in cardiogenic shock, possibly because of impaired pressure diffusion of what are typically large molecules,[16] and observational data suggest that blood pressure of less than 80 mm Hg is associated with lower angiographic (TIMI) grades of flow. It should be recalled that coronary perfusion pressure is influenced by aortic diastolic pressure but also by left ventricular diastolic pressure.[17,18]

Percutaneous Coronary Intervention

Observational data associated successful percutaneous transluminal coronary angioplasty (PTCA) or percutaneous coronary intervention (PCI) with dramatically improved outcomes, but selection bias is inherent. Unsuccessful PCI is a marker of more extensive coronary disease and more disease patients.

The majority of data on the role of PCI in cardiogenic shock derive from a single study, the SHOCK multicenter trial, whose hypothesis was that emergency or early revascularization results in 20% absolute reduction in all-cause 30-day mortality compared with initial medical stabilization.[19] Cardiogenic shock was defined as prolonged chest pain or equivalent symptoms, ST elevation, systolic blood pressure of less than 90 mm Hg for more than 30 minutes or IABP or inotropes to maintain systolic blood pressure above 90 mm Hg, decreased end-organ perfusion, PCWP above 15 mm Hg, and CI below 2.2 L/min/m². Patients were enrolled if they were less than 36 hours from symptom onset of infarction and less than 12 hours since the onset of shock. The primary endpoint was 30-day all-cause mortality; the secondary endpoints were 6- and 12-month all-cause mortality, change in left ventricular function at 2 weeks, quality of life, and functional status.

The SHOCK trial concluded that early revascularization offers benefit (secondary endpoint) for cardiogenic shock in patients younger than 75 years and that cardiogenic shock continues to be a highly lethal diagnosis with a mortality of more than 50% (Table 1-5).[19] At 1 year, 83% of survivors were in NYHA class I or II.[20]

Table 1-5. SHOCK Trial

	Early Intervention	Delayed Intervention	Absolute Difference	Relative Difference
Survival				
30 days (primary endpoint)[19]	46.7%	50.3%	NS	
6 months (secondary endpoint)[19]	56%	63%		
1 year[20]	46.7%	33.6%	13%	
6 years[21]	62.4%	44.4%	13%	67%
Annualized mortality, 1-year survivors[21]	8.0%	10.7%		
Annualized mortality, 6-year survivors[21]	8.3%	14.3%		

From Hochman JS, Sleeper LA, Webb JG, et al: Early revascularization in acute myocardial infarction complicated by cardiogenic shock. SHOCK Investigators. Should We Emergently Revascularize Occluded Coronaries for Cardiogenic Shock? N Engl J Med 1999;341:625-634.

American College of Cardiology/American Heart Association Recommendations for Percutaneous Coronary Intervention for Cardiogenic Shock[22]

Class I Primary PCI is recommended for patients younger than 75 years with ST elevation or left bundle branch block who develop shock within 36 hours of infarction and are suitable for revascularization that can be performed within 18 hours of shock, unless further support is futile because of the patient's wishes or contraindications or the unsuitability for further invasive care. (*Level of Evidence: A*)

Class IIa Primary PCI is reasonable for selected patients 75 years or older with ST elevation or left bundle branch block who develop shock within 36 hours of myocardial infarction and are suitable for revascularization that can be performed within 18 hours of shock. Patients with good prior functional status who are suitable for revascularization and agree to invasive care may be selected for such an invasive strategy. (*Level of Evidence: B*)

Aortocoronary Bypass Grafting

Coronary artery bypass surgery is an option for revascularization of cardiogenic shock cases. The average mortality for aortocoronary bypass surgery observed in the SHOCK registry was 28%,[2] which is similar to an average of 30% to 35% in the literature. Thirty-day survival rates were 55.6% for early revascularization patients undergoing PCI and 57.4% for those undergoing aortocoronary bypass surgery (*P* = .86). At 1 year, survival was 51.9% for PCI and 46.8% for surgery (*P* = .71). Eighty-eight percent of

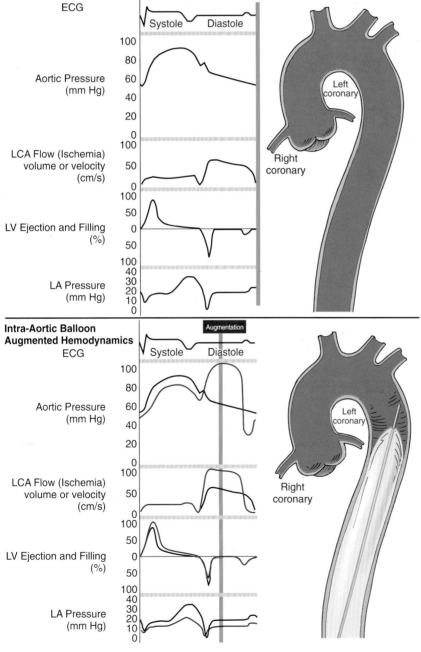

Figure 1-7. TOP, Cardiogenic shock native state hemodynamics. The mean, systolic, and diastolic arterial blood pressures are low—60% of usual. Left coronary artery (LCA) flow is reduced because of the lowered perfusion pressure (aortic diastolic pressure minus [elevated] left ventricular diastolic pressure). Left coronary flow, though, is diastole predominant because the perfusion pressure is positive only in diastole. Left ventricular (LV) ejection is an early systolic phenomenon, and left ventricular filling is predominantly an early diastolic occurrence because of the elevated left atrial pressure. Left atrial (LA) pressure is elevated, and the waveform is revealing of the overload of the left atrium—a V wave occurs. BOTTOM, IABP-augmented hemodynamics. Intra-aortic balloon inflation at the dicrotic notch increases intra-aortic volume and pressure. With deflation, late diastolic pressure falls beneath the native level, such that the next systolic ejection occurs against an initially lower pressure—"assisting" ejection. This lessening of afterload to the left ventricle results in a 10% to 15% increase in ejection and a lowering of ventricular volumes and pressure. Consequently, left atrial pressure is reduced. MI, myocardial infarction.

surgery patients were deemed completely revascularized.[23] Emergency or urgent aortocoronary bypass grafting with coronary anatomy suitable for surgery is an ACC/AHA class IIa indication.[13]

Intra-aortic Balloon Counterpulsation

Intra-aortic balloon counterpulsation (IABP) is a supportive device, not an intervention. In GUSTO I, its use correlated with better outcomes (Figs. 1-7 to 1-12).[7,24] Major complications can be as infrequent as 2.7%.[25]

IABP increases mean aortic pressure by diastolic augmentation; and by deflating before systole, it lowers end-diastolic and systolic pressure and thereby "assists" left ventricular ejection by lessening afterload. The predominant hemodynamic effect is an increase in mean blood pressure; cardiac index modestly increases approximately 0.5 L/min/m^2, sometimes up to 0.8 L/min/m^2. The effect of reducing afterload, though, may be physiologically prominent in cases of septal rupture, severe mitral regurgitation, and papillary muscle rupture, in which a significant proportion of shunt volume or regurgitant volume can be redirected to become forward stroke volume, reducing left-sided heart volume and filling pressures.

The anti-ischemic benefit of IABP is predominantly through reduction of myocardial oxygen demand by lowering of systolic pressure and often by lowering of heart rate as well. Cases with left mainstem coronary lesions and myocardial ischemia (which eliminates coronary autoregulation and confers a linear relation of myocardial blood flow to aortic diastolic pressure) experience an increase in coronary blood flow with IABP.[26] The effect of IABP on coronary flow across other lesions is unclear, although IABP may increase flow to myocardium through collaterals.

Nonrandomized data in anterior infarction cases suggest that the combination of fibrinolytics (streptokinase) and IABP achieves superior coronary reperfusion (TIMI III flow).[27] Randomized data in small trials have not shown 6-month mortality benefit, although in the TACTICS trial, among patients assigned to Killip classes III and IV, there was a trend toward benefit ($P = .05$), 39% mortality for the combination of fibrinolysis and IABP versus 80% for fibrinolysis alone.[28]

Assist Devices

Percutaneous cardiopulmonary bypass affords short-lived benefit but may be lifesaving.[29] Left ventricular assist devices (LVADs) afford longer benefit,[30] but their availability is limited.

Ventilation

Noninvasive ventilation can be used with success to avoid the complications of intubation and mechanical ventilation in several scenarios, including heart failure. However, in severe heart failure and in cardiogenic shock, noninvasive ventilation may be associated with more rapid deterioration,[31] and the safety of noninvasive ventilation for the management of acute cardiogenic pulmonary edema is unknown.[32]

Airway intubation and mechanical ventilation afford protection to the airway, although with some risks at the time of intubation. Because cardiogenic shock is not a short-course problem, and also because it is expected to be progressive, definitive ventilatory support rather than a trial of attempted noninvasive ventilation is usually appropriate. Ventilatory support lessens the respiratory stress and lowers the heart rate, which is a significant benefit in the setting of acute infarction. Last, for patients who appear to be in shock and will undergo early PCI, a strong case can be made for intubation and ventilation before arrival in the catheterization laboratory to maximize stability in lying supine and to avoid jeopardizing safety or interruption of angiography, PCI, or IABP insertion.

Left Main Coronary Stenosis

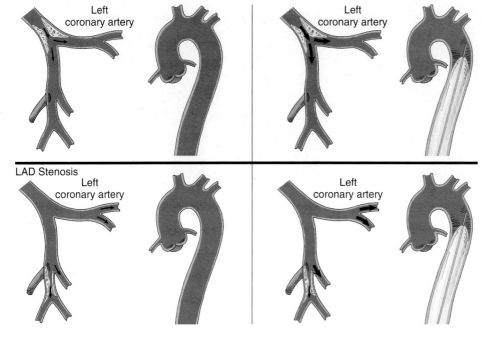

LAD Stenosis

Figure 1-8. TOP ROW, Left mainstem disease. BOTTOM ROW, More distal LAD disease. LEFT IMAGES, Native state. RIGHT IMAGES, IABP-augmented state. IABP augmentation increases flow across left mainstem lesions, especially in the presence of left coronary ischemia. More distal LAD stenoses do not receive the same augmentation of flow from IABP counterpulsation, as augmented pressure and flow run off through proximal vessels.

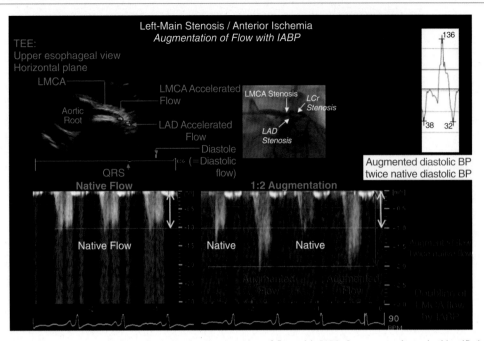

Figure 1-9. Left coronary mainstem stenosis and anterior ischemia: augmentation of flow with IABP. Coronary angiography identified a distal left mainstem stenosis that extended into the proximal LAD and left circumflex arteries. TEE color Doppler images reveal a small lumen and flow acceleration in the distal left mainstem coronary artery (LMCA) and LAD. IABP augmentation, doubling diastolic blood pressure, doubles left coronary flow velocity, as revealed by the 2:1 augmentation pattern.

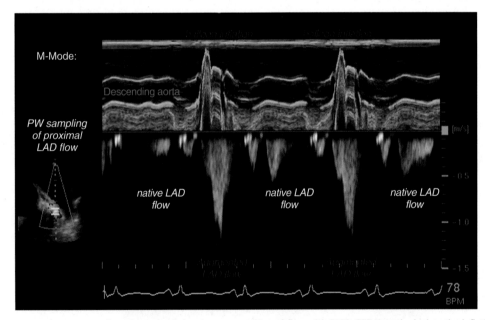

Figure 1-10. Left coronary mainstem stenosis and anterior ischemia: augmentation of flow with IABP. TEE M-mode depicts the inflation of the intra-aortic balloon each second cardiac cycle, and pulsed wave Doppler depicts the doubling of diastolic blood flow velocity from IABP-induced doubling of aortic diastolic pressure.

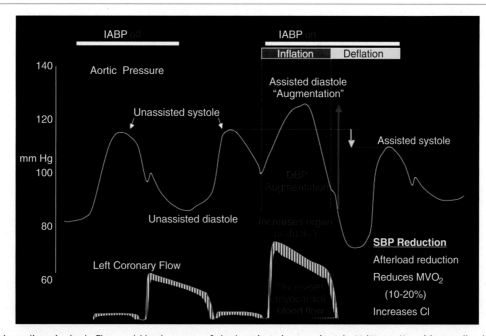

Figure 1-11. IABP in cardiogenic shock. The usual blood pressure of shock patients is approximately 85/60 mm Hg, with a small pulse pressure due to a small forward stroke volume. The left ventricular perfusion pressure is the aortic diastolic pressure minus the left ventricular diastolic pressure: typically 60 − 25 mm Hg = 35 mm Hg or half normal. Left coronary flow to the left ventricular myocardium is diastolic predominant as there is no driving perfusion pressure gradient in systole. The dicrotic notch of the aortic pressure contour indicates the onset of diastole. With intra-aortic balloon inflation in diastole timed to start after the dicrotic notch, the increase in aortic volume (34 or 40 mL) increases or "augments" aortic pressure because of limited compliance of the aorta. The older the patient, the greater the augmentation because the aortic compliance is less. The increase in perfusion gradient (aortic diastolic pressure rises and LV diastolic pressure falls slightly) increases coronary flow. The balloon deflates before the onset of systole, so aortic end-diastolic pressure is lower than native state, and the left ventricular ejection occurs against a lower aortic pressure (afterload), assisting ejection and reducing myocardial oxygen consumption by the proportion that the systolic blood pressure × heart rate product reduces. Assisting ejection enables a small increase in cardiac output.

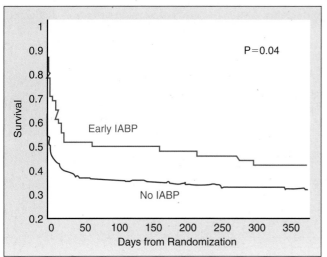

Figure 1-12. Nonrandomized study data reveal that early IABP use in STEMI is associated with improved survival. (From Anderson RD, Ohman EM, Holmes DR Jr, et al: Use of intraaortic balloon counterpulsation in patients presenting with cardiogenic shock: observations from the GUSTO-I Study. Global Utilization of Streptokinase and TPA for Occluded Coronary Arteries. J Am Coll Cardiol 1997;30:708-715, with permission from Elsevier.)

CASE 1

History

▸ 65-year-old woman presented to local emergency department "feeling unwell"
▸ Mild chest pains, variable descriptions
▸ Short of breath for 12 hours
▸ No fevers, chills
▸ Active (walked 5 km/day until 2 days before)
▸ "Upper respiratory tract infection" 3 weeks before
▸ Past medical history is significant for mild hypertension.

Physical Examination

▸ Appeared fit for age, weak and diaphoretic, respiratory distress
▸ BP 80/50 mm Hg, HR 110 bpm, RR 30/min
▸ Venous distention
▸ Heart sounds muffled, S_3 gallop
▸ No murmurs or pericardial rub
▸ Crepitations >50% of lung fields

Initial Management

▸ Recurrent episodes of sustained ventricular tachycardia (VT) began 10 minutes after she reached the emergency department.
▸ Transfer was requested because of suspected myocardial infarction with hemodynamic and electrical instability.

Clinical Impression

▸ Impression on arrival was that of cardiogenic shock due to acute infarction, pseudoinfarction-type presentation of myocarditis, or cardiomyopathy with aggravating factors.
▸ Given the unsure diagnosis of myocardial infarction, fibrinolytics were considered but not given.
▸ IABP was inserted at bedside for hemodynamic support.
▸ Echocardiography, coronary angiography, and catheterization were ordered.

Evolution

▸ Balloon flotation pulmonary artery hemodynamics (with inotropes) confirmed cardiogenic shock parameters (CI <2.2 L/min/m² despite PCWP >20 mm Hg):
  ▸ CI: 2.0 L/min/m²
  ▸ PCWP: 30 mm Hg
  ▸ RAP: 14 mm Hg
  ▸ PAP: 45/20 mm Hg

Management

▸ Clinical impression was that of cardiogenic shock due to acute myocarditis, with a pseudoinfarction presentation.
▸ Supportive measures: mechanical ventilation, IABP and inotropes for hemodynamics, IV administration of amiodarone for VT storm
▸ Ongoing shock hemodynamics, marginal urine output
▸ Deliberation of immunosuppression: IV high-dose steroids given because hemodynamics were not improving and were marginal
▸ Improvement in blood pressure, not in filling pressures
▸ Stable for 4 days, still receiving inotropes and IABP

Evolution and Outcome

▸ Another series (20) of recurrent VT episodes
▸ Ongoing shock state, unsure of neurologic status
▸ During 3 weeks, multiple medical comorbidities developed (recurrent GI bleed, worsening respiratory status, pulmonary sepsis)
▸ Died after 4 weeks in hospital

Comments

▸ Pseudoinfarction presentation of fulminant myocarditis, complicated by cardiogenic shock from severe biventricular dysfunction and VT storm, which may be seen in almost any disease of the myocardium
▸ The ECG pattern, low voltages, and lack of evolution were suggestive of pseudoinfarction, but coronary angiography was necessary to exclude coronary artery disease as a possible cause.
▸ Angiography excluded coronary artery stenosis, and endomyocardial biopsy established a positive diagnosis.
▸ Antiarrhythmics caused hypotension that increased pressor and inotrope needs, which may have perpetuated a cycle of ventricular arrhythmia.

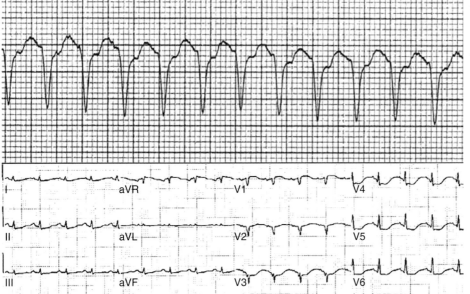

Figure 1-13. TOP, VT storm: monomorphic VT (recurrent—45 defibrillations). BOTTOM, ECG shows sinus tachycardia, low voltages, Q waves, and ST depression without evolution during 3 hours. CK (only), 310; TnI, 50.

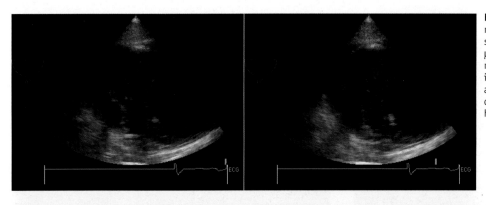

Figure 1-14. TEE transgastric views of the mid–left ventricle in diastole (LEFT) and systole (RIGHT) (study performed with 30 µg/min/m² dobutamine). The ventricular myocardium is mildly thickened. Despite inotropic support, there is extremely little apparent systolic function. The LVH is out of proportion to the history of mild hypertension.

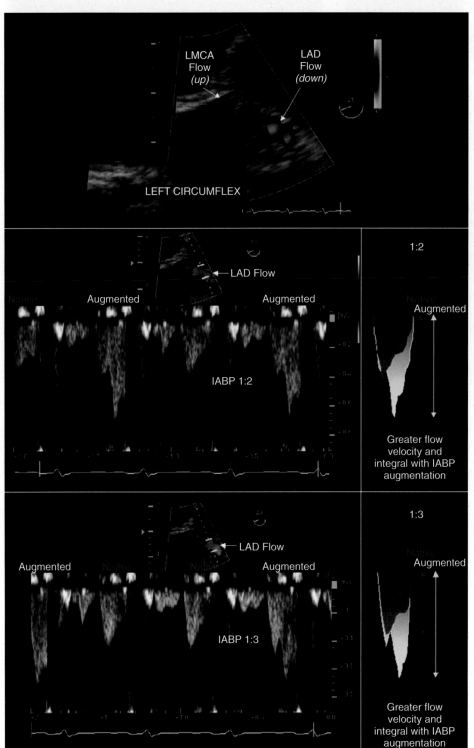

Figure 1-15. Left coronary flow sampling and the effect of IABP visualized by TEE. TOP, Color Doppler flow mapping of the left main coronary artery (LMCA). The left main diameter is large, and there is no aliasing or other signs of stenosis. The left circumflex is also imaged in cross section and also has (at the site of sampling) a large lumen. MIDDLE, Coronary flow (LAD coronary artery) augmentation with 1:2 IABP; 100% augmentation of every second LAD diastolic coronary artery flow velocity spectral occurred with IABP in the 1:2 mode. BOTTOM, Coronary flow (LAD coronary artery) augmentation with 1:3 IABP; 100% augmentation of every third LAD diastolic coronary artery flow velocity spectral occurred with IABP in the 1:3 mode.

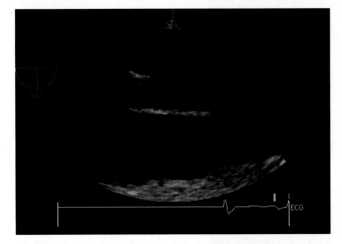

Figure 1-16. TEE longitudinal view of the proximal descending aorta. The intra-aortic balloon pump tip resides several centimeters too low in the descending aorta. There is no atheroma apparent by TEE, which is unusual for patients with severe coronary artery disease.

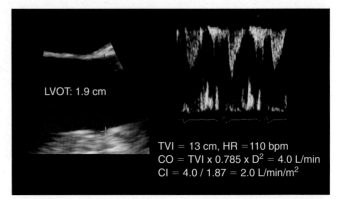

LVOT: 1.9 cm

TVI = 13 cm, HR =110 bpm
CO = TVI x 0.785 x D^2 = 4.0 L/min
CI = 4.0 / 1.87 = 2.0 L/min/m^2

Figure 1-17. TEE study of cardiac output (study performed with 30 µg/min/m^2 dobutamine).

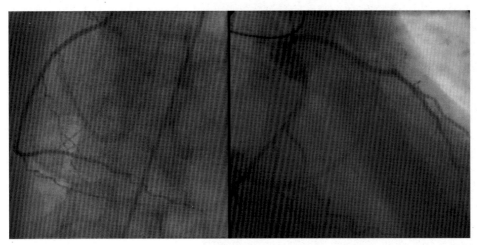

Figure 1-18. Coronary angiography of the RCA (LEFT) and the LCA (RIGHT). The angiographic appearance and pattern of the right and left coronary arteries are normal.

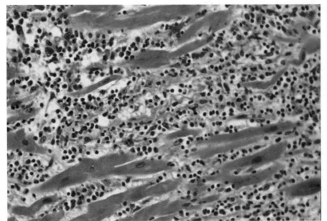

Figure 1-19. Myocardial biopsy. Marked lymphocytic infiltration and myocellular necrosis.

CASE 2

History

- 55-year-old man accepted in transfer in cardiogenic shock with acute myocardial infarction, after the administration of tPA
- Past medical history is significant for type 2 diabetes and a myocardial infarction in 1995 (no details).
- No habitual angina or heart failure symptoms
- On the day of presentation: 08:00 nausea; 08:20 chest pain; 09:00 presented to emergency department; 09:15 diagnosed with acute myocardial infarction and Killip I

Physical Examination

- BP 80/50 mm Hg, HR 115 bpm, ventilated
- Venous distention, no edema
- S_1, S_2 normal; gallop
- No murmurs or rubs
- Apex distant, not displaced

Initial Management

- Received tPA less than 1 hour after onset of chest pain
- Ongoing nausea and chest pain
- Systolic BP fell from 110 to 80 to 60 mm Hg
- Received fluids with little BP response
- Developed acute pulmonary edema, intubated
- Dopamine for pressor support
- Transfer accepted, but 8 hours elapsed before arrival

Subsequent Management

- Clinical impression was that of cardiogenic shock due to acute myocardial infarction with the backdrop of prior infarction.
- IABP inserted for blood pressure support

- 12 hours after onset of pain, electrocardiographically no longer in ST elevation, had formed Q waves, and only minimal residual pain
- Angiography indicated as revascularization strategy (<36 hours) in cardiogenic shock
- PTCA of infarct-related vessel performed

Evolution and Outcome

- Massive CK washout: 8000+
- No mechanical complications developed
- Falling blood pressure, requiring higher pressor-inotropes—dilation of the infarct territory (infarct expansion, early aneurysm) occurred
  - CI 1.3 L/min/m²
  - PCWP 20 mm Hg
  - PAP 50/13 mm Hg
- Repeated echocardiography and oximetry exclude mechanical complications
- Transfer for maximal pretransplantation resources
- LVAD not inserted because of spontaneous hemodynamic improvement
- Further spontaneous hemodynamic improvement during the next 2 weeks
- Discharged angina free, NYHA class III CHF 5 weeks later

Comments

- Cardiogenic shock due to cumulative left ventricular systolic dysfunction from coronary artery disease due to the combination of large acute infarction, previous moderate-sized myocardial infarction, acute myocardial infarction, and myocardial stunning (given the spontaneous improvement after reperfusion)
- The patient survived, but with resting hypotension and considerable CHF symptoms. Late investigations showed no evidence of viability; therefore, coronary revascularization was not performed.
- The patient remains a candidate for cardiac transplantation.

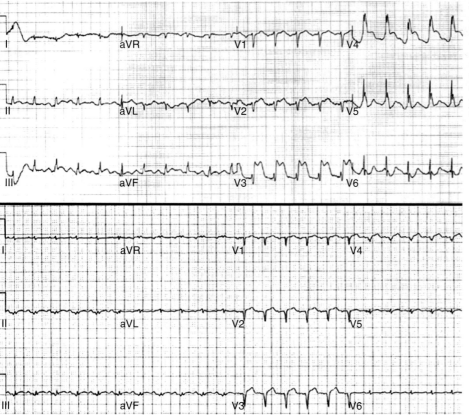

Figure 1-20. TOP, ECG at presentation to community hospital shows sinus tachycardia, precordial ST elevation (V_2-V_4), and inferior (III, aVF) as well as acute anteroapical infarction. BOTTOM, ECG at time of transfer shows sinus tachycardia, low voltages, and Q waves (V_2-V_5, III, aVF) as well as extensive anterior infarction. Low voltages may be the result of myopathic disease, effusion, or a large infarction.

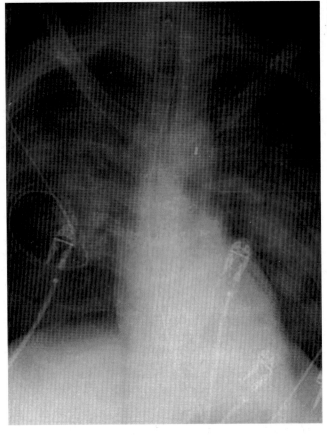

Figure 1-21. Chest radiograph shows small heart, acute "bat-wing" pulmonary edema, and endotracheal tube and intra-aortic balloon tip in correct position.

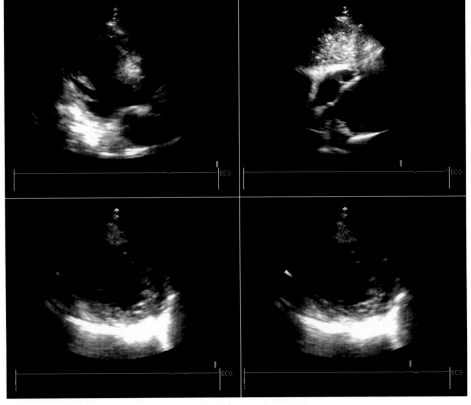

Figure 1-22. TTE. TOP LEFT, Parasternal long-axis view shows intact posteromedial papillary muscles. TOP RIGHT, Subcostal view shows no pericardial effusion and no tamponade signs. BOTTOM, Diastole (LEFT). Systole (RIGHT). There is very little contraction of the left ventricle.

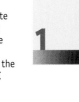

Figure 1-23. TOP ROW, Coronary angiography. LCA injection reveals a small-caliper left main, left LAD, and left circumflex coronary artery, with moderate to severe disease throughout, including extensive branch and distal disease. The left circumflex coronary artery is also proximally occluded. BOTTOM ROW, PCI of the occluded left circumflex artery: TIMI III flow.

CASE 3

History

▸ 63-year-old man collapsed walking across the street from the hospital coffee shop
▸ Brought to emergency department 10 minutes after collapse
▸ Had chest pain that he could not describe
▸ No known coronary artery disease, peripheral vascular disease, or cardiovascular disease
▸ Cigarettes were found in his pocket.

Physical Examination

▸ Agitated, barely responsive, in respiratory distress
▸ BP 60/– mm Hg, HR 120 bpm, RR 40/min, sat 70% on 100% O_2, afebrile
▸ Venous distention, no edema
▸ Muffled heart sounds, gallop present
▸ No murmurs
▸ Crepitations over all lung fields

Initial Management

▸ Intubated for shock
▸ Vasopressors started with poor response
▸ Suspected myocardial infarction

Clinical Impression

▸ Echocardiography was performed to establish wall motion abnormality and to exclude other cardiac diseases and aortic dissection. It revealed large anterior, anterolateral, septal, and apical wall motion abnormalities (akinesis); nondilated heart, low output; no valvular pathologic processes; and no ruptures or tamponade.
▸ Presumed acute massive anterolateral myocardial infarction

Subsequent Management

▸ Dopamine, norepinephrine, BP 60/–, falling HR
▸ Episodes of electromechanical dissociation and cardiopulmonary resuscitation
▸ IABP and urgent angiography were ordered.

Evolution and Outcome

▸ Flow restored in left coronary system, but "no reflow" phenomenon
▸ IABP 1:1, high doses of epinephrine
▸ Despite all these measures, BP fell to 45/–, falling heart rate, worsening acidosis despite bicarbonate, anuria
▸ Asystole developed, unresponsive to epinephrine, epinephrine boluses, and pacing
▸ Died less than 3 hours after initial collapse, before LVAD insertion could be arranged

Comments

▸ Massive acute myocardial infarction without prodromal symptoms in a male smoker
▸ Early (immediate) cardiogenic shock due to left main occlusion
▸ Poor electrocardiographic depiction of such a large acute infarction
▸ Poor reflow after PTCA followed by death

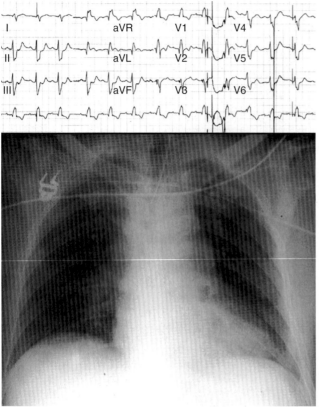

Figure 1-24. TOP, ECG shows sinus rhythm, first-degree aortic valve block, right bundle branch block, Q waves in V_1-V_3, abnormal septal repolarization, and ST elevation in lead aVR. Subtle findings of anterior ST elevation are partially obscured by the right bundle branch block pattern. BOTTOM, Chest radiograph shows normal-sized CPS and interstitial pulmonary edema.

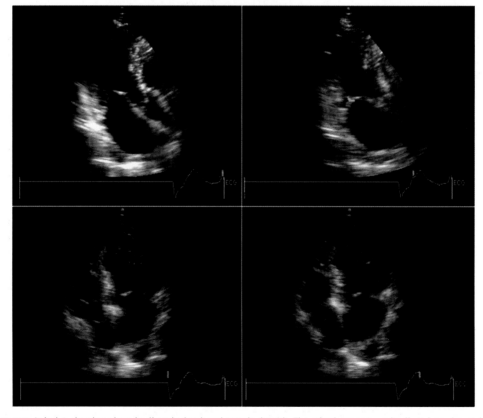

Figure 1-25. TTE. TOP ROW, Apical 3-chamber views in diastole (LEFT) and systole (RIGHT). The mitral appearance in diastole and systole is unremarkable—there is no apparent disruption or prolapse, and there is very little MR. There is only contraction (hypokinesis) of the posterior wall. BOTTOM ROW, Apical 4-chamber views show that the distal inferior septum, apex, and lateral walls are akinetic. Only the basal inferior septum is contracting, but it is hypokinetic. Again, the mitral valve appearance is unremarkable, and there is no pericardial effusion.

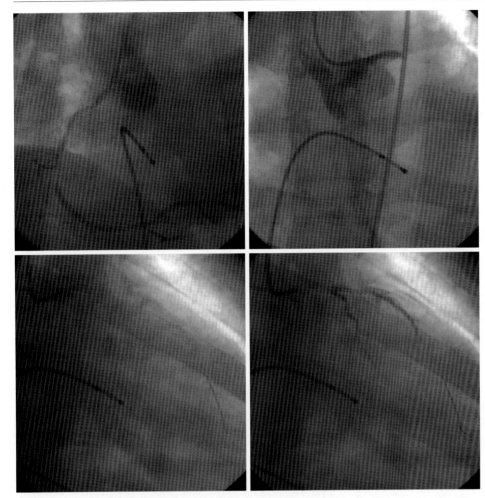

Figure 1-26. Coronary angiography. TOP LEFT, RCA injection reveals dominance of the artery and significant disease at multiple sites. TOP RIGHT, LCA injection reveals a small and short, occluded left main coronary artery. BOTTOM ROW, The LMCA is wired (LEFT) and angioplastied (RIGHT), but the restoration of flow is poor.

CASE 4

History

▸ 61-year-old man, manual laborer
▸ Chest pain and shortness of breath in the following sequence: 8:00 am, sudden onset of severe chest pain, radiating to both arms and the back; 8:30 am, ongoing chest pain, developing dyspnea; 9:00 am, presented to community hospital
▸ No known coronary artery disease, peripheral vascular disease, or cardiovascular disease
▸ Past medical history is significant for hypertension with monotherapy.

Physical Examination

▸ BP 80/50 mm Hg, HR 110 bpm, ventilated
▸ No venous distention, no edema
▸ Quiet heart sounds, gallop
▸ Short decrescendo murmur at left sternal border
▸ No rub

Initial Management

▸ Hypotensive at presentation, in pulmonary edema
▸ Ventricular fibrillation arrest shortly after arrival at local emergency department
▸ Successfully defibrillated
▸ Intubated for airway protection and mechanically ventilated for severe pulmonary edema
▸ Transferred in cardiogenic shock

Clinical Impression

▸ Initial clinical impression was that of cardiogenic shock from myocardial ischemia/non–ST elevation myocardial infarction.
▸ Although cardiogenic shock from extensive left coronary ischemia was possible, there were several inconsistent details: (1) abrupt onset of chest pain is more typical of aortic dissection than of infarction; (2) there was an aortic insufficiency (AI) murmur, potentially consistent with complication from a type A (proximal) aortic dissection.
▸ Echocardiography was performed urgently and revealed proximal aortic dissection, complicated by cardiogenic shock, due to either acute severe AI and myocardial ischemia or cardiac arrest secondary to myocardial ischemia.
▸ Neurologic status was unclear—there were no focal deficits, but responsiveness was impaired, possibly due to hypoxic brain damage, sedation, or impaired carotid flow.

Evolution and Management

▸ Although neurologic status was poor, waiting for improvement was not tenable.

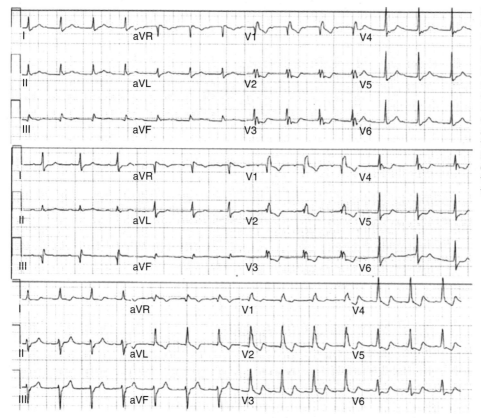

Figure 1-27. ECGs at presentation (TOP), at 30 minutes (MIDDLE), and at 60 minutes (BOTTOM). At presentation, notable findings are sinus rhythm, first-degree aortic valve block, and right bundle branch block. At 30 minutes, findings are sinus rhythm, right bundle branch block, downsloping ST depression V_1-V_3 secondary to the right bundle branch block, and horizontal ST depression V_4-V_6, aVL, indicating probable anterolateral ischemia. At 60 minutes, findings are sinus rhythm, right bundle branch block, and downsloping ST depression worsening in V_1-V_6, I, aVL, indicative of anterolateral ischemia or infarction.

▸ Patient was referred for emergent cardiac surgery that revealed (1) proximal dissection, (2) prolapsing flap and aortic valve, and (3) flap at left main coronary artery.
▸ Bentall repair was performed (composite prosthetic valve and tube graft replacement of the aortic valve and ascending aorta).

Outcome

▸ Uneventful operation
▸ No postoperative hemodynamic problems
▸ Never woke up; died 4 weeks later

Comments

▸ This patient suffered from cardiogenic shock and pulmonary edema secondary to acute AI and anterolateral ischemia from left coronary obstruction by the intimal flap. The pulmonary edema resulted from the excess volume load into the LV, which was noncompliant as a result of the ischemia.
▸ The murmur was subtle but present and a significant finding when coupled with the abnormal aortic appearance on the chest radiograph.
▸ Most patients with acute aortic dissection are chronically hypertensive, particularly when they are under stress or in pain. Cardiogenic shock combined with a dissection implies one or more major complications of the dissection (rupture, tamponade, acute AI, or coronary occlusion).
▸ The etiology of cardiogenic shock must be established in all cases to ensure appropriate treatment and to avoid inappropriate treatment.

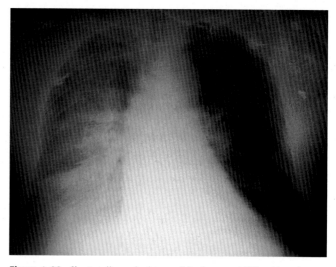

Figure 1-28. Chest radiograph shows mildly increased CPS, widened mediastinum, and asymmetric pulmonary edema.

1

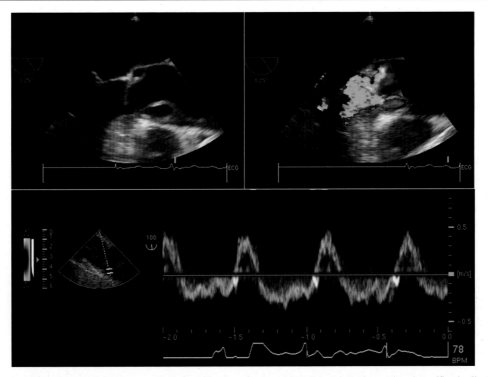

Figure 1-29. TEE longitudinal views of the aortic root. The intimal flap is extensive and prolapses into the aortic valve orifice in diastole, as does a leaflet of the aortic valve. There is a regurgitant jet filling the height of the LVOT. Pulsed wave recording of flow in the descending aorta reveals holodiastolic reversal consistent with severe AI.

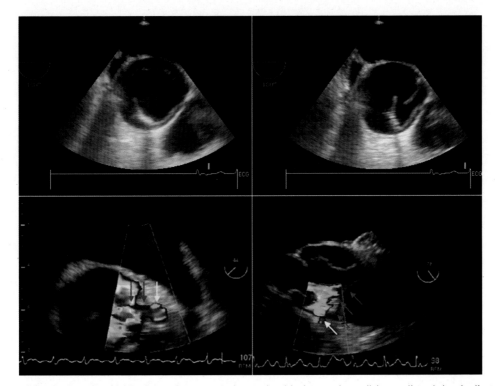

Figure 1-30. The intimal flap is circumferential in the aortic root, seen in systole with the true (central) lumen distended or in diastole (TOP LEFT) with the true lumen collapsed, probably for several reasons, including its decompression into the LV by the AI (TOP RIGHT). In the lower views, the flap is seen to extend to the left main ostium (BOTTOM LEFT) and the right ostium (BOTTOM RIGHT).

CASE 5

History

‣ 87-year-old woman presented with 6 hours of severe chest pressure and worsening shortness of breath
‣ Uncommonly well and active for her age
‣ Past medical history is significant for hypertension.
‣ Chronic stable angina CCS class I perfusion study a year before demonstrated a medium-sized reversing lateral wall defect.

Physical Examination

‣ Distressed with dyspnea and pain
‣ BP 100/65 mm Hg, HR 95 bpm, RR 21/min
‣ Crepitations 50% bilaterally
‣ S_3; 2/6 SEM at the base, 2/6 pansystolic murmur at the apex
‣ Warm extremities
‣ Urine output 25 mL/hr

Initial Management

‣ Initially, she was supported with noninvasive ventilation; but during 90 minutes, her breathing became more labored and the blood pressure fell to 80/50 mm Hg.
‣ She was intubated and mechanically ventilated and referred for angiography and IABP support.
‣ Inotropes were started.

Evolution and Outcome

‣ She was ventilated for 5 days but extubated once heart failure had cleared sufficiently.
‣ Initial pulmonary artery hemodynamic data were a CI (unassisted) of 1.4 L/min/m² and a PCWP of 30 mm Hg.
‣ Mild renal insufficiency developed, but not oliguria.
‣ Mild hepatic dysfunction also occurred and resolved within a week.
‣ The patient remained in the hospital 4 more weeks but made a full recovery.
‣ Post discharge: CCS class I and NYHA class II

Comments

‣ Early cardiogenic shock from STEMI from left mainstem disease
‣ Noninvasive ventilation in cardiogenic shock is less successful and sometimes less safe. Intubation with mechanical ventilation is more secure.
‣ Successful PCI and survival
‣ Although female gender and her age are strong predictors of adverse outcome, her excellent premorbid functional status, amenability of the culprit lesion to PCI, and absence of peripheral organ failure enabled survival.
‣ The flow recording from the left mainstem revealed the coronary hemodynamic augmentation effect of IABP on ischemic left main coronary disease.

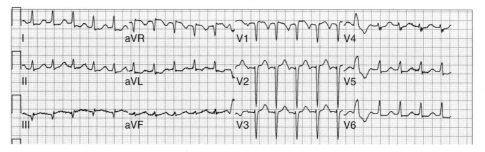

Figure 1-31. Sinus tachycardia. There is ST elevation in leads aVR and V_1, which is consistent with ischemia (80% sensitive) of left mainstem origin (if the ST elevation in aVR exceeds that of V_1). There is ST depression in leads I, aVL, V_5-V_6.

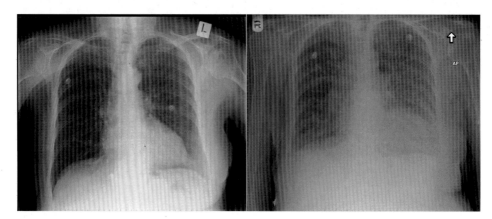

Figure 1-32. LEFT, Chest radiograph taken 3 weeks before presentation with chest pain (chest radiography was prompted by external dyspnea). RIGHT, Chest radiograph at presentation with chest pain and dyspnea. The CPS is not larger. There is interstitial edema and enlarged pulmonary veins.

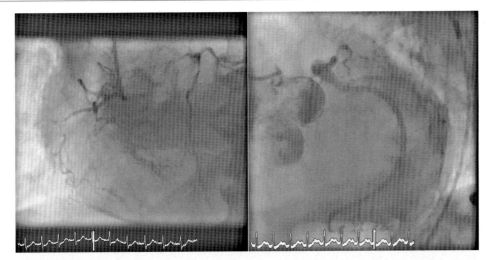

Figure 1-33. Selective coronary angiography. LEFT, Injection of the RCA shows that it is nondominant and collateralizing to the LAD. RIGHT, LCA injection shows that the left circumflex artery is dominant. There is an ostial left mainstem stenosis and a distal left main aneurysm.

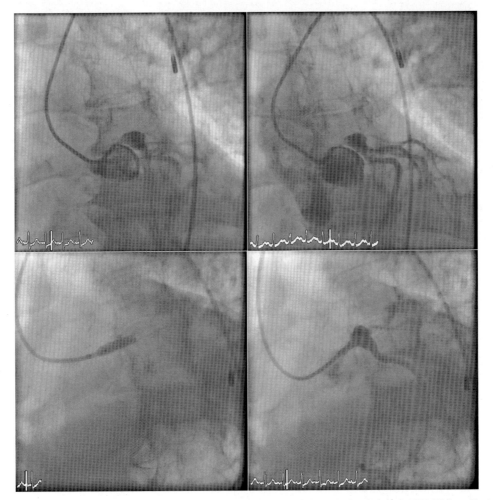

Figure 1-34. PCI of the ostial left mainstem stenosis. After stenting, the angiographic result is good and there is TIMI III flow. The intra-aortic balloon tip is seen in the descending aorta.

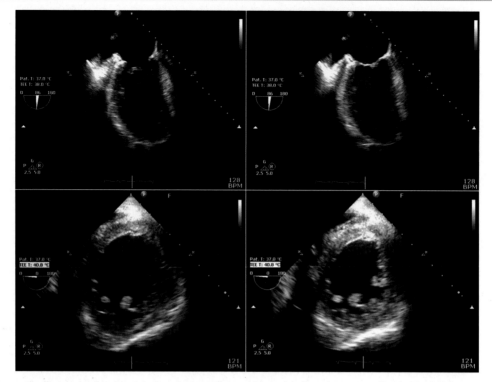

Figure 1-35. TEE images in diastole (LEFT) and systole (RIGHT). The anterior and lateral walls and apex are akinetic. The inferior wall is hypokinetic, EF 20% to 30%. Mitral leaflet coaptation is slightly apically displaced. No pericardial effusion.

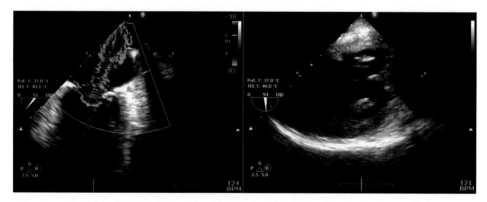

Figure 1-36. TEE. LEFT, There is moderate 3+ mitral insufficiency. The coaptation line is displaced apically. RIGHT, TEE transgastric long-axis view through the papillary muscle bodies, which are intact; the anterolateral papillary muscle is well seen on this plane.

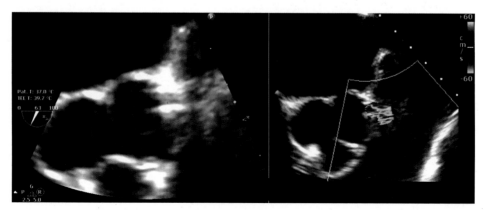

Figure 1-37. TEE. LEFT, The stent is sticking out into the sinus of Valsalva. RIGHT, Color flow mapping of the flow in the left main coronary artery.

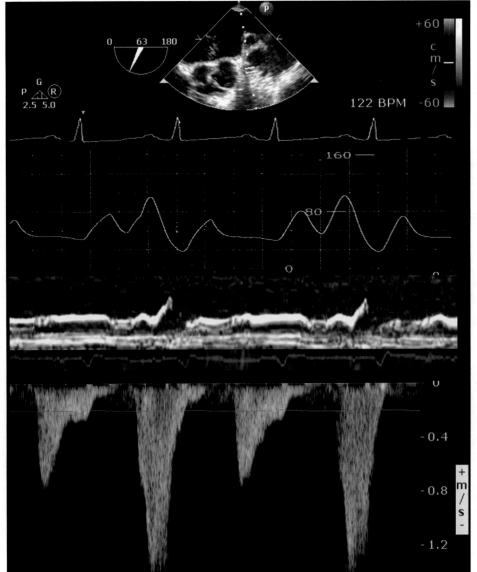

Figure 1-38. Composite TTE and pressure waveform image. The IABP is on 1:2 augmentation. The upper image shows that the pulsed wave sample volume is placed over the aneurysm of the distal left main coronary artery. The ECG and arterial pressure tracing reveal 1:2 augmentation, with good augmentation effect. The M-mode tracing depicts the IABP balloon opening every second cardiac cycle. The lower image reveals the left main coronary flow (velocity) augmentation from the aortic pressure augmentation. The presence of ischemia within the vascular territory facilitates a direct pressure:flow relationship.

References

1. Becker RC, Gore JM, Lambrew C, et al: A composite view of cardiac rupture in the United States National Registry of Myocardial Infarction. J Am Coll Cardiol 1996;27:1321-1326.

2. Hochman JS, Buller CE, Sleeper LA, et al: Cardiogenic shock complicating acute myocardial infarction—etiologies, management and outcome: a report from the SHOCK Trial Registry. SHould we emergently revascularize Occluded Coronaries for cardiogenic shocK? J Am Coll Cardiol 2000;36(Suppl A):1063-1070.

3. Wong SC, Sanborn T, Sleeper LA, et al: Angiographic findings and clinical correlates in patients with cardiogenic shock complicating acute myocardial infarction: a report from the SHOCK Trial Registry. SHould we emergently revascularize Occluded Coronaries for cardiogenic shocK? J Am Coll Cardiol 2000;36(Suppl A):1077-1083.

4. Fincke R, Hochman JS, Lowe AM, et al: Cardiac power is the strongest hemodynamic correlate of mortality in cardiogenic shock: a report from the SHOCK trial registry. J Am Coll Cardiol 2004;44:340-348.

5. Holmes DR Jr, Berger PB, Hochman JS, et al: Cardiogenic shock in patients with acute ischemic syndromes with and without ST-segment elevation. Circulation 1999;100:2067-2073.

6. Webb JG, Sleeper LA, Buller CE, et al: Implications of the timing of onset of cardiogenic shock after acute myocardial infarction: a report from the SHOCK Trial Registry. SHould we emergently revascularize Occluded Coronaries for cardiogenic shocK? J Am Coll Cardiol 2000;36(Suppl A):1084-1090.

7. Anderson RD, Ohman EM, Holmes DR Jr, et al: Use of intraaortic balloon counterpulsation in patients presenting with cardiogenic shock: observations from the GUSTO-I Study. Global Utilization of Streptokinase and TPA for Occluded Coronary Arteries. J Am Coll Cardiol 1997;30:708-715.

8. Goldberg RJ, Samad NA, Yarzebski J, et al: Temporal trends in cardiogenic shock complicating acute myocardial infarction. N Engl J Med 1999;340:1162-1168.

9. Forrester JS, Diamond GA, Swan HJ: Correlative classification of clinical and hemodynamic function after acute myocardial infarction. Am J Cardiol 1977;39:137-145.

10. Killip T III, Kimball JT: Treatment of myocardial infarction in a coronary care unit. A two year experience with 250 patients. Am J Cardiol 1967;20:457-464.

11. Menon V, White H, LeJemtel T, et al: The clinical profile of patients with suspected cardiogenic shock due to predominant left ventricular failure:

a report from the SHOCK Trial Registry. SHould we emergently revascularize Occluded Coronaries in cardiogenic shocK? J Am Coll Cardiol 2000;36(Suppl A):1071-1076.

12. Joseph MX, Disney PJ, Da CR, Hutchison SJ: Transthoracic echocardiography to identify or exclude cardiac cause of shock. Chest 2004;126:1592-1597.

13. Ryan TJ, Antman EM, Brooks NH, et al: 1999 update: ACC/AHA Guidelines for the Management of Patients With Acute Myocardial Infarction: Executive Summary and Recommendations: A report of the American College of Cardiology/American Heart Association Task Force on Practice Guidelines (Committee on Management of Acute Myocardial Infarction). Circulation 1999;100:1016-1030.

14. Mechanisms for the early mortality reduction produced by beta-blockade started early in acute myocardial infarction: ISIS-1. ISIS-1 (First International Study of Infarct Survival) Collaborative Group. Lancet 1988;1:921-923.

15. Indications for fibrinolytic therapy in suspected acute myocardial infarction: collaborative overview of early mortality and major morbidity results from all randomised trials of more than 1000 patients. Fibrinolytic Therapy Trialists (FTT) Collaborative Group. Lancet 1994;343:311-322.

16. Prewitt RM, Gu S, Garber PJ, Ducas J: Marked systemic hypotension depresses coronary thrombolysis induced by intracoronary administration of recombinant tissue-type plasminogen activator. J Am Coll Cardiol 1992;20:1626-1633.

17. Sabol MB, Luippold RS, Hebert J, et al: Association between serial measures of systemic blood pressure and early coronary arterial perfusion status following intravenous thrombolytic therapy. J Thromb Thrombolysis 1994;1:79-84.

18. Herlitz J, Hartford M, Aune S, Karlsson T: Occurrence of hypotension during streptokinase infusion in suspected acute myocardial infarction, and its relation to prognosis and metoprolol therapy. Am J Cardiol 1993;71:1021-1024.

19. Hochman JS, Sleeper LA, Webb JG, et al: Early revascularization in acute myocardial infarction complicated by cardiogenic shock. SHOCK Investigators. Should We Emergently Revascularize Occluded Coronaries for Cardiogenic Shock? N Engl J Med 1999;341:625-634.

20. Hochman JS, Sleeper LA, White HD, et al: One-year survival following early revascularization for cardiogenic shock. JAMA 2001;285:190-192.

21. Hochman JS, Sleeper LA, Webb JG, et al: Early revascularization and long-term survival in cardiogenic shock complicating acute myocardial infarction. JAMA 2006;295:2511-2515.

22. Smith SC Jr, Feldman TE, Hirshfeld JW Jr, et al: ACC/AHA/SCAI 2005 guideline update for percutaneous coronary intervention: a report of the American College of Cardiology/American Heart Association Task Force on Practice Guidelines (ACC/AHA/SCAI Writing Committee to Update the 2001 Guidelines for Percutaneous Coronary Intervention). J Am Coll Cardiol 2006;47:e1-121.

23. White HD, Assmann SF, Sanborn TA, et al: Comparison of percutaneous coronary intervention and coronary artery bypass grafting after acute myocardial infarction complicated by cardiogenic shock: results from the Should We Emergently Revascularize Occluded Coronaries for Cardiogenic Shock? (SHOCK) trial. Circulation 2005;112:1992-2001.

24. Sanborn TA, Sleeper LA, Bates ER, et al: Impact of thrombolysis, intra-aortic balloon pump counterpulsation, and their combination in cardiogenic shock complicating acute myocardial infarction: a report from the SHOCK Trial Registry. SHould we emergently revascularize Occluded Coronaries for cardiogenic shocK? J Am Coll Cardiol 2000;36(Suppl A):1123-1129.

25. Stone GW, Ohman EM, Miller MF, et al: Contemporary utilization and outcomes of intra-aortic balloon counterpulsation in acute myocardial infarction: the benchmark registry. J Am Coll Cardiol 2003;41:1940-1945.

26. Hutchison SJ, Thaker KB, Chandraratna PA: Effects of intraaortic balloon counterpulsation on flow velocity in stenotic left main coronary arteries from transesophageal echocardiography. Am J Cardiol 1994;74:1063-1065.

27. Kumbasar SD, Semiz E, Sancaktar O, et al: Concomitant use of intraaortic balloon counterpulsation and streptokinase in acute anterior myocardial infarction. Angiology 1999;50:465-471.

28. Ohman EM, Nanas J, Stomel RJ, et al: Thrombolysis and counterpulsation to improve survival in myocardial infarction complicated by hypotension and suspected cardiogenic shock or heart failure: results of the TACTICS Trial. J Thromb Thrombolysis 2005;19:33-39.

29. Delgado DH, Rao V, Ross HJ, et al: Mechanical circulatory assistance: state of art. Circulation 2002;106:2046-2050.

30. Rose EA, Gelijns AC, Moskowitz AJ, et al: Long-term mechanical left ventricular assistance for end-stage heart failure. N Engl J Med 2001;345:1435-1443.

31. Sharon A, Shpirer I, Kaluski E, et al: High-dose intravenous isosorbide-dinitrate is safer and better than Bi-PAP ventilation combined with conventional treatment for severe pulmonary edema. J Am Coll Cardiol 2000;36:832-837.

32. Pang D, Keenan SP, Cook DJ, Sibbald WJ: The effect of positive pressure airway support on mortality and the need for intubation in cardiogenic pulmonary edema: a systematic review. Chest 1998;114:1185-1192.

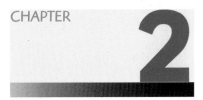

CHAPTER 2

Assessment of the Infarcted Left Ventricle

KEY POINTS

▸ Although it is imperfect, the physical examination is the most rapid and the most cost-effective method to evaluate ventricular function. Diligent and repeated history taking and physical examination are critical in establishing a basis and pretest probability for the direction of subsequent testing.

▸ Echocardiography, the most commonly performed test to determine left ventricular systolic function, can describe most functional and anatomic complications of infarction.

▸ Pulmonary artery catheterization allows accurate determinations of filling pressures and cardiac index and can be used to confirm a septal rupture.

▸ Contrast ventriculography is the second most commonly performed test to assess left ventricular systolic

function and the test most commonly performed for emergency cases that are initially assessed in the catheterization laboratory.

▸ Blood pool scanning is a reproducible test to establish ejection fraction.

▸ Cardiac MR, a test more useful for postinfarction cases than for acute infarction cases, is highly accurate for determination of ventricular geometry and systolic function.

▸ Left ventricular dysfunction is the dominant postinfarction clinical problem and determines the majority of in-hospital and postdischarge deaths. Although bedside clinical assessment is imperfect, it is a critical foundation of subsequent testing.

Multiple diagnostic tests are available to assess the postinfarction ventricle, but no single test alone is adequate or well enough suited to address all of the aspects of anatomic and functional assessment that may be needed. Proficiency with and efficient integration of bedside assessment (history and physical examination), electrocardiography, echocardiography, left- or right-sided heart catheterization, nuclear techniques, and cardiac magnetic resonance (MR) currently allow better clinical assessment than ever before; but some problems, such as suspected subacute rupture, may require definitive surgical inspection. Although many tests currently afford anatomic and functional detail, recording of pressure waveforms remains available only through catheterization—hence, its regular use in almost all cases of complicated infarction.

HISTORY AND PHYSICAL EXAMINATION

Many cardiac physical diagnosis findings are useful, although knowledge of the limitations of physical diagnosis is as important

as awareness of their utility. Physical examination should be performed repeatedly during admission for myocardial infarction to recognize left- or right-sided heart failure, onset of shock, development of mechanical complications, respiratory failure, and other conditions that require specific treatment. Important physical diagnosis signs and their possible causes are listed in Table 2-1.

Symptoms of left-sided heart failure (left atrial pressure elevation), such as dyspnea, orthopnea, and paroxysmal nocturnal dyspnea, are probably more meaningful in chronic heart disease cases than among acutely ill cardiac patients, particularly among shock cases (see Chapter 1). There is systematic tendency to underestimate the severity of left-sided heart failure, both pulmonary congestion and low systemic output or hypoperfusion. Key physical findings of left-sided heart failure are listed in Table 2-2. One of the important findings is the left ventricular third heart sound, S_3 (Figs. 2-1 and 2-2). The third heart sound is predictive of the following[1]:

Death from pump failure	1.40 [1.14-1.71]
Hospitalization for heart failure	1.42 [1.21-1.66]
Death or hospitalization for heart failure	1.22 [1.08-1.38]

Table 2-1. Physical Diagnosis Signs and Possible Causes

Sign	Possible Causes
Appearance of shock	
Agitation, poor mentation	Impaired perfusion, hypoxemia, hypercarbia, acidosis
Cool	Impaired perfusion, high SVR
Clammy	Vagal, impaired perfusion
Vitals	
Tachypnea	Pulmonary congestion, acidosis
Tachycardia	Pain, pulmonary congestion, respiratory distress, small forward stroke volume
Hypotension	Small forward stroke volume, vasodepression—acidosis, vagal, pharmacologic
Tachycardia and hypotension	Small forward stroke volume
Fever	Endocarditis, infarction, tachypnea
Pulsus paradoxus	Tamponade, pulmonary congestion
Venous distention	Tamponade, RV infarction, RV failure, tricuspid insufficiency, septal rupture
Gallop	
S$_3$	Elevated filling pressures
S$_4$	Stiff ventricle
Rub	Pericarditis, early rupture
Murmur	
Holosystolic	MR, septal rupture, papillary muscle rupture, TR, false aneurysm
Short systolic murmur	Papillary muscle rupture
To-and-fro	False aneurysm
Thrill	Septal rupture, papillary rupture
Apex	
Enlarged apex	Anteroapical dilation, anterolateral false aneurysm
Displaced apex	Anteroapical dilation, anteroapical displacement
Sustained apex	Dyskinetic anteroapex, pressure overload, low ejection fraction, anterolateral false aneurysm
Mesoapical impulse	Septal aneurysm
Parasternal impulse	RV enlargement, RV overload, severe MR
Rales	Pulmonary congestion

MR, mitral regurgitation; RV, right ventricular; SVR, systemic vascular resistance; TR, tricuspid regurgitation.

Table 2-2. Key Physical Findings of Left-Sided Heart Failure

Elevated left atrial pressure	Tachypnea
	Increased respiratory effort
	Fatigued respiratory effort
	Rales, rhonchi
	Left ventricular third heart sound (S$_3$)
Presence of a regurgitant lesion (MR, false aneurysm)	Thrill
	Systolic murmur
	Holosystolic murmur most typical of MR
	Mid to late murmur characteristic of ischemic MR
	Short murmur of papillary rupture
	Absent murmur of complete papillary rupture
	To-and-fro murmur of false aneurysm
	In some patients, only a systolic murmur may be audible.
	Small, especially inferior false aneurysms may not generate a murmur.
	Large false aneurysms with a wide neck may not cause murmurs.
Presence of a shunt lesion	Thrill (present in only half of septal rupture cases)
	Systolic murmur
	Holosystolic in most
	Present at right lower sternal border with radiation to right side of chest
	May be absent if the rent is large
Left ventricular aneurysms	Apex enlargement, displacement, sustained quality
	Anteroseptal aneurysm
	Mesoapical impulse (halfway between the sternum and the apex)
Possibility that the left ventricle is not intact	Presence of a pericardial rub
	Systolic murmur (may be present in papillary rupture, septal rupture, false aneurysm, or free wall rupture—or may be absent)
	Shock
	Electromechanical dissociation

MR, mitral regurgitation.

Recognition of the signs of cardiogenic shock remains difficult; only overt cases are obvious. Prominent elevation of heart rate and low blood pressure are valuable observations but ones confounded by both beta-blocker use and hypertensive and hyperadrenergic traits and responses. A small pulse pressure bespeaks a small stroke volume—a sign of left ventricular failure or a regurgitant or shunt lesion detracting from forward stroke volume. Obvious signs of shock, such as severely low blood pressure, poor mentation, agitation, and cool extremities, indicate severe, often advanced shock.

The limitations of the physical examination are related to experience, learning, and persistence. About 25% of cases of very low output (CI < 2.2 L/min/m^2) and 15% to 20% of cases of pulmonary congestion are not recognized by bedside examination; the latter percentage is higher in cardiogenic shock. Papillary muscle rupture may be present without a murmur when there is equilibration of left ventricular and left atrial systolic pressures. Free wall rupture may be present without a pulsus paradoxus, and false aneurysms may be inaudible. Right ventricular infarction and tamponade have similar findings.

ELECTROCARDIOGRAPHIC ASSESSMENT OF THE INFARCTED LEFT VENTRICLE

The presence of Q waves suggests transmural infarction, the antecedent of aneurysms and false aneurysms and most forms of myocardial rupture. Electrocardiography (ECG) is relatively insensitive to posterior left ventricular infarction. Sensitivity for right ventricular infarction falls after 12 hours. Discernible Q waves may be absent in the presence of posterior wall infarction and its complications, such as posteromedial papillary muscle rupture and posterior false aneurysms.

ST elevation is far more useful to localize infarction than is ST depression, which is almost useless toward infarction territory localization. ST elevation is also seen in pericarditis and aneurysms. Few patterns of ST elevation response to fibrinolytics are reliable other than prompt normalization of the ST segment with preservation of R waves without development of Q waves. Most other patterns have intermediate predictiveness of reperfusion.

ECG lacks sensitivity for infarction in the presence of left bundle branch block, ventricular paced rhythm, prior significant infarction in the same territory, posterior infarction, severe left ventricular hypertrophy, and right ventricular infarction (after hour 12).

ECG and rhythm strips remain the best test to record and to analyze rhythm disturbances related to infarction.

Some Q waves resolve postinfarction, consistent with electrocardiographic stunning.

ECHOCARDIOGRAPHIC ASSESSMENT OF THE INFARCTED LEFT VENTRICLE

The value of echocardiography in assessing various complications of infarction is summarized in Table 2-3. Echocardiography is the most commonly employed test to assess the left ventricle after infarction. Echocardiography is portable and versatile, but its greater contribution in assessing acutely infarcted ventricles is to identify structural and functional complications (mitral regurgitation; effusions, tamponade, ventricular septal rupture; papillary muscle rupture; false aneurysms), regional wall motion abnormalities, and cardiac output rather than to precisely determine ejection fraction or to determine left atrial pressure. Advantages and drawbacks of echocardiography in assessing left ventricular function are summarized in Table 2-4 and examples provided in Figures 2-3 and 2-4.

Echocardiographic Description of Systolic Parameters

Regional Wall Motion Assessment
Regional wall motion assessment by the ACC/AHA 17-segment model of the left ventricle (Fig. 2-5) should describe the severity and extent of the wall motion abnormalities. The usual standardized terminology of regional systolic function should be used:

1 = normal to hyperdynamic
2 = mild to moderate hypokinesis
3 = severe hypokinesis

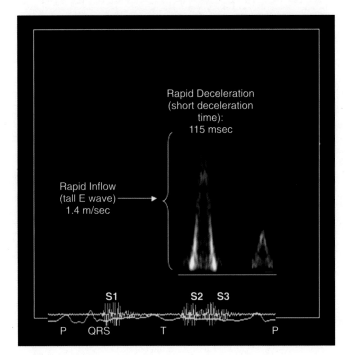

Figure 2-1. Combined LV inflow spectral profile and phonocardiogram. The early inflow (E) is rapid and the deceleration time is short—restrictive filling. The abrupt deceleration of the inflow generates the third heart sound.

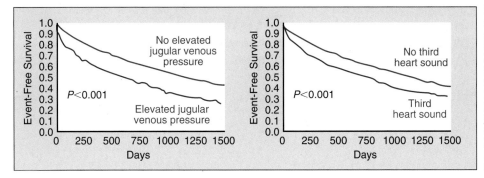

Figure 2-2. Kaplan-Meier analysis of event-free survival according to the presence or absence of elevated jugular venous pressures or third heart sound. Jugular venous pressure elevation and a third heart sound are findings associated with a significantly worse prognosis. (From Drazner MH, Rame JE, Stevenson LW, Dries DL: Prognostic importance of elevated jugular venous pressure and a third heart sound in patients with heart failure. N Engl J Med 2001;345:574-581. Copyright © [2001] Massachusetts Medical Society. All rights reserved.)

Table 2-3. Value of Echocardiography in Assessing Complications of Myocardial Infarction

Infarct expansion	Without use of endocardial surface mapping techniques, echocardiographic recognition of an increase in a wall motion area relies on subjective impression and is prone to lesser accuracy and recognition of only more severe instances of expansion.
Infarct extension	Same as above
Ischemia at distance	Recognition of wall motion abnormalities in opposite vascular territories (such as LAD and RCA) is usually straightforward. Recognition of left circumflex disease as distinct from LAD disease is more difficult as diagonal branches and obtuse marginal branches have unpredictable relation, and the lateral wall of the left ventricle is often imperfectly imaged by transthoracic echocardiography.
Aneurysms	Echocardiographic recognition of aneurysms, anterior or inferior, is good. The presence of a laminated thrombus within an anterior aneurysm may lessen the recognition of the size of the aneurysm and sometimes its presence.
False aneurysms	Other than poor-quality studies, the ability of echocardiography to recognize false aneurysms is good, and Doppler flow mapping is useful. Imaging of the full lateral extent of the body of a false aneurysm may be limited.
Effusions	Echocardiography is a good test to establish the presence of an effusion.
Tamponade	Echocardiographic recognition of tamponade is very good; however, acute tamponade cases are more difficult, especially with an underlying abnormal (infarcted) heart and especially when intrapericardial clot is present.
MR, nonpapillary muscle rupture	Echocardiography is a good test to establish the presence and severity of MR and its cause.
MR, papillary muscle rupture	Echocardiography, particularly TEE, is a good test to establish the presence and severity of MR and its origin due to partial or complete papillary muscle rupture.
Ventricular septal rupture	Echocardiography is a good test to establish the presence of ventricular septal rupture and associated complications.
Free wall rupture	Echocardiography is a useful test to build the case of free wall rupture (large effusion with clot, elevated CVP findings).
Right ventricular infarction	Echocardiography is a good test to identify right ventricular infarction and its complications.
Thrombi	Echocardiography is a good test to establish the presence and severity of intracavitary thrombi, but small thrombi, especially nonprotuberant ones, are difficult to recognize and to distinguish from trabeculations.
Dynamic LVOT obstruction	Echocardiography is a good test to establish the presence and severity of LVOT outflow obstruction.

CVP, central venous pressure; LAD, left anterior descending coronary artery; LVOT, left ventricular outflow tract; MR, mitral regurgitation; RCA, right coronary artery; TEE, transesophageal echocardiography.

Table 2-4. Value of Echocardiography in Assessing Left Ventricular Function

Advantages	Disadvantages	Common Problems
Widely available, portable, rapid bedside technique	Cannot accurately predict left atrial pressure per case	Assuming that the absence of a wall motion abnormality excludes a recent ischemic syndrome
When supplemented with TEE, offers the single best overall test to assess the acutely infarcted left ventricle for function, hemodynamics, and mechanical complications	Hemodynamic quantitation (stroke volume, cardiac index, RVSP) is underused	Underuse of TEE in inconclusive cases with potential mechanical complications
	Quantitative ejection fraction techniques are not that accurate or reproducible	Lack of familiarity with echo signs of specific diagnoses, such as intramyocardial hematomas and ruptures
Offers cardiac output, RVSP	Interpretation skills are critical	Describing that mitral insufficiency is present but not establishing the cause
	Inability to resolve a new versus old wall motion abnormality	Inability to visualize the entire left ventricle
		Inability to visualize a small thrombus or one obscured by artifact

RVSP, right ventricular systolic pressure; TEE, transesophageal echocardiography.

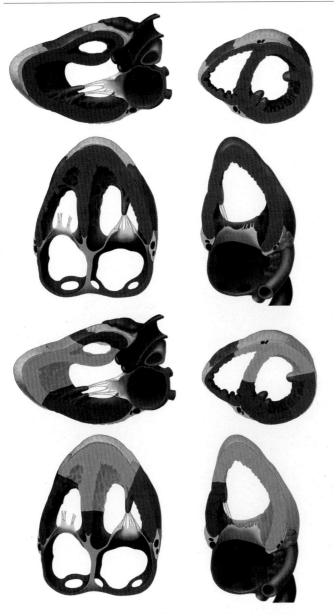

Figure 2-3. TOP TWO ROWS, Standard echocardiographic views of the left ventricle: parasternal long-axis view (TOP ROW, LEFT); parasternal short-axis view at the mid-ventricular level, denoted by the bodies of the papillary muscles (TOP ROW, RIGHT); apical 4-chamber view (SECOND ROW, LEFT); apical 2-chamber view (SECOND ROW, RIGHT). BOTTOM TWO ROWS, Usual conferred coronary anatomy: yellow, LAD-supplied perfusion; red, RCA-supplied perfusion; and purple, left circumflex coronary artery–supplied perfusion (assuming left dominance).

4 = dyskinesis (systolic outward motion)
5 = aneurysm (systolic and diastolic outward position)

The wall motion score index (wall motion segment sum/number of segments visualized) is useful because it is predictive of adverse events (Fig. 2-6). A WMSI of 1.76, 2, or 2.3 predicts a higher complication (congestive heart failure, ventricular tachycardia, ventricular fibrillation, septal rupture, and death) rate (79% versus 18%) after infarction.[2-4] Death in patients with lower wall motion score indices is often due to myocardial rupture.[2]

Ejection Fraction

Ejection fraction (EF), which correlates inversely with postinfarction survival (Fig. 2-7),[5] is a useful but imperfect descriptor of left ventricular systolic function that is available through numerous modalities (echocardiography, angiography, gated blood pool scanning, sestamibi imaging, cardiac computed tomography [CT], and cardiac MR). Calculated ejection fraction is regularly used (1) to describe predicted mortality risk,[3,5,6] (2) to predict operative (aortocoronary bypass) risk, (3) to indicate ACE inhibitor use (e.g., EF < 40%,[7] although clinical heart failure may also be used[8]), and (4) to determine ICD need (= 40 days after infarction, EF < 30%).[9]

Linear dimension formulae should never be used to calculate ejection fraction after infarction; they assume uniformity to the ventricle, which is virtually never the case in the postinfarction setting. Similarly, M-mode determined volumes should not be used; they correlate poorly with angiographic volumes ($r = 0.49$ to 0.64).[10]

Ejection fraction calculation is not the strength of echocardiography—Doppler interrogation and anatomic detailing are. The biplane Simpson techniques should be employed in postinfarction cases, but even the best echocardiographic technique is imperfect to describe many ventricles with chamber distortion. Biplane Simpson estimates correlate well with angiographic estimates of end-systolic volume ($r = 0.90$), quite well with ejection fraction ($r = 0.87$), but less well with end-diastolic volume ($r = 0.80$).[10] More important, echocardiography underestimates left ventricular diastolic volumes and overestimates ejection fraction by 10% compared with angiography.[10] In carefully performed studies, the standard error of the estimate of echocardiographic calculation of ejection fraction is 8%[10]; in the real world, it is unlikely to be better than 10%.

Interobserver and intraobserver variability of echocardiographic visual estimates (13.4% and 17.4%, respectively) are far worse than for equilibrium radionuclide angiography (1.8% and 3.6%, respectively) (Fig. 2-8).[11] The interobserver and intraobserver variability of echocardiographic visual estimates and calculated ejection fraction are far greater than those of quantitative contrast ventrculography[10] or gated blood pool scanning. Hence, some centers retain use of a grading system for categorization of left ventricular systolic function:

Grade 1 (normal):	EF% > 60%
Grade 2 (mild systolic dysfunction):	EF% 40% to 60%
Grade 3 (moderate systolic dysfunction):	EF% 20% to 40%
Grade 4 (severe systolic dysfunction):	EF% < 20%

End-Systolic Volume

End-systolic volume[5] and end-systolic volume index (ESVI)[12] are the best predictors of postinfarction systolic dysfunction and mortality (Figs. 2-9 to 2-11). GUSTO I data[12] described linear risk of 30-day mortality after infarction and after fibrinolytic use according to ESVI that was superior to location of infarction:

ESVI = 30 mL/m^2: 2.4
ESVI = 35 mL/m^2: 3.0
ESVI = 40 mL/m^2: 3.4

Three-dimensional echocardiographic determinations of left ventricular volume compare favorably with those of cardiac MR but are more variable and less available at present (Fig. 2-12).[13]

Text continued on p. 36.

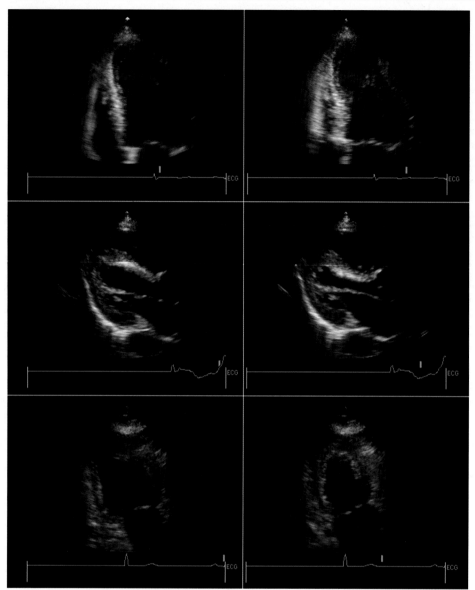

Figure 2-4. Transthoracic echocardiography. TOP IMAGES, Shallow apical 4-chamber view for LV function assessment in diastole (LEFT) and systole (RIGHT). The regionality of the wall motion abnormality is evident, with dilation of the left ventricular cavity at the apex and the distal septum. This degree of distortion is difficult for algorithms such as the biplane Simpson technique to describe accurately. MIDDLE IMAGES, Parasternal long-axis views in systole (LEFT) and diastole (RIGHT). The right ventricle is dilated as a result of infarction; the elevated right ventricular diastolic pressure has shifted the septum to the left in diastole. In systole, the distal septum has a peculiar hinge to it, which is usually due to adjacent hyperkinesis and dyskinesis but in this case was also due to a septal rupture off the plane of imaging. BOTTOM IMAGES, Apical 2-chamber views in diastole (LEFT) and systole (RIGHT). The rounder appearance of the apex in systole and the far shorter long axis of the left ventricle bespeak foreshortening of the LV due to translational artifact.

Figure 2-5. ACC/AHA 17-segment model.

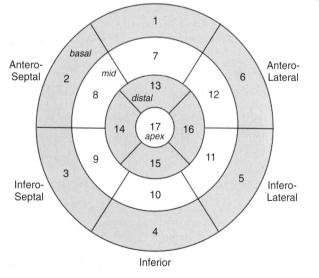

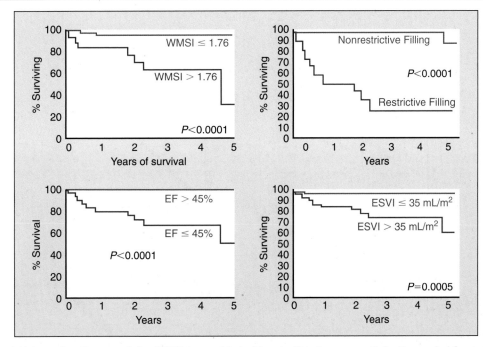

Figure 2-6. TOP LEFT, A higher wall motion score index (WMSI) is associated with a significantly worse postinfarction survival for up to 5 years. TOP RIGHT, A transmitral restrictive filling pattern is associated with a significantly worse postinfarction survival up to 5 years. BOTTOM LEFT, An ejection fraction (EF) threshold of 45% is associated with significantly different postinfarction survival, as is an end-systolic volume index (ESVI) greater than 35 mL/m² (BOTTOM RIGHT). (From Nijland F, Kamp O, Karreman AJ, et al: Prognostic implications of restrictive left ventricular filling in acute myocardial infarction: a serial Doppler echocardiographic study. J Am Coll Cardiol 1997;30:1618-1624, with permission from Elsevier.)

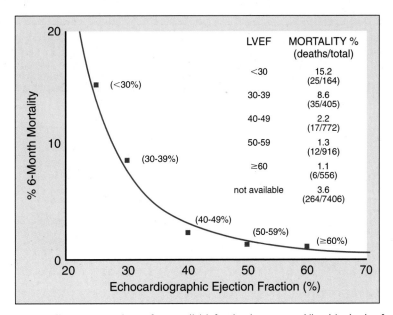

Figure 2-7. Six-month postinfarction mortality among survivors of myocardial infarction increases rapidly with ejection fraction less than 40%. LVEF, left ventricular ejection fraction. (From Volpi A, De Vita C, Franzosi MG, et al: Determinants of 6-month mortality in survivors of myocardial infarction after thrombolysis. Results of the GISSI-2 data base. The Ad hoc Working Group of the Gruppo Italiano per lo Studio della Sopravvivenza nell'Infarto Miocardico [GISSI]–2 Data Base. Circulation 1993;88:416-429.)

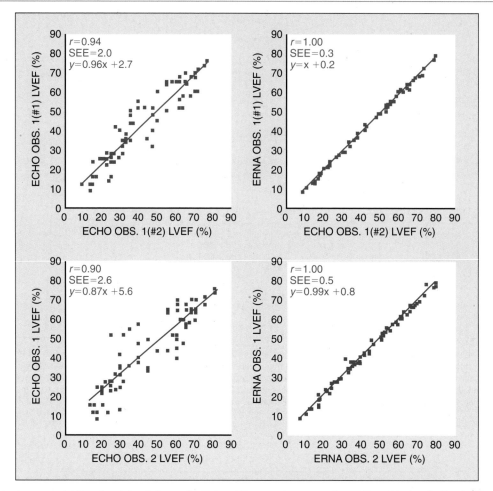

Figure 2-8. TOP, Intraobserver variability. Correlation between the first and the second assessments of left ventricular ejection fraction (LVEF) by echocardiographer 1 (LEFT) and between the first and the second assessments of LVEF by nuclear technologist 1 (RIGHT). Mean intraobserver variability is 2% for equilibrium radionuclide angiography (ERNA) and 15.3% for 2-dimensional echocardiography (ECHO). BOTTOM, Correlation between the assessment of LVEF by echocardiographers 1 and 2 (LEFT) and by nuclear technologists 1 and 2 (RIGHT). Mean interobserver variability is 3.8% for ERNA and 18.1% for ECHO. (From van Royen N, Jaffe CC, Krumholz HM, et al: Comparison and reproducibility of visual echocardiographic and quantitative radionuclide left ventricular ejection fractions. Am J Cardiol 1996;77:843-850, with permission from Elsevier.)

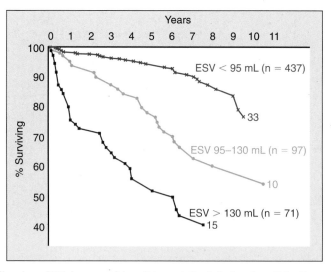

Figure 2-9. Left ventricular end-systolic volume (ESV) is a powerful predictor and discriminator of postinfarction mortality. (From White HD, Norris RM, Brown MA, et al: Left ventricular end-systolic volume as the major determinant of survival after recovery from myocardial infarction. Circulation 1987;76:44-51.)

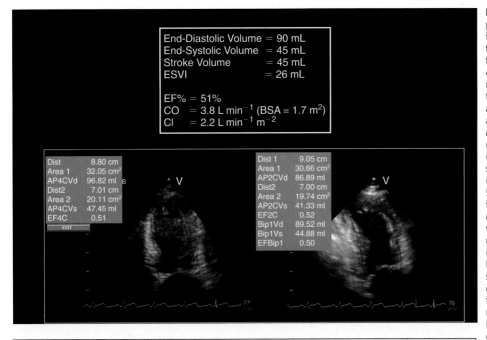

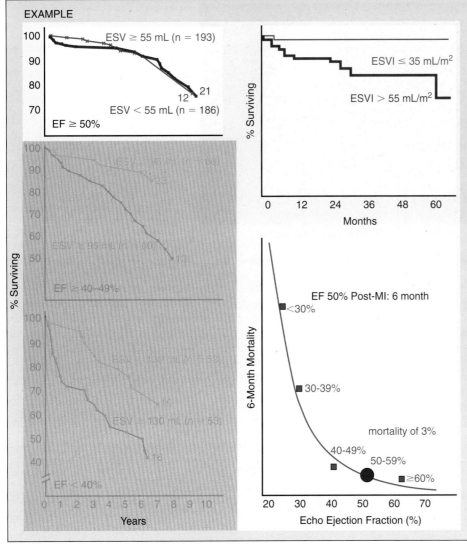

Figure 2-10. Postinfarction prognostication by echo-derived systolic indices using the biplane Simpson technique. In this example, the ejection fraction is 50%, the end-systolic volume is 45 mL, and the cardiac index is 2.2 L/min/m². All good prognostic factors, except for the lower cardiac index, as can be seen by associating these indices with the applicable survival curves (*yellow backgrounds*): survival by ejection fraction (EF) percentage and end-systolic volume (ESV) (*three left plots*), this patient's survival curve is predicted by the red line (ESV < 55 mL) of the *top left plot* (EF ≥ 50%); survival by end-systolic volume index (ESVI), the red line of the *upper right plot* (ESVI < 35 mL/m²); and survival versus ejection fraction percentage, the red circle of the *lower right plot* (EF 50%). (Three left graphs from White HD, Norris RM, Brown MA, et al: Left ventricular end-systolic volume as the major determinant of survival after recovery from myocardial infarction. Circulation 1987;76:44-51. Top right graph from Niijland F, Kamp O, Karreman AJ, et al: Prognostic implications of restrictive left ventricular filling in acute myocardial infarction: a serial Doppler echocardiographic study. J Am Coll Cardiol 1997;30:1618-1624. Lower right graph from Volpi A, De Vita C, Franzosi MG, et al: Determinants of 6-month mortality in survivors of myocardial infarction after thrombolysis. Results of the GISSI-2 data base. The Ad hoc Working Group of the Gruppo Italiano per lo Studio della Sopravvivenza nell'Infarto Miocardico [GISSI]-2 Data Base. Circulation 1993;88:416-429.)

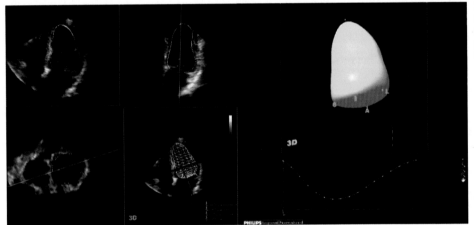

Figure 2-11. LEFT, The relationship between biplane 2-dimensional echocardiographic LV end-diastolic volumes indexed to body surface area, on the ordinate, and biplane cineventriculographic end-diastolic volumes indexed to body surface area, on the abscissa, is shown. MIDDLE, A similar comparison is shown for LV end-systolic volumes. RIGHT, A similar comparison is shown for LV ejection fractions. The outer limit lines represent 95% confidence intervals for the data. (From Schiller NB, Acquatella H, Ports TA, et al: Left ventricular volume from paired biplane two-dimensional echocardiography. Circulation 1979;60:547-555.)

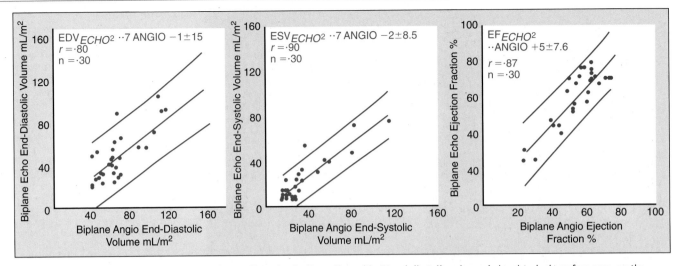

Figure 2-12. Three-dimensional echocardiography. LEFT, Standard echocardiographic views enabling endocardial tracing. RIGHT, Rendered 3D image and time:volume curve.

Echocardiographic Description of Diastolic Parameters

Numerous echocardiographic diastolic parameters correlate with indices of left ventricular dysfunction and pulmonary capillary wedge pressure and have been shown to predict risk (Figs. 2-13 to 2-16). The majority of these parameters are readily obtained; however, few have translated to clinically reliable descriptions of mean left atrial pressure or of pulmonary capillary wedge pressure. Mitral inflow deceleration time is lower among patients with left ventricular dilation than among those without.[14] There is an inverse relationship ($r = 0.90$; $P < .01$) of mitral inflow deceleration time and pulmonary capillary wedge pressure in patients after infarction but substantially lesser correlation of E/A and pulmonary capillary wedge pressure ($r = 0.65$; $P < .01$).[15] A problematic aspect of inflow patterns is that infarction-related loss of compliance of the left ventricle and elevated left atrial pressure result in competing effects that cause a pseudonormal pattern. Nevertheless, pseudonormal and restrictive left ventricular inflow patterns are more predictive of cardiac death than wall motion score index, peak creatine kinase, and age and are slightly more predictive than Killip class (Table 2-5).[3,4]

Left Atrial Volume Index

Left atrial volume index is influenced by the diastolic and systolic function of the left ventricle, the presence of atrial fibrillation, and mitral insufficiency. Whereas many diastolic parameters exhibit variability, left atrial volume has been suggested as a more stable reflection of the extent of dysfunction of the left side of the heart and has been established as another independent predictor of survival after infarction. The predictive value of left atrial volume is incremental to that of clinical parameters, left ventricular systolic function, and usual diastolic parameters.[16]

CARDIAC CATHETERIZATION TECHNIQUES FOR ASSESSMENT OF THE INFARCTED LEFT VENTRICLE

Uncomplicated infarction cases do not require left- or right-sided heart catheterization, but patients with any significant or persistent hemodynamic problems or suspected mechanical

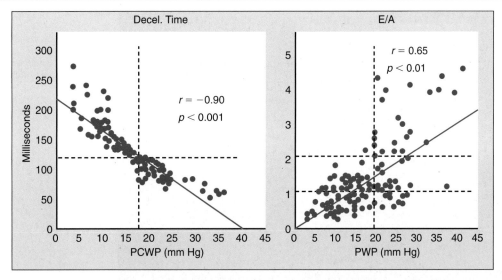

Figure 2-13. LEFT, Mitral inflow deceleration time correlates with pulmonary capillary wedge pressure (PCWP) in postinfarction patients. RIGHT, Mitral inflow E/A ratio correlates poorly with pulmonary capillary wedge pressure in postinfarction patients. (From Giannuzzi P, Imparato A, Temporelli PL, et al: Doppler-derived mitral deceleration time of early filling as a strong predictor of pulmonary capillary wedge pressure in postinfarction patients with left ventricular systolic dysfunction. J Am Coll Cardiol 1994;23:1630-1637.)

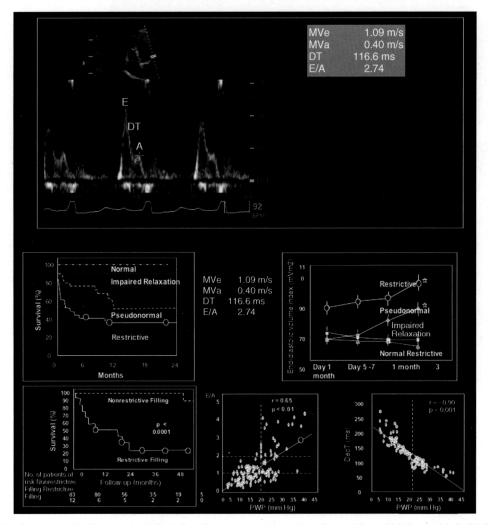

Figure 2-14. Postinfarction prognostication by echo-derived diastolic parameters. The pattern is restrictive, which is associated with higher mortality, higher PCWP, and higher end-diastolic volume index.

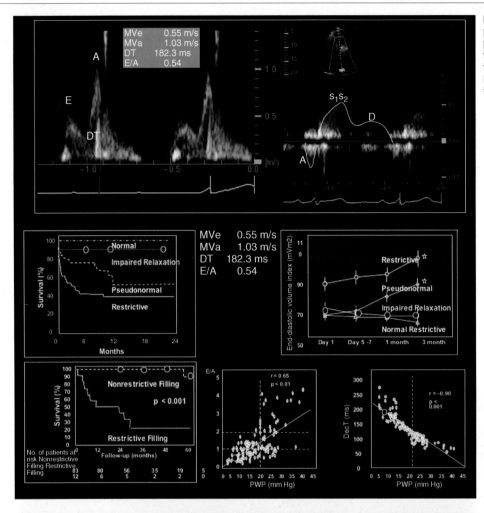

Figure 2-15. Postinfarction prognostication by echo-derived diastolic parameters. The overall pattern is of impaired relaxation (nonrestrictive), which is associated with lower mortality, lower PCWP, and lower end-diastolic volume index.

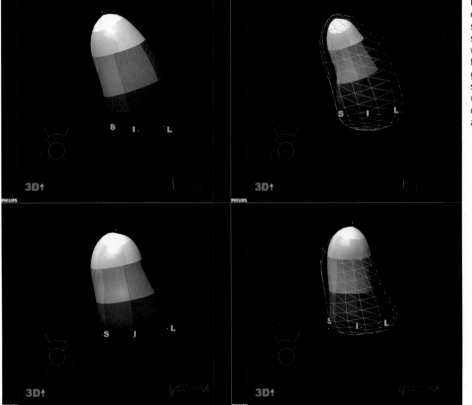

Figure 2-16. Three-dimensional real-time echo images during diastole (TOP) and systole (BOTTOM) of a patient with normal systolic function (TOP) and of a patient with an apical infarction. The wire mesh frame serves to render the end-diastolic geometry of the LV. Conventional wall segments are depicted in different colors with the corresponding segment denoted on the bullet plot. Ejection fraction is automatically yielded.

Table 2-5. Univariate Predictors of Cardiac Death

	Survivors (n = 92)	Cardiac Death (n = 33)	P Value
Age (years)	65 ± 12	76 ± 9	<.0005
Anterior MI	42 (46%)	16 (48%)	NS
Q-wave MI	28 (30%)	16 (48%)	NS
Hypertension	31 (34%)	13 (39%)	NS
Killip class ≥II	29 (32%)	31 (94%)	<.0005
Use of fibrinolytic therapy	52 (57%)	12 (36%)	.04
Peak creatine kinase (U/L)	1895 ± 1408	2955 ± 1153	.001
Ejection fraction	0.57 ± 0.14	0.43 ± 0.14	<.0005
Wall motion score index	1.40 ± 0.26	1.68 ± 0.34	<.0005
End-systolic volume index	29 ± 16	41 ± 20	<.0005
End-diastolic volume index	64 ± 18	68 ± 23	NS
Restrictive or pseudonormal filling pattern	21 (23%)	28 (85%)	<.0005

MI, myocardial infarction.
From Moller JE, Sondergaard E, Poulsen SH, Egstrup K: Pseudonormal and restrictive filling patterns predict left ventricular dilation and cardiac death after a first myocardial infarction: a serial color M-mode Doppler echocardiographic study. J Am Coll Cardiol 2000;36:1841-1846, with permission from Elsevier.

complications should undergo right-sided heart catheterization.[17] Left-sided heart catheterization is available through coronary angiography procedures but may be separately indicated to assess for complications of infarction. Pulmonary artery catheterization is also useful in recognizing systolic dysfunction (Table 2-6). Contrast ventriculography is the second most commonly used test to assess left ventricular function and has a number of advantages and disadvantages (Table 2-7; Figs. 2-17 to 2-19).

NUCLEAR TECHNIQUES FOR ASSESSMENT OF THE INFARCTED LEFT VENTRICLE

Blood Pool Scanning: Multiple Gaited Acquisition

Multiple gaited acquisition (MUGA) is probably the most reproducible test for estimating LVEF % (±3% to 5%), although it is seldom available at the bedside (Figs. 2-20 to 2-22). It is rarely done, given the utility of contrast ventriculography in patients undergoing early invasive assessment and echocardiography in the remainder. It is an excellent test to prognosticate the basis of left ventricular dysfunction[19] and to determine eligibility for ICDs. It is also a good test for evaluation of regional systolic function as long as cardiac rhythm is regular and there are no conduction disturbances.

Sestamibi Imaging

Sestamibi imaging can yield LVEF, but it is the least accurate nuclear method to assess regional or global systolic function (Fig. 2-23).

Table 2-6. Signs of Severe Systolic (Right or Left Ventricular) Dysfunction on Pulmonary Artery Catheterization

Cardiac index <2.2 L/min/m²

Sign of elevated left atrial pressure

Elevated pulmonary artery pressure

Elevated pulmonary capillary wedge pressure

Signs of left ventricular mechanical complications or disruption

O_2 saturation step-up consistent with septal rupture

V waves are consistent with mitral insufficiency but are also seen with septal rupture and left-sided heart failure and are not present in all cases of papillary rupture.

Elevated or equilibrated diastolic pressures are consistent with both tamponade and right ventricular infarction.

Technetium Pyrophosphate Imaging

Technetium pyrophosphate (TPP) scanning offered hope to establish the presence and site of infarction, but it lacks sensitivity, specificity, and availability.

CARDIAC MAGNETIC RESONANCE AND CARDIAC COMPUTED TOMOGRAPHY FOR ASSESSMENT OF THE INFARCTED LEFT VENTRICLE

Cardiac MR (Figs. 2-24 to 2-28) is accepted as probably the most accurate means to assess left or right ventricular regional systolic

Text continued on p. 47.

Table 2-7. Usefulness of Contrast Ventriculography in Assessing Left Ventricular Function

Advantages	Disadvantages
A standard test (the second most common test to assess left ventricular function)	Inaccurate with highly irregular rhythm (atrial fibrillation, PVCs, VT)
Integral to early invasive assessment	Poor opacification yields uncertain depictions of cavitary borders, especially in larger cavities.
Complementary *biplane* (RAO + LAO) projections depict ventricular geometry and systolic function. The RAO projection approximates the echocardiographic 2-chamber view, and the LAO projection approximates the parasternal short-axis image.	If it is performed only in the RAO projection, the lack of representation of the septal and lateral wall systolic function systematically and significantly underestimates ejection fraction in the presence of an anterior wall motion abnormality, as the RAO projection overemphasizes LAD-related dysfunction.[18]
Depicts mitral insufficiency and septal rupture (if the LAO projection is used) and false aneurysms and aneurysms (if the optimal plane of depiction is achieved)	Often subjective assessment of wall motion alone is offered, despite availability of computer-assisted endocardial planimetry.
If good opacification is achieved, the apex is probably better (more completely) seen by contrast ventriculography than it is by echocardiography, as foreshortening is avoided.	Interobserver and intraobserver variability is low (SD ± 5%-7%), but only if computer-assisted techniques are employed. "Eye-ball" determinations are as inexact and poorly reproducible as those of echocardiography.
On occasion, ventriculography (by any technique) can visualize larger and protruding thrombi.	Incurs contrast dye risks, puncture risks, and aortic catheterization risks
Catheterization allows diastolic and systolic pressure waveform recording.	

LAD, left anterior descending coronary artery; LAO, left anterior oblique; PVCs, premature ventricular contractions; RAO, right anterior oblique; VT, ventricular tachycardia.

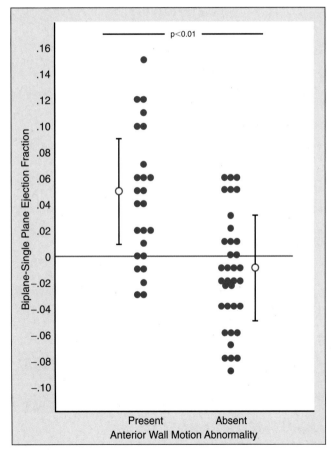

Figure 2-17. In the presence of an anterior wall motion abnormality, biplane contrast ventriculography establishes a significantly higher ejection fraction than does single-plane RAO ventriculography, which is weighted by overrepresentation of the anterior wall systolic function. (From Tate DA, Weaver D, Dehmer GJ: Effect of an anterior wall motion abnormality on the results of single-plane and biplane left ventriculography. Am J Cardiol 1992;70:791-796, with permission from Elsevier.)

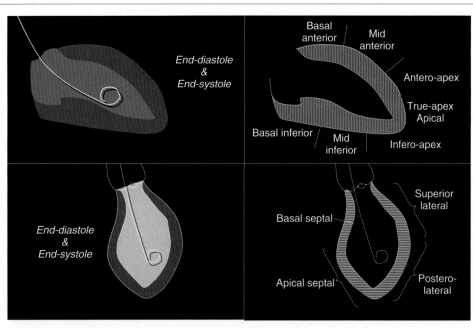

Figure 2-18. Biplane ventriculography enables tracing of left ventricular end-diastolic and end-systolic borders. The nomenclature of wall motion assessment is different from that of the 17-segmentation model.

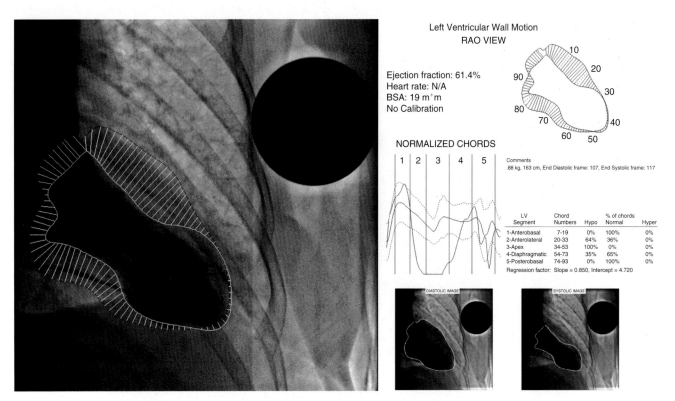

Left Ventricular Wall Motion
RAO VIEW

Ejection fraction: 61.4%
Heart rate: N/A
BSA: 19 m⁺m
No Calibration

NORMALIZED CHORDS

Comments
.88 kg, 163 cm, End Diastolic frame: 107, End Systolic frame: 117

LV Segment	Chord Numbers	Hypo	% of chords Normal	Hyper
1-Anterobasal	7-19	0%	100%	0%
2-Anterolateral	20-33	64%	36%	0%
3-Apex	34-53	100%	0%	0%
4-Diaphragmatic	54-73	35%	65%	0%
5-Posterobasal	74-93	0%	100%	0%

Regression factor: Slope = 0.850, Intercept = 4.720

DIASTOLIC IMAGE   SYSTOLIC IMAGE

Figure 2-19. This single-plane (RAO) contrast ventriculogram has been planimetered at both end-diastole and end-systole. A calibration disk was placed at the patient's left side. Regional function is denoted by the chord length, which is plotted. Ejection fraction is automatically yielded. The impact of LAD-generated LV dysfunction is understandably overweighted by use of the RAO projection alone, without an LAO projection as well.

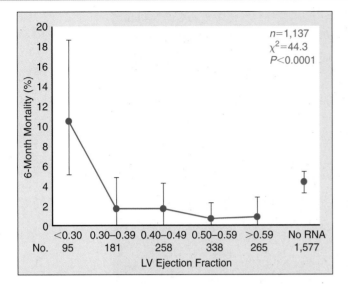

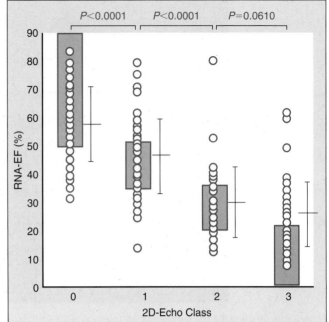

Figure 2-20. Nuclear assessment of left ventricular ejection fraction predicts 6-month mortality after infarction. (From Burns RJ, Gibbons RJ, Yi Q, et al: The relationships of left ventricular ejection fraction, end-systolic volume index and infarct size to six-month mortality after hospital discharge following myocardial infarction treated by thrombolysis. J Am Coll Cardiol 2002;39:30-36, with permission from Elsevier.)

Figure 2-21. The MUGA LV ejection fractions *(solid bars)* and the mean and standard deviation for the visual 2-dimensional echocardiographic LV ejection fraction estimates are shown. Echocardiographic scores are as follows: 0, normal; 1, slightly reduced; 2, moderately reduced; and 3, severely reduced. Note the broad standard deviations and wide range of visual estimates for LV ejection fraction from the 2-dimensional echocardiographic images in each category. (With kind permission from Springer Science + Business Media: Gottsauner-Wolf M, Schedlmayer-Duit J, Porenta G, et al: Assessment of left ventricular function: comparison between radionuclide angiography and semiquantitative two-dimensional echocardiographic analysis. Eur J Nucl Med 1996;23:1613-1618.)

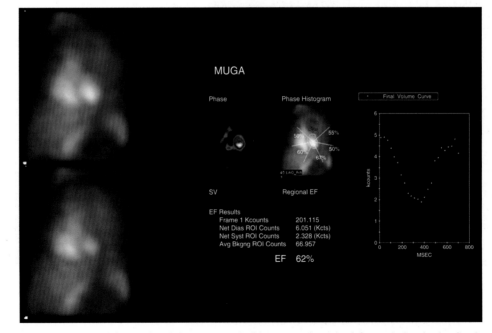

Figure 2-22. Gated blood pool scanning (MUGA) is one of the most reproducible tests to determine left ventricular ejection fraction and diastolic filling curves.

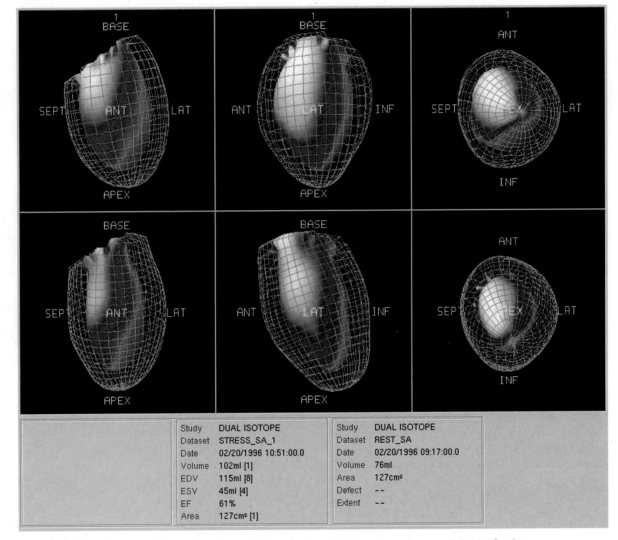

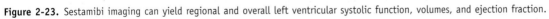

Figure 2-23. Sestamibi imaging can yield regional and overall left ventricular systolic function, volumes, and ejection fraction.

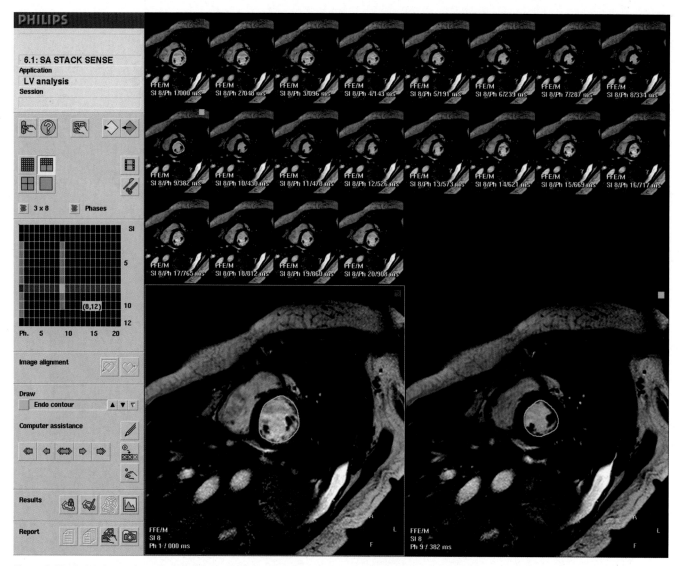

Figure 2-24. Serial short-axis cardiac MR images of the heart, with endocardial planimetry at end-diastole and end-systole. The high quality of endocardial definition is the basis of the cardiac MR modality's ability to establish ventricular volume and ejection fraction.

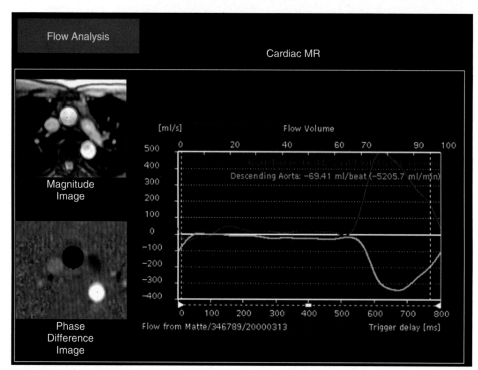

Figure 2-25. By use of the phase-contrast technique, cardiac MR can measure volumetric flow in large, round, nonmoving structures such as the aorta and pulmonary artery.

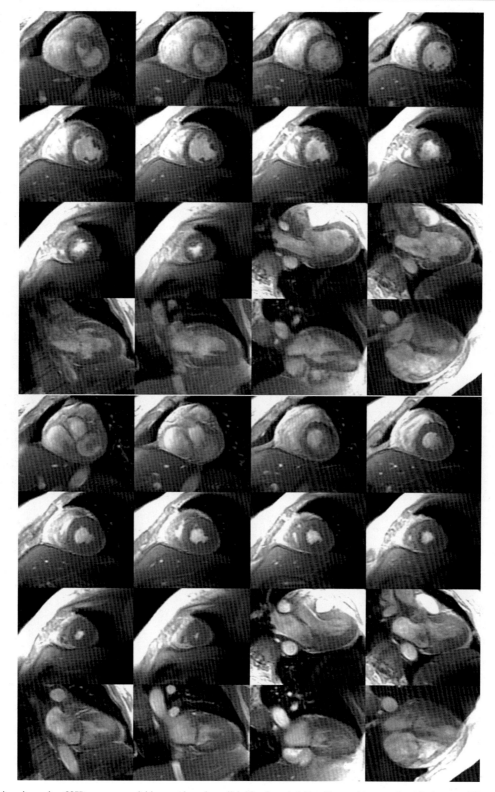

Figure 2-26. Cine imaging using SSFP sequences yields superb endocardial:blood pool delineation and temporal resolution, providing superb wall motion assessment. Also, note the completeness of the endocardial definition, especially over the lateral wall—a problem area for echocardiography.

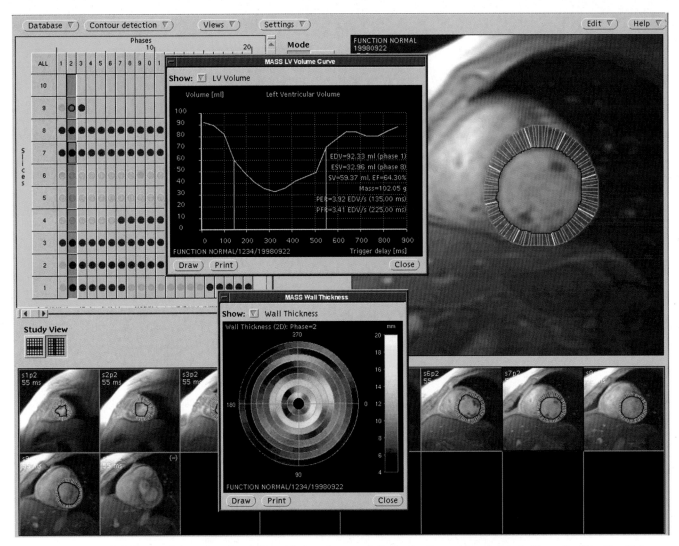

Figure 2-27. By use of planimetry of the endocardium, left ventricular volumes and ejection fraction can be calculated with cardiac MR with a high degree of reproducibility. By use of planimetry of the epicardium as well, left ventricular mass can be calculated with a reproducibility greater than by any other technology.

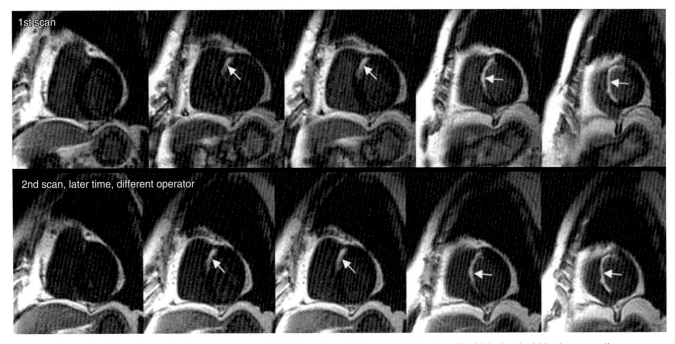

Figure 2-28. Cardiac MR: gradient echo inversion recovery/gadolinium delayed enhancement technique. The high signal within the myocardium reproducibly localizes to scar tissue, enabling determination of anatomic territory and of degree of transmurality in this chronic infarction case. (From Mahrholdt H, Wagner A, Holly TA, et al: Reproducibility of chronic infarct size measurement by contrast-enhanced magnetic resonance imaging. Circulation 2002;106:2322-2327.)

function, overall systolic function, and geometry (volumes, masses) and to localize infarction by delayed gadolinium enhancement inversion recovery technique (territory, subendocardial infarction versus transmural). Significant drawbacks of cardiac MR in critically ill patients include its lack of on-site availability at most centers, its challenges in ventilated cases and lesser monitoring ability, and its risks in patients with implanted pacemakers or implantable defibrillators.

Cardiac MR reproducibly localizes and quantifies (chronic) myocardial infarction with a bias (0.1% versus −1.3%) and coefficient of repeatability superior to SPECT imaging (±2.4% versus ±4.0%). Cardiac MR is also more sensitive than echocardiography in the detection of thrombi.[20]

ECG-gated cardiac CT can retrospectively or prospectively acquire through a cardiac cycle and approximate end-diastolic and end-systolic areas and volumes and thereby ejection fraction. Cardiac CT yields highly reproducible determinations of left ventricular volumes, but ones that are significantly greater than by cardiac MR.[13]

References

1. Drazner MH, Rame JE, Stevenson LW, Dries DL: Prognostic importance of elevated jugular venous pressure and a third heart sound in patients with heart failure. N Engl J Med 2001;345:574-581.
2. Nishimura RA, Tajik AJ, Shub C, et al: Role of two-dimensional echocardiography in the prediction of in-hospital complications after acute myocardial infarction. J Am Coll Cardiol 1984;4:1080-1087.
3. Nijland F, Kamp O, Karreman AJ, et al: Prognostic implications of restrictive left ventricular filling in acute myocardial infarction: a serial Doppler echocardiographic study. J Am Coll Cardiol 1997;30:1618-1624.
4. Moller JE, Sondergaard E, Poulsen SH, Egstrup K: Pseudonormal and restrictive filling patterns predict left ventricular dilation and cardiac death after a first myocardial infarction: a serial color M-mode Doppler echocardiographic study. J Am Coll Cardiol 2000;36:1841-1846.
5. White HD, Norris RM, Brown MA, et al: Left ventricular end-systolic volume as the major determinant of survival after recovery from myocardial infarction. Circulation 1987;76:44-51.
6. Volpi A, De Vita C, Franzosi MG, et al: Determinants of 6-month mortality in survivors of myocardial infarction after thrombolysis. Results of the GISSI-2 data base. The Ad hoc Working Group of the Gruppo Italiano per lo Studio della Sopravvivenza nell'Infarto Miocardico (GISSI)–2 Data Base. Circulation 1993;88:416-429.
7. Pfeffer MA, Braunwald E, Moye LA, et al: Effect of captopril on mortality and morbidity in patients with left ventricular dysfunction after myocardial infarction. Results of the survival and ventricular enlargement trial. The SAVE Investigators. N Engl J Med 1992;327:669-677.
8. Effect of ramipril on mortality and morbidity of survivors of acute myocardial infarction with clinical evidence of heart failure. The Acute Infarction Ramipril Efficacy (AIRE) Study Investigators. Lancet 1993;342: 821-828.
9. Moss AJ, Hall WJ, Cannom DS, et al: Improved survival with an implanted defibrillator in patients with coronary disease at high risk for ventricular arrhythmia. Multicenter Automatic Defibrillator Implantation Trial Investigators. N Engl J Med 1996;335:1933-1940.
10. Schiller NB, Acquatella H, Ports TA, et al: Left ventricular volume from paired biplane two-dimensional echocardiography. Circulation 1979;60: 547-555.
11. van Royen N, Jaffe CC, Krumholz HM, et al: Comparison and reproducibility of visual echocardiographic and quantitative radionuclide left ventricular ejection fractions. Am J Cardiol 1996;77:843-850.
12. Migrino RQ, Young JB, Ellis SG, et al: End-systolic volume index at 90 to 180 minutes into reperfusion therapy for acute myocardial infarction is a strong predictor of early and late mortality. The Global Utilization of Streptokinase and t-PA for Occluded Coronary Arteries (GUSTO)–I Angiographic Investigators. Circulation 1997;96:116-121.
13. Sugeng L, Mor-Avi V, Weinert L, et al: Quantitative assessment of left ventricular size and function: side-by-side comparison of real-time three-dimensional echocardiography and computed tomography with magnetic resonance reference. Circulation 2006;114:654-661.
14. Cerisano G, Bolognese L, Carrabba N, et al: Doppler-derived mitral deceleration time: an early strong predictor of left ventricular remodeling after reperfused anterior acute myocardial infarction. Circulation 1999;99:230-236.
15. Giannuzzi P, Imparato A, Temporelli PL, et al: Doppler-derived mitral deceleration time of early filling as a strong predictor of pulmonary capillary wedge pressure in postinfarction patients with left ventricular systolic dysfunction. J Am Coll Cardiol 1994;23:1630-1637.
16. Moller JE, Hillis GS, Oh JK, et al: Left atrial volume: a powerful predictor of survival after acute myocardial infarction. Circulation 2003;107:2207-2212.
17. Ryan TJ, Antman EM, Brooks NH, et al: 1999 update: ACC/AHA Guidelines for the Management of Patients With Acute Myocardial Infarction: Executive Summary and Recommendations: a report of the American College of Cardiology/American Heart Association Task Force on Practice Guidelines (Committee on Management of Acute Myocardial Infarction). Circulation 1999;100:1016-1030.
18. Tate DA, Weaver D, Dehmer GJ: Effect of an anterior wall motion abnormality on the results of single-plane and biplane left ventriculography. Am J Cardiol 1992;70:791-796.
19. Burns RJ, Gibbons RJ, Yi Q, et al: The relationships of left ventricular ejection fraction, end-systolic volume index and infarct size to six-month mortality after hospital discharge following myocardial infarction treated by thrombolysis. J Am Coll Cardiol 2002;39:30-36.
20. Mahrholdt H, Wagner A, Holly TA, et al: Reproducibility of chronic infarct size measurement by contrast-enhanced magnetic resonance imaging. Circulation 2002;106:2322-2327.

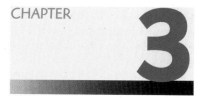
Myocardial Dysfunction, Aneurysm Formation, and Left Ventricular Remodeling

Left ventricular dysfunction is responsible for the large majority of postinfarction heart failure states and of cardiogenic shock. The SHOCK registry observed that 78.5% of cardiogenic shock cases were due to pump failure and that the mortality of this group was 59%.[1]

In the setting of myocardial infarction, myocardial contractile dysfunction is due to different causes. Infarction or necrosis, hibernation, stunning, ischemia within the infarct territory, ischemia at distance (ischemia in a separate vascular territory), infarct extension (infarction of myocardium adjacent to acutely infarcted myocardium within the penumbra of the initial infarct), infarct expansion (dilation or stretching of the infarct segment), and remodeling all confer systolic and diastolic dysfunction or failure and may contribute to heart failure. Transmural infarction and necrosis in a minority of unfortunate individuals will serve as the substrate for myocardial rupture, usually when the noninfarcted myocardium retains enough mechanical function to disrupt the tissue integrity of the infarct zone.

POSTINFARCTION MYOCARDIAL DYSFUNCTION

Infarct extension (infarction of myocardium adjacent to acutely infarcted myocardium)[2] is associated with a 2.5-fold increase in in-hospital mortality and a 30% decrease of 1-year survival. Infarct extension is identified by a larger wall motion abnormality. Although echocardiography would be the test most commonly used to recognize an increase in the extent of wall motion abnormalities and has some validation (sensitivity, 70%; specificity, 100%),[3] more sophisticated and comprehensive mapping techniques, such as cardiac magnetic resonance, are likely to be superior.

Ischemia at distance refers to ischemia or infarction at a site remote from the acute infarction. The anatomic implication is of multivessel coronary artery disease (CAD), and the clinical implication is of a greatly increased risk of cardiogenic shock and death

(78% versus 7%). The diagnosis can be made by recognition of a new wall motion abnormality by echocardiography[4] at a site remote from the acute infarction or potentially by perfusion evidence.

Infarct expansion refers to progressive thinning and dilation (stretching) of the infarct segment into an aneurysm.[2]

POSTINFARCTION VENTRICULAR REMODELING

Ventricular geometric remodeling is an adaptive but also a pathologic process. Dilation of the left ventricle will achieve partial normalization of stroke volume, which declined abruptly with acute myocardial infarction.[5] Hence, from the perspective of the circulation, ventricular dilation is adaptive. From the perspective of the heart, it places a greater stress and strain on residual myocardium and is adaptation with cost, conferring a burden similar to volume overload on a heart with depressed systolic function. Some aspects of infarct expansion and ventricular dilation remain poorly understood in the era of reperfusion. The factors that determine limited, adaptive dilation and remodeling and those that determine progressive detrimental dilation and remodeling are not well understood. Patency of the infarct-related artery may be less important, in the era of reperfusion, than factors intrinsic to the remodeling process.[6]

Progressive dilation and remodeling occur in some patients, characterized by dilation of the infarct segment, dilation of the remainder of the heart (typically conferring a globular shape to the left ventricular cavity), and elevation of the filling pressures. Radial and longitudinal dilation of the left ventricular cavity commonly results in functional mitral insufficiency, which is usually mild or moderate, but it is a marker of more severe left ventricular dysfunction and worse prognosis.[7] Even if the mitral insufficiency is not severe, it compromises forward stroke volume, facilitates further left-sided heart dilation, and augments heart failure, including backpressure to the right side of the heart. The combination of elevated left ventricular diastolic pressure and mitral insufficiency leads to globular dilation of the left atrium. Postinfarction left atrial volume is a significant predictor of adverse outcome as it integrates several adverse parameters (left atrial pressure, mitral insufficiency, and atrial fibrillation).[8] Elevated left atrial pressure, septal dysfunction or right ventricular free wall dysfunction, and volume overload may incite right-sided heart failure, resulting in an ischemic cardiomyopathy picture that resembles dilated cardiomyopathy.

Infarct expansion predicts excess in-hospital events (50% versus 0%), is seen in most fatal cases of cardiogenic shock (70%),[2] and is associated with an increased frequency of myocardial rupture.[9] Infarct expansion is diagnosed by identification of a thinned and dilated infarct segment, usually by echocardiography or ventriculography,[10] although cardiac magnetic resonance is probably the best tool for serial quantification and comparisons. Remodeling is essentially an area increase and volume increase; therefore, linear dimensional measurements, as with M-mode echocardiography, are prone to error and misrepresentation of the overall geometry of distorted ventricles. Volume measurement is the preferred means to describe remodeling.[11]

Expansion begins in days and typically occurs during several weeks (Fig. 3-1).[9] Anterior infarctions are far more likely

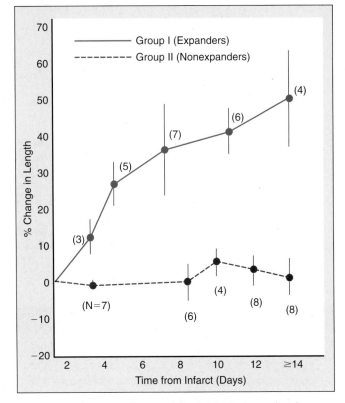

Figure 3-1. Infarct expansion-remodeling begins in days and evolves during weeks to months. (From Eaton LW, Weiss JL, Bulkley BH, et al: Regional cardiac dilatation after acute myocardial infarction: Recognition by two-dimensional echocardiography. N Engl J Med 1979; 300:57-62. Copyright © [2001] Massachusetts Medical Society. All rights reserved.)

to expand than are inferior infarctions[12] because of their size, the relative thinness of the normal apex, and the lack of adjacent diaphragm to buttress the infarct segment (Fig. 3-2).

Dilation of the infarct segment invariably occurs with and due to loss of contractile function. Dyskinesis of the expanded infarct segment consumes a proportion of the stroke volume, which functions as regurgitant volume, reducing the efficiency of the noninfarcted myocardium. The greater the thinning, dilation, and dyskinesis of the infarct segment into an aneurysm, the greater the regurgitant volume wasted into it.

There is poor correlation of infarct sizing (by biomarker rise) with postinfarction ejection fraction (Fig. 3-3). There is better correlation of postinfarction end-systolic volume with ejection fraction.[13]

The noninfarcted myocardium acutely and chronically functions to compensate for the loss of contractile function due to the infarction and the further loss of function due to inefficiency imparted by functional mitral regurgitation and loss of stroke volume into a dyskinetic aneurysm (Table 3-1). Infarct expansion leads to dilation of the left ventricular cavity, increasing wall stress that increases the proportion of internal workload and reduces the proportion of external work achieved, resulting in a fall in ejection. The left ventricular cavity will dilate (enlarge) by an average of 50 mL among first-infarction middle-aged patients with left anterior descending (LAD) coronary artery occlusions.

Initially, the noninfarcted segments of the left ventricle compensate by hypercontractile function and at a higher cardiac

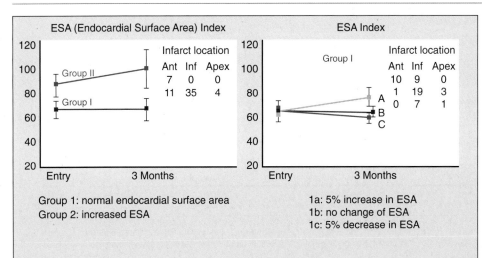

Figure 3-2. Most cases of ventricular dilation occur in anterior infarction. (From Picard MH, Wilkins GT, Ray PA, Weyman AE: Natural history of left ventricular size and function after acute myocardial infarction. Assessment and prediction by echocardiographic endocardial surface mapping. Circulation 1990;82:484-494.)

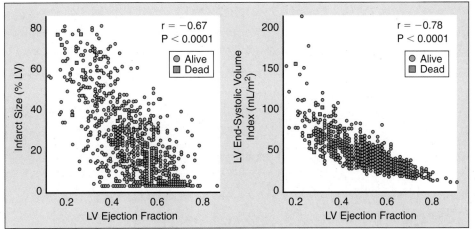

Figure 3-3. LEFT, Infarct size and left ventricular (LV) ejection fraction in the 872 patients with both measurements. There is a highly significant correlation ($r = -0.67$, $P <.0001$) between the two but substantial variability to the relation. RIGHT, LV end-systolic volume index and LV ejection fraction in 909 patients with both measurements. There is a highly significant correlation ($r = -0.78$, $P <.0001$) between the two, but again, variability to the relation. (From Burns RJ, Gibbons RJ, Yi Q, et al; CORE Study Investigators: The relationships of left ventricular ejection fraction, end-systolic volume index and infarct size to six-month mortality after hospital discharge following myocardial infarction treated by thrombolysis. J Am Coll Cardiol 2002;39:30-36, with permission from Elsevier.)

Table 3-1. Example of Serial Effects of Adverse Remodeling Compromising Stroke Volume

		Residual SV
Normal stroke volume (SV)	100 mL	
Loss of contractility from MI	−30 mL	70 mL
Loss of stroke volume into dyskinetic aneurysm	−10 mL	60 mL
Further loss of contractility	−5 mL	55 mL
Development of MR from LV dilation, leading to loss of stroke volume as a regurgitant volume	−20 mL	35 mL

MI, myocardial infarction; MR, mitral regurgitation; LV, left ventricular.

frequency. Prior infarction, or acute ischemia in other vascular territories, attenuates the compensatory response, resulting in a higher incidence of early heart failure, pump failure, and death. Chronically, compensatory hypertrophy of noninfarcted myocardial segments occurs in survivors.

Infarct expansion and remodeling can be significantly attenuated by successful timely reperfusion and by ACE inhibitor afterload reduction after infarction (Figs. 3-4 to 3-9).[14-16] Some patients (30%) who undergo successful reperfusion still experience left ventricular dilation (>20% increase in volume).[17]

POSTINFARCTION ANEURYSM FORMATION

The term *aneurysm* to anatomists means dilation of a cavity with all histologic layers of the wall present. Although aneurysm to an imaging clinician implicitly means the same, in a more practical sense it means a wide-necked extension of the cavity that can be imaged. Even state-of-the-art cardiac magnetic resonance and computed tomography cannot establish wall composition, especially in areas of wall thinning. Thrombus formation within an aneurysm is common but not universal (Fig. 3-10).

If the infarct expansion or aneurysm involves the bases of the papillary muscles, the spatial relation of the papillary muscles and their chordae will likely affect mitral leaflet coaptation because of the apical and radial displacement of the papillary muscles, their chordae, and the leaflets. The development of functional mitral insufficiency is another factor disadvantaging the left ventricle and heart after infarct expansion.

Although it is a widely held belief that aneurysms do not rupture, early aneurysms may rupture because fibrosis, which confers strength to the aneurysm, takes weeks to form. Hence, chronic aneurysms rarely rupture, but a subset of early postinfarction ruptures do occur through early, acute aneurysms.

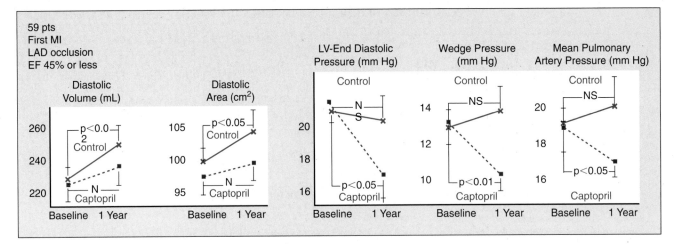

Figure 3-4. ACE inhibitors reduce postinfarction left ventricular dilation and left ventricular filling pressures. (From Pfeffer MA, Lamas GA, Vaughan DE, et al: Effect of captopril on progressive ventricular dilatation after anterior myocardial infarction. N Engl J Med 1988;319:80-86. Copyright © [2001] Massachusetts Medical Society. All rights reserved.)

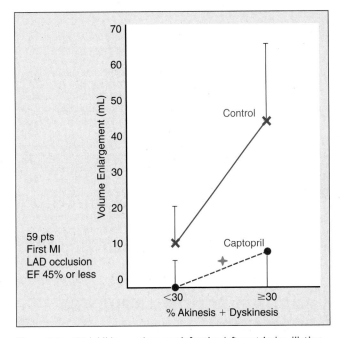

Figure 3-5. ACE inhibitors reduce postinfarction left ventricular dilation and left ventricular infarct territory systolic dysfunction. (From Pfeffer MA, Lamas GA, Vaughan DE, et al: Effect of captopril on progressive ventricular dilatation after anterior myocardial infarction. N Engl J Med 1988;319:80-86. Copyright © [2001] Massachusetts Medical Society. All rights reserved.)

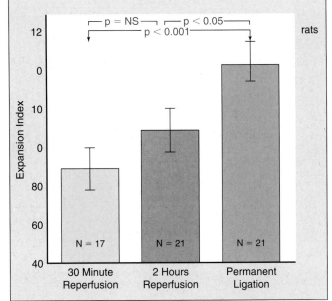

Figure 3-6. Reperfusion has a graded effect on infarct expansion. (From Hochman JS, Choo H: Limitation of myocardial infarct expansion by reperfusion independent of myocardial salvage. Circulation 1987;75:299-306.)

Figure 3-7. Irrespective of the enzymatic size of infarction, patients with occluded arteries are more likely to experience postinfarction left ventricular dilation. (From Jeremy RW, Hackworthy RA, Bautovich G, et al: Infarct artery perfusion and changes in left ventricular volume in the month after acute myocardial infarction. J Am Coll Cardiol 1987;9:989-995.)

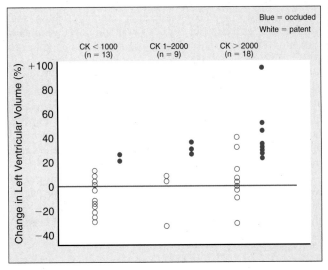

3

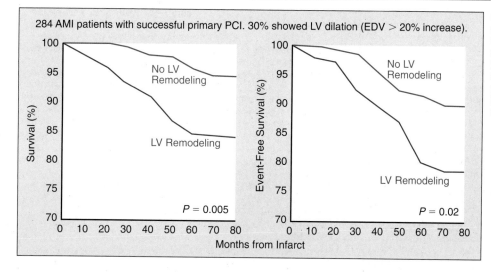

284 AMI patients with successful primary PCI. 30% showed LV dilation (EDV > 20% increase).

Figure 3-8. Left ventricular remodeling after infarction is associated with significantly lower survival and event-free survival. (From Bolognese L, Neskovic AN, Parodi G, et al: Left ventricular remodeling after primary coronary angioplasty: patterns of left ventricular dilation and long-term prognostic implications. Circulation 2002;106:2351-2357.)

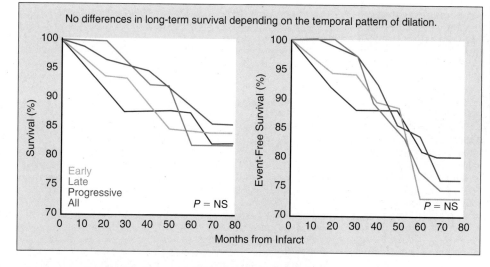

No differences in long-term survival depending on the temporal pattern of dilation.

Figure 3-9. The temporal pattern of remodeling (dilation)—early, late, or progressive does not influence survival or event-free survival. (From Bolognese L, Neskovic AN, Parodi G, et al: Left ventricular remodeling after primary coronary angioplasty: patterns of left ventricular dilation and long-term prognostic implications. Circulation 2002;106:2351-2357.)

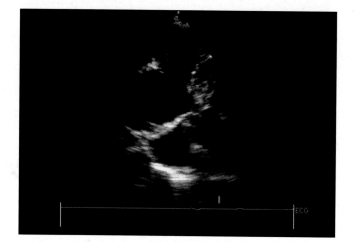

Figure 3-10. A crescentic laminated thrombus is present within the body of a basal posterior left ventricular aneurysm.

Early (Acute) Postinfarction Aneurysm

An area of early postinfarction myocardial dysfunction, with distinct diastolic deformity (dilation), may exhibit systolic akinesis or dyskinesis. Mortality is substantially increased among patients in whom aneurysms develop early (<48 hours), who typically experience severe, progressive, and ultimately fatal pump failure (Fig. 3-11).[18]

Management of Acute Left Ventricular Aneurysm
- Establish reperfusion (primary percutaneous coronary intervention preferable)
- Pharmacologic (inotropic ± vasopressor support)
- Intra-aortic balloon counterpulsation (IABP) may be needed
- Consider assist device if needed, if available
- Transplant if needed, if available

Late (Chronic) Postinfarction Aneurysm

Chronic postinfarction aneurysm is a late postinfarction myocardial dysfunction with distinct diastolic deformity (dilation) that may exhibit systolic akinesis or dyskinesis (Fig. 3-12). On micro-

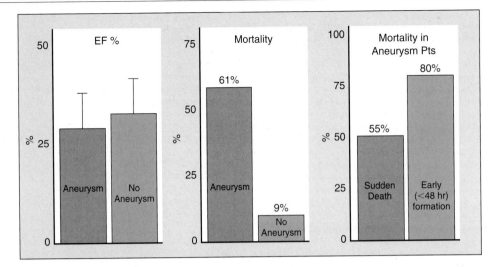

Figure 3-11. Postinfarction aneurysm formation has a dramatic effect on mortality, particularly when it occurs early. (Data from Meizlish JL, Berger HJ, Plankey M, et al: Functional left ventricular aneurysm formation after acute anterior transmural myocardial infarction. Incidence, natural history, and prognostic implications. N Engl J Med 1984;311:1001-1006.)

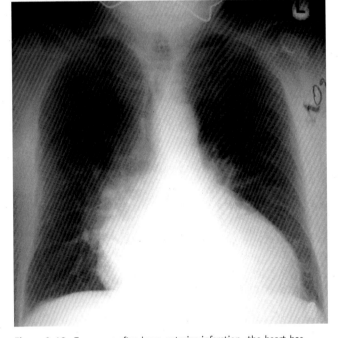

Figure 3-12. Two years after large anterior infarction, the heart has significantly dilated.

Table 3-2. Clinical Profile of Patients with Left Ventricular Aneurysm[20]

	Aneurysm	No Aneurysm	P Value
Significant variables			
Previous infarction	92%	56%	<.01
EF < 50%	68%	26%	<.01
Angina	70%	84%	<.01
LVEDP > 21 mm Hg	29%	12%	<.01
CHF	27%	9%	<.01
S₃ gallop	23%	5%	<.01
Mural thrombus	13%	1%	<.01
Nonsignificant variables			
Number of diseased vessels			
CCS class			
Creatine			
LVEDVI			
Cardiac index			

CCS, Canadian Cardiovascular Society; CHF, congestive heart failure; EF, ejection fraction; LVEDVI , left ventricular end-diastolic volume index; LVEDP, left ventricular end-diastolic pressure.

scopic examination, it is composed of "scar" with dense fibrotic tissue largely replacing myocardium and may or may not contain calcification. On macroscopic examination, it is thinned, tough, and dense and dilated at both end-diastole and end-systole. Lacking sufficient surviving myocytes, it is noncontractile and often dyskinetic unless heavily calcified. The overall left ventricular ejection fraction of patients with chronic left ventricular aneurysms is typically in the 25% to 30% range. Mortality among those with postinfarction aneurysms is substantially increased; a high percentage experience sudden death.[18] Most aneurysms are apical, but 5% are inferior and a few are lateral (Figs. 3-13 and 3-14). First infarction, no prior angina (collaterals), and inadequate reperfusion (occlusion) underlie most aneurysms. Chronic aneurysm formation occurs in 10% to 30% of patients experiencing first infarction.[19]

Clinical associations of chronic postinfarction aneurysms include (1) heart failure (systolic heart failure; diastolic dysfunction), (2) intracavitary thrombi with or without systemic embolism, (3) arrhythmias (ventricular arrhythmias; atrial tachyarrhythmias associated with heart failure), and (4) angina. The clinical profile of patients with left ventricular aneurysm is summarized in Table 3-2.[20]

Management consists of medical heart failure drug regimens (ACE inhibitors, angiotensin receptor blockers, diuretics including aldactone ± digoxin), consideration of ICD, consideration of warfarin, and consideration of surgical aneurysmectomy (Figs. 3-15 to 3-17; Table 3-3)[21-23] if the patient is to undergo aortocoronary bypass grafting.

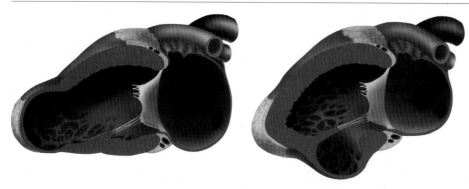

Figure 3-13. Aneurysms may be located in any region of the left ventricle but are most commonly seen at the left ventricular apex (LEFT). Aneurysms may also arise off the posterior wall of the left ventricle. On pathologic examination, an aneurysm has all layers of the wall present, but the wall is invariably thinned. Aneurysms are identified clinically by the diastolic dilation and wall thinning. Aneurysms commonly exhibit dyskinesis, but so may nonaneurysmal infarcted myocardium; therefore, dyskinesis is not a clinical criterion.

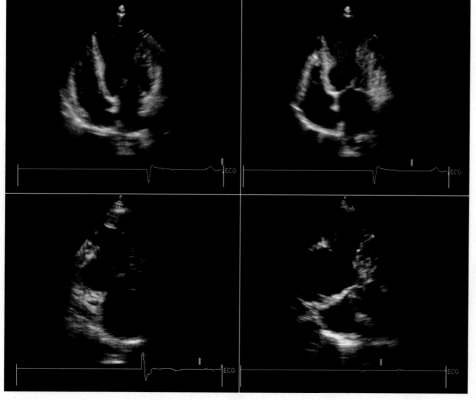

Figure 3-14. Transthoracic echocardiography. LEFT IMAGES, Diastole. RIGHT IMAGES, Systole. TOP IMAGES, Anteroapical aneurysm—dilation in diastole and dyskinesis in systole. BOTTOM IMAGES, Inferior aneurysm also with diastolic dilation and systolic dyskinesis and mural thrombus as well.

Table 3-3. Surgical Aneurysmectomy for Late (Chronic) Left Ventricular Aneurysm

Indications	Intractable heart failure
	Recurrent embolization despite therapeutic anticoagulation
	In patients otherwise undergoing aortocoronary bypass surgery
Key surgical considerations	Well-defined margins
	Margins do not involve papillary muscles
	Good to excellent systolic function of the nonaneurysm segments
Risk	10%-15% mortality
Outcomes	Symptom improvement: NYHA class, greater exercise tolerance
	Objective improvement: improves resting EF% in most (but not all) cases; residual or recurrent aneurysm occurs in 5%
	Left ventricular aneurysmectomy does not reduce mortality, after adjustment for CHF

CHF, congestive heart failure; EF, ejection fraction; NYHA, New York Heart Association.

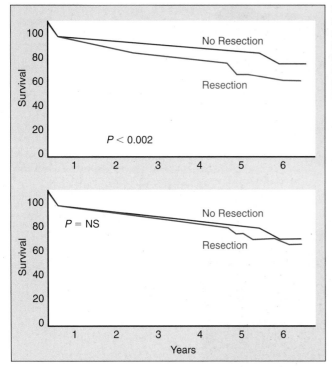

Figure 3-15. Without adjustment for congestive heart failure status, aneurysmectomy appears to be associated with better survival (UPPER PLOT). It can therefore seldom be recommended as a primary indication. However, after adjusting for congestive heart failure status, aneurysmectomy does not appear to be associated with better survival (LOWER PLOT). (From Faxon DP, Ryan TJ, Davis KB, et al: Prognostic significance of angiographically documented left ventricular aneurysm from the Coronary Artery Surgery Study [CASS]. Am J Cardiol 1982;50:157-164, with permission from Elsevier.)

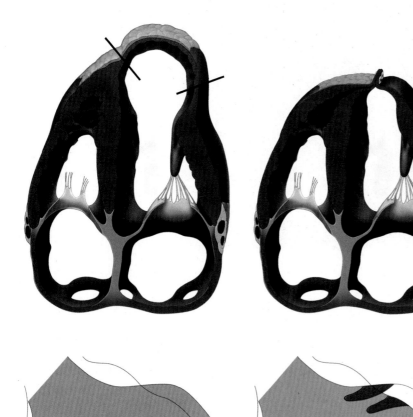

Figure 3-16. Surgical resection of left ventricular aneurysms is intended to reduce the volume of the aneurysm (which wastes stroke volume if it is dyskinetic) and of the ventricle, which reduces wall stress and thereby myocardial oxygen consumption. The margins of the resection are approximated and usually held by pledget sutures to distribute the tension of the sutures.

Figure 3-17. Resection of left ventricular aneurysm must be attuned to the location of the papillary muscles. LEFT, The left ventricle at end-diastole and end-systole revealing the margins of the aneurysm and its dyskinesis. RIGHT, The left ventricle with papillary muscles in two positions with respect to the margins of the aneurysm. The closer the papillary muscles are to the margins of resection, the more likely the components of the mitral valve and its competence are affected.

OTHER TYPES OF POSTINFARCTION MYOCARDIAL DYSFUNCTION

Myocardial stunning is a term used for postischemic myocardial contractile dysfunction (Fig. 3-18). After reperfusion, contractile function remains impaired for a time (minutes, hours, days, or weeks) until spontaneous recovery occurs. By definition, the culprit (infarct-related) artery is patent.

Myocardial hibernation is chronic ischemic contractile dysfunction. By definition, the relevant artery is severely stenosed, and resting flow is reduced. Because the myocardium is not infarcted, when revascularization is conferred and chronic ischemia alleviated, contractile function recovers.

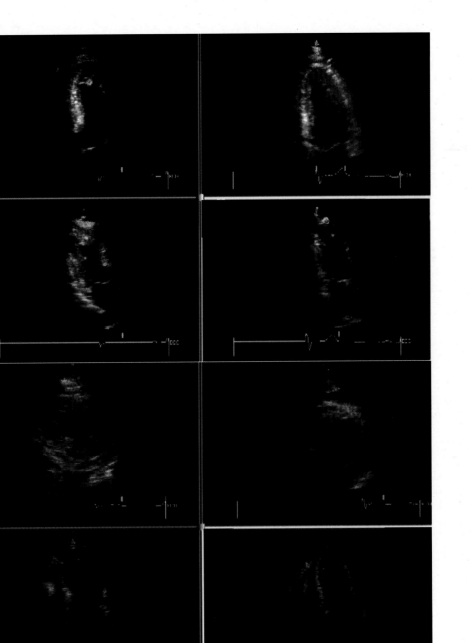

Figure 3-18. Transthoracic echocardiography, systolic frames. LEFT, In the hospital after anterior infarction. RIGHT, Two months later. In the hospital, there was anterior and apical akinesis and apical thrombi. Two months later, the wall motion has normalized, the apical cavitary dilation has normalized, and the thrombi are no longer present. Although this acute infarction was unequivocal (CK 1100 U), stunning was the predominant cause of left ventricular dysfunction. The most accurate predictor of what is predominantly stunned and what is predominantly infarcted is the retrospective perspective of time.

CASE 1

History

- 79-year-old man, active, living alone
- Presyncopal episodes lasting 15 seconds to 10 minutes associated with palpitations, without exertion or chest pain
- Past medical history is significant for anterior ST elevation myocardial infarction (STEMI) 8 years before. No angiography was performed at that time.
- Since then, NYHA class II congestive heart failure, CCS class I angina, hypertension

Physical Examination

- Robust for his age
- BP 145/65 mm Hg, HR 62 bpm (regular), RR 13/min (comfortable breathing)
- Normal pulse volume, upstroke, and contour
- Venous pressure 2 cm above the sternal angle, no edema
- S_1, S_2 normal; S_4 present
- Apical holosystolic murmur 2/6 with radiation into the axilla; no thrill; no diastolic murmurs, no rubs
- Enlarged and sustained apex, consistent with reduced ejection fraction
- No crepitations

Impression

- Adverse remodeling after remote anteroseptal myocardial infarction with functional mitral regurgitation
- Marked cavitary dilation and severe biventricular systolic dysfunction

Management

- ICD (secondary prevention strategy), antiarrhythmics to minimize VT frequency and rate
- Maximal anti–heart failure medications
- Angiography revealed inoperable three-vessel disease

Points

- Adverse remodeling ("ischemic cardiomyopathy") more than a decade after a large anterior myocardial infarction
- Marked cavitary dilation and severely reduced systolic function, with few heart failure symptom complaints
- LV dilation resulting in ischemic (functional) mitral regurgitation (3+)
- Multivessel CAD probably contributed to the adverse remodeling

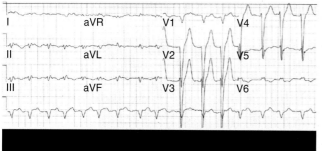

Figure 3-19. TOP, ECG shows sinus rhythm, left bundle branch block. The site of infarction is not able to be determined. BOTTOM, The chest radiograph shows marked cardiomegaly, globular heart, no heart failure.

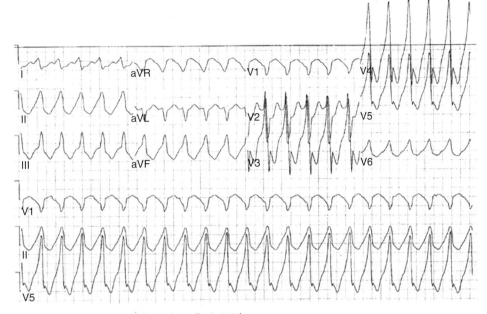

Figure 3-20. ECG during presyncope shows ventricular tachycardia at 140 bpm.

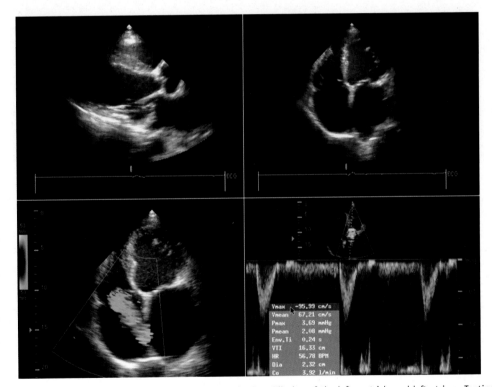

Figure 3-21. Transthoracic echocardiography. TOP LEFT, Parasternal long-axis view. Dilation of the left ventricle and left atrium. Tenting of the mitral valve. Thinning and akinesis of the posterior wall (near akinesis of the septum). TOP RIGHT, Apical 4-chamber view. Globular enlargement of all four cardiac chambers. Severe left ventricular systolic dysfunction. Tenting of the mitral apparatus. Tricuspid tenting and annular dilation. BOTTOM LEFT, Color Doppler flow mapping: severe tricuspid regurgitation from annular dilation and leaflet tenting. Similarly, there was 3+ mitral insufficiency. BOTTOM RIGHT, Calculation of cardiac output by the left ventricular outflow tract method ($0.785 \times$ diameter squared $\times$ VTI $\times$ HR); CI = CO/BSA = $3.9/1.9 = 2.05$ L/min/m^2.

CASE 2

History

- 72-year-old man transferred with post–anterior STEMI angina and heart failure
- Five days before, he had presented to a community hospital at hour 3 of an anterior STEMI, with severe hypertension (240/135 mm Hg). Blood pressure was controlled with IV nitroglycerin, before administration of tPA. A nonhemorrhagic ischemic stroke occurred during the tPA administration, attributed to the rapid control of the blood pressure.
- Large CK washout (6500 U). Early heart failure resolved during the next 36 hours. Complete neurologic recovery occurred during 4 days. Episodes of recurrent angina began on the third day after infarction.
- Past medical history is significant for untreated hypertension of at least a decade.
- No history of CAD, cardiovascular disease, or peripheral vascular disease

Management and Follow-up

- Underwent uneventful aortocoronary bypass
- Discharged heart failure free and angina free
- At follow-up 2 months later, presented with class IV shortness of breath, orthopnea, paroxysmal nocturnal dyspnea, and 11 kg of weight gain
- No angina, chest pain, or syncope

Physical Examination

- Dyspneic at rest
- BP 155/90 mm Hg, HR 85 bpm, RR 23/min
- Large-volume pulses, normal upstroke, normal contour

- Warm extremities, alert
- Anasarca—pitting edema to the thighs, scrotal edema
- Venous pressure to angle of the jaw with a prominent V wave
- S_1, S_2 normal; S_3 present
- Apical holosystolic murmur 4/6 with radiation into the axilla; anterograde flow rumble
- Lower parasternal holosystolic murmur 3/6 increasing with inspiration
- No thrill; no diastolic murmurs; no rubs
- Apex enlarged, displaced, and sustained
- Dull to percussion over the lower third of the lung fields
- Crepitations at midlung zones

Impression and Management

- Adverse remodeling resulting in biventricular heart failure and functional mitral and tricuspid insufficiency
- Managed by diuretics, ACE inhibitors, and beta-blockers once euvolemic

Evolution

- Improved during 8 days
- Discharged NYHA class II, CCS class I
- Died of a massive myocardial infarction 6 years later

Points

- Adverse remodeling during 2 months after anterior myocardial infarction despite complete surgical revascularization
- Left ventricle dilation resulting in ischemic (functional) mitral regurgitation
- Right-sided heart failure from left ventricle failure and severe mitral regurgitation

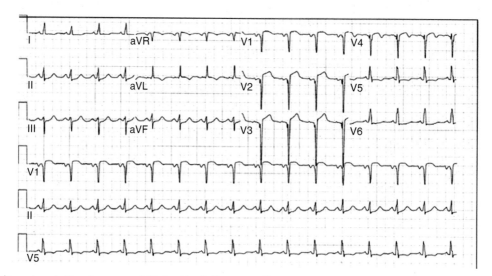

Figure 3-22. ECG shows sinus rhythm, Q waves, and ST elevation V_1-V_4; nonspecific repolarization abnormalities V_5, V_6, I, aVL; and anteroseptal infarction. Persistent ST elevation may indicate aneurysm formation.

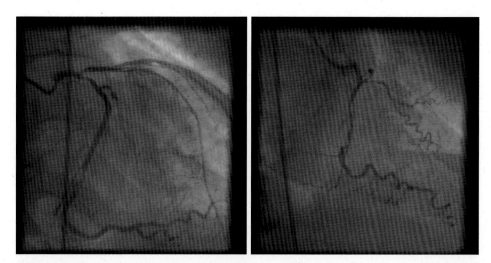

Figure 3-23. Selective coronary angiography. LEFT, Left coronary artery injection. No stenoses of the left main coronary artery. Significant proximal and mid LAD stensoses. Significant stenosis of the midportion of the dominant left circumflex artery. RIGHT, Right coronary artery injection. Nondominant. Diseased before the acute marginal branch. Collateral vessels from the conus branch to the LAD and from an acute marginal branch to the posterior descending artery.

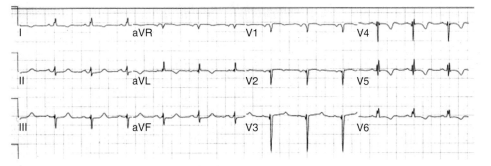

Figure 3-24. ECG taken 2 months later shows sinus rhythm; no atrial fibrillation to explain heart failure; Q waves V_1-V_4; and widespread repolarization abnormalities. There are no major acute changes since the ECGs 2 months before.

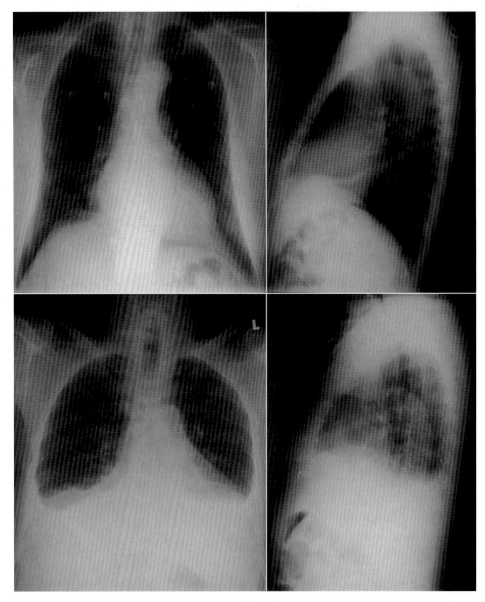

Figure 3-25. Chest radiography. TOP, Postoperative chest radiographs show mild cardiomegaly, sternotomy wires; no left-sided heart failure; and fluid in the lower right major fissure. BOTTOM, Chest radiographs taken more than 2 months later show worsened cardiomegaly, and the adverse development of bilateral pleural effusions of at least moderate size and interstitial edema.

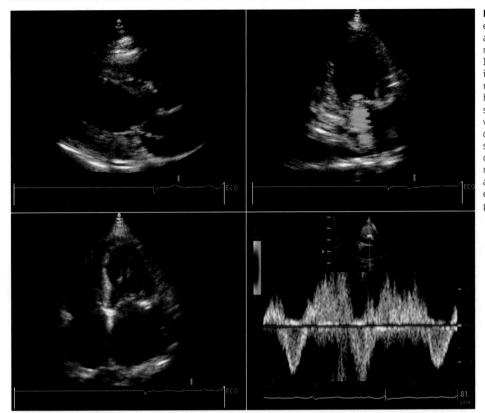

Figure 3-26. Transthoracic echocardiography. TOP LEFT, Images taken after infarction: some leaflet tenting; mild mitral regurgitation. TOP RIGHT AND BOTTOM, Images taken on re-presentation. There is now moderate to severe mitral regurgitation. All four cardiac chambers have become dilated with a globular shape. The systolic function of both ventricles is moderately to severely depressed. The spectral flow pattern reveals systolic flow reversal in the hepatic veins consistent with severe tricuspid regurgitation. The calculated cardiac index after infarction was 2.4 L/min/m^2 at an elevated heart rate of 95 bpm; on re-presentation, it was 1.7 L/min/m^2.

CASE 3

History

- 63-year-old woman with postinfarction heart failure
- Three days before, she had presented with a non-STEMI, initially without heart failure. Treated medically, she had progressively falling blood pressure and congestive heart failure. No recurrences of angina or arrhythmias developed.
- Past medical history is significant for hypertension and type 2 diabetes.

Physical Examination

- Mildly distressed with dyspnea, warm extremities, alert
- BP 80/50 mm Hg, HR 110 bpm, RR 18/min
- Low volume pulse, normal upstroke
- Venous pressure 7 cm above the sternal angle, no edema
- S$_1$, S$_2$ normal; S$_3$ present
- Blowing apical holosystolic murmur 4/6 with radiation to the axilla; no thrill; anterograde diastolic flow rumble; no rubs
- Crepitations in two thirds of lungs
- Urine output (initially): 40 mL/hr

Evolution

- Intubated for shock
- Vasopressors started with poor response
- Suspected myocardial infarction

- Echocardiography was performed to establish wall motion abnormality and to exclude other cardiac pathologic processes, such as aortic dissection

Clinical Impression

- Inferoposterior subendocardial infarction complicated by
  - Severe mitral regurgitation; no evidence of papillary rupture, thus presumed to be "ischemic" mitral regurgitation from adverse ventricular geometry
  - Severe tricuspid regurgitation
  - Right ventricular dysfunction from infarction and mitral regurgitation
  - Three-vessel CAD with poor distal targets for bypass surgery
  - Severe left ventricular dysfunction, generalized hypokinesis—possible ongoing ischemia
  - Killip class IV (cardiogenic shock hemodynamics)

Management and Outcome

- IABP for stabilization, inotropes as tolerated
- Mitral repair or replacement surgery was considered and assessed as high risk. The patient was not stabilizing well, and further delay was anticipated to incur further worsening and even higher risk.
- The patient declined surgery.
- Died 12 days later from progressive multiorgan failure

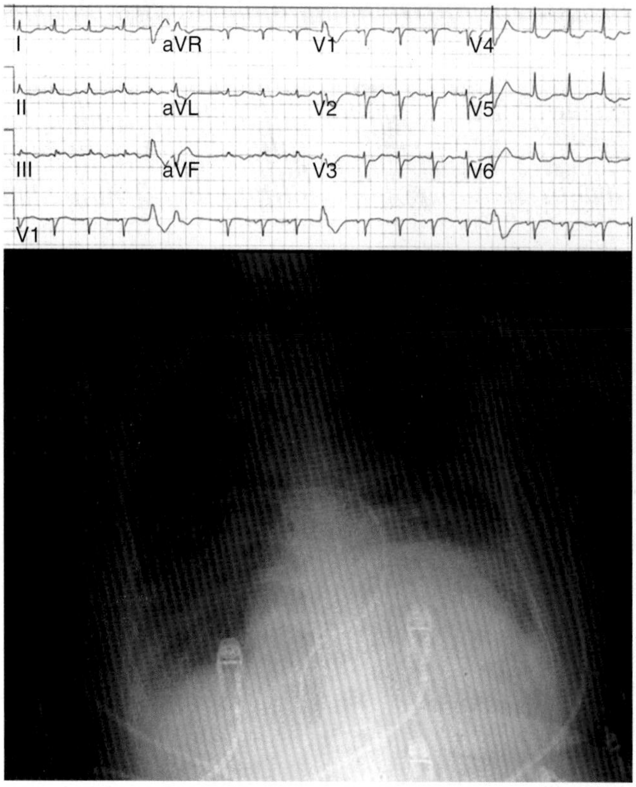

Figure 3-27. TOP, ECG shows sinus rhythm, first-degree aortic valve block, right bundle branch block, Q waves in V_1-V_3, abnormal septal repolarization, and ST elevation aVR. Subtle findings of anterior ST elevation are partially obscured by the right bundle branch block pattern. BOTTOM, Chest radiograph shows normal-sized cardiopericardial silhouette and interstitial pulmonary edema.

Comments

- Early adverse remodeling (days), with inexorable hemodynamic failure
- Associated with torrential postinfarction mitral regurgitation
- Mitral regurgitation not due to papillary rupture (confirmed at autopsy) but due to early left ventricle remodeling with loss of coaptation from apical tenting
- Common association of severe postinfarction mitral regurgitation (no papillary rupture) with underlying three-vessel CAD

- Pattern of left ventricular systolic dysfunction was regional (inferoposterior infarct) and global (as seen with multivessel CAD), leading to global dilation
- Concurrent right ventricular infarction aggravating worsening hemodynamics
- Tricuspid regurgitation from right ventricular infarction (dilation and annular dilation), not right ventricular papillary muscle rupture

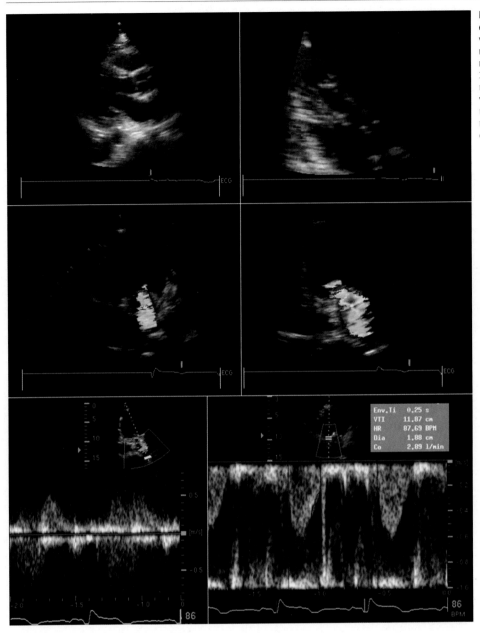

Figure 3-28. Transthoracic echocardiography. TOP LEFT, Mild left ventricle dilation and apical tenting of the mitral leaflets. TOP RIGHT, Intact papillary muscles; tenting of the leaflets. MIDDLE LEFT, 3+ tricuspid regurgitation; MIDDLE RIGHT, 3+ mitral regurgitation. BOTTOM LEFT, Pulmonary venous flow reversal indicative of severe mitral insufficiency. BOTTOM RIGHT, Severely reduced LVOT VTI, stroke volume, and cardiac output.

References

1. Hochman JS, Buller CE, Sleeper LA, et al: Cardiogenic shock complicating acute myocardial infarction: etiologies, management and outcome: a report from the SHOCK Trial Registry. SHould we emergently revascularize Occluded Coronaries for cardiogenic shocK? J Am Coll Cardiol 2000;36(Suppl A):1063-1070.

2. Hutchins GM, Bulkley BH: Infarct expansion versus extension: two different complications of acute myocardial infarction. Am J Cardiol 1978 June;41(7):1127-32.

3. Isaacsohn JL, Earle MG, Kemper AJ, Parisi AF: Postmyocardial infarction pain and infarct extension in the coronary care unit: role of two-dimensional echocardiography. J Am Coll Cardiol 1988;11:246-251.

4. Gibson RS, Bishop HL, Stamm RB, et al: Value of early two dimensional echocardiography in patients with acute myocardial infarction. Am J Cardiol 1982;49:1110-1119.

5. Gaudron P, Eilles C, Kugler I, Ertl G: Progressive left ventricular dysfunction and remodeling after myocardial infarction. Potential mechanisms and early predictors. Circulation 1993;87:755-763.

6. Kern MJ: Patterns of left ventricular dilatation with an opened artery after acute myocardial infarction: missing links to long-term prognosis. Circulation 2002;106:2294-2295.

7. Grigioni F, Enriquez-Sarano M, Zehr KJ, et al: Ischemic mitral regurgitation: long-term outcome and prognostic implications with quantitative Doppler assessment. Circulation 2001;103:1759-1764.

8. Moller JE, Hillis GS, Oh JK, et al: Left atrial volume: a powerful predictor of survival after acute myocardial infarction. Circulation 2003;107:2207-2212.

9. Eaton LW, Weiss JL, Bulkley BH, et al: Regional cardiac dilatation after acute myocardial infarction: recognition by two-dimensional echocardiography. N Engl J Med 1979;300:57-62.

10. Schuster EH, Bulkley BH: Expansion of transmural myocardial infarction: a pathophysiologic factor in cardiac rupture. Circulation 1979;60:1532-1538.

11. Dujardin KS, Enriquez-Sarano M, Rossi A, et al: Echocardiographic assessment of left ventricular remodeling: are left ventricular diameters suitable tools? J Am Coll Cardiol 1997;30:1534-1541.

12. Picard MH, Wilkins GT, Ray PA, Weyman AE: Natural history of left ventricular size and function after acute myocardial infarction. Assessment and prediction by echocardiographic endocardial surface mapping. Circulation 1990;82:484-494.

13. Burns RJ, Gibbons RJ, Yi Q, et al; CORE Study Investigators: The relationships of left ventricular ejection fraction, end-systolic volume index and infarct size to six-month mortality after hospital discharge following myocardial infarction treated by thrombolysis. J Am Coll Cardiol 2002; 39:30-36.

14. Pfeffer MA, Lamas GA, Vaughan DE, et al: Effect of captopril on progressive ventricular dilatation after anterior myocardial infarction. N Engl J Med 1988;319:80-86.

15. Hochman JS, Choo H: Limitation of myocardial infarct expansion by reperfusion independent of myocardial salvage. Circulation 1987;75:299-306.

16. Jeremy RW, Hackworthy RA, Bautovich G, et al: Infarct artery perfusion and changes in left ventricular volume in the month after acute myocardial infarction. J Am Coll Cardiol 1987;9:989-995.

17. Bolognese L, Neskovic AN, Parodi G, et al: Left ventricular remodeling after primary coronary angioplasty: patterns of left ventricular dilation and long-term prognostic implications. Circulation 2002;106:2351-2357.

18. Meizlish JL, Berger HJ, Plankey M, et al: Functional left ventricular aneurysm formation after acute anterior transmural myocardial infarction. Incidence, natural history, and prognostic implications. N Engl J Med 1984;311:1001-1006.

19. Shen WF, Tribouilloy C, Mirode A, et al: Left ventricular aneurysm and prognosis in patients with first acute transmural anterior myocardial infarction and isolated left anterior descending artery disease. Eur Heart J 1992;13:39-44.

20. Faxon DP, Ryan TJ, Davis KB, et al: Prognostic significance of angiographically documented left ventricular aneurysm from the Coronary Artery Surgery Study (CASS). Am J Cardiol 1982;50:157-164.

21. Taylor NC, Barber R, Crossland P, et al: Does left ventricular aneurysmectomy improve ventricular function in patients undergoing coronary bypass surgery? Br Heart J 1985;54:145-152.

22. Olearchyk AS: Recurrent (residual?) left ventricular aneurysm. A report of 11 cases. J Thorac Cardiovasc Surg 1984;88:554-557.

23. Faxon DP, Myers WO, McCabe CH, et al: The influence of surgery on the natural history of angiographically documented left ventricular aneurysm: the Coronary Artery Surgery Study. Circulation 1986;74:110-118.

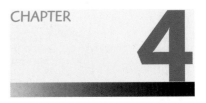

Postinfarction Dynamic Left Ventricular Outflow Tract Obstruction

Acute systolic dysfunction of the left ventricular apex, in the context of a small dynamic cavity, may result in compensatory hyperdynamic function of the basal segments and thereby dynamic systolic outflow tract obstruction. The combination of acute apical systolic and diastolic dysfunction, with or without an outflow tract obstruction, may result in pulmonary edema, hypotension, or shock. Thus, a few patients with cardiogenic shock have a unique syndrome of apical dysfunction and dynamic left ventricular outflow tract (LVOT) obstruction.

A small left ventricular cavity that experiences severe apical stunning appears to be the substrate. The basal segments of the left ventricle, driven by adrenergic response, become hypercontractile. Typically, the apex experiences both severe systolic dysfunction (akinesis or dyskinesis) and also transient apical aneurysm with an unusually symmetric shape ("balloon"). The balloon-shaped apex and small base attracted the Japanese name for the similar-shaped octopus pot, *tako-tsubo*. The apical systolic dysfunction and ballooning appear to be the primary process because only a minority of such cases develop an outflow tract obstruction.[1,2] Pulmonary edema, hypotension, and cardiogenic shock may be due to apical stunning alone or apical stunning with an outflow tract obstruction. Mitral insufficiency may occur from systolic anterior motion (SAM) of the mitral leaflets (Fig. 4-1).

Despite suggestions, the etiology of transient apical ballooning with LVOT obstruction is unclear in some cases. Some cases have the profile of acute coronary syndromes/small myocardial infarctions and underlying coronary artery disease that plausibly serve as the substrate; however, other cases are without angiographically apparent coronary artery disease.[3-5]

Related variants of midventricular ballooning have been described.[6] The presence of a systolic ejection murmur is an invaluable clue to the presence of a dynamic LVOT obstruction. Other common causes of a systolic ejection murmur include underlying aortic stenosis and sclerosis.

Echocardiography and contrast ventriculography are able to depict both the apical ballooning–wall motion abnormality and the LVOT gradient.

The gradient's lability is an important issue and should guide therapeutic interventions. Preload reducing, afterload reducing, and inotropic agents will worsen the LVOT gradient, sometimes precipitously lowering the blood pressure. Afterload-increasing agents and volume infusion will lessen the gradient.

The syndrome generally evolves with the clinical profile of prominent myocardial stunning, such as discordance of electrocardiographic and biomarker results, gradual recovery (often normalization) of left ventricular systolic function, resolution of the outflow tract gradient, and higher than expected survival for the initial degree of left ventricular systolic dysfunction and hemodynamic disturbance.[2,5]

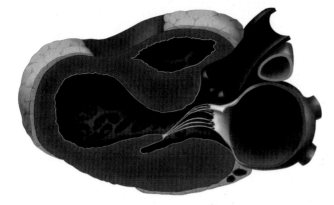

Figure 4-1. The typical heart that develops a postinfarction LVOT obstruction previously had a small cavity, often was previously hypertensive, and develops extensive and symmetric apical ballooning and akinesis or dyskinesis and compensatory hypercontractile systolic function of the basal segments. The small basal cavity and hypercontractile basal systolic function incite an outflow obstruction characterized by SAM of the mitral leaflets, LVOT turbulence and gradient, and often mitral insufficiency due to the SAM of the mitral leaflets.

CASE 1

History

▸ 66-year-old woman presented with chest pain and shortness of breath
▸ Past medical history is significant for hypertension, spinal tumor treated with radium implants, severe kyphoscoliosis, and restrictive lung disease.

Physical Examination

▸ BP 140/60 mm Hg, HR 80 bpm, RR 32/min, afebrile
▸ No venous distention or edema
▸ S_1, S_2 normal; 4th heart sound
▸ 3/6 SEM at the base and a 3/6 apical holosystolic murmur; no murmur of aortic insufficiency
▸ No thrill
▸ Apex enlarged and sustained
▸ Troponins 3.5; CK 210, positive MB

Initial Clinical Impression

▸ Acute coronary syndrome and acute left-sided heart failure due to left ventricular dysfunction and mitral regurgitation (MR) of unknown origin
▸ Dyspnea due to acute left-sided heart failure and chronic restrictive chest disease
▸ Unknown basis of the ejection murmur
▸ Initial treatment included ASA, heparin, and diuresis for pulmonary edema

Clinical Impression After Echocardiography

▸ Anteroapical wall motion abnormality consistent with the ECG territory of involvement
▸ Dynamic LVOT obstruction due to a small cavity with hyperdynamic basal systolic function
▸ MR secondary to LVOT obstruction
▸ Referred for early coronary angiography
▸ Ongoing diuresis (only 1 dose of lasix, 40 mg IV): 0.5 → 1.0 → 1.5 L

Evolution

▸ Hemodynamic deterioration on the catheterization laboratory table
▸ Fall in systolic BP: 100 → 90 → 80 → 70 → 60 mm Hg

▸ Cause was supposed to be the left ventricular dysfunction and LVOT obstruction.
▸ Volume sensitivity of the gradient was clearly established by the effect of diuresis on the gradient and the therapeutic effect of volume infusion.
▸ Volume depletion was avoided, and the patient was stable.
▸ That evening, her usual nighttime BiPAP was started; but BP again started falling, reaching 60 mm Hg, and the murmur recurred.
▸ BiPAP presumably unmasked inadequate volume (relative underfilling for the infarction).
▸ With a small dose of esmolol, the murmur diminished and the BP normalized.

Management

▸ Avoidance of preload reduction (diuretics)
▸ Avoidance of afterload reduction (vasodilators)
▸ Small dose of a beta-blocker
▸ Usual BiPAP

Outcome

▸ Discharged stable

Comments

▸ Dynamic LVOT obstruction and MR after anterior wall infarction, with extreme sensitivity to volume status
▸ Severe hypotension and pulmonary edema occurred at times, and near cardiac arrest at one point.
▸ Murmurs of MR and outflow obstruction
▸ Predisposing factors include a small, previously hypertensive heart and the dynamic compensatory response of the basal segments to the acute apical systolic dysfunction.
▸ The chest deformity and history of hypertension may have contributed to predisposition by abnormally aligning the ascending aorta and basal septum.
▸ Maneuvers that reduced preload and afterload narrowed the LVOT and facilitated obstruction.
▸ MR was secondary to the SAM from the LVOT obstruction, as it resolved in tandem with resolution of SAM.

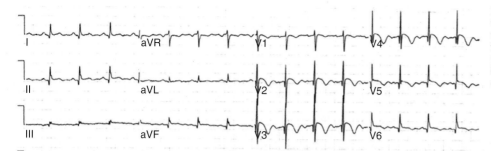

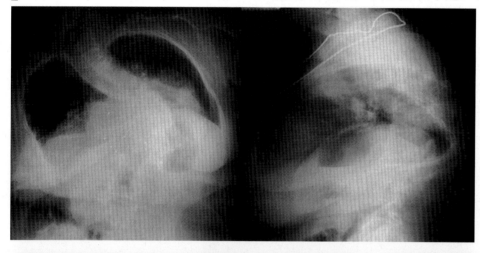

Figure 4-2. TOP, ECG shows sinus tachycardia. Precordial ST elevation and T-wave inversion are consistent with anterior infarction. BOTTOM, Chest radiograph shows marked thoracic deformity due to kyphoscoliosis and mild interstitial edema (old radium pellets).

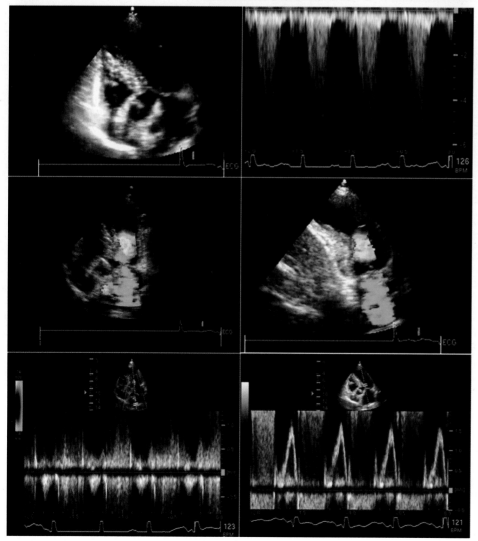

Figure 4-3. Transthoracic echocardiography. TOP LEFT, There is left ventricular hypertrophy with a small cavity at the base, severe SAM of the mitral valve across the LVOT. TOP RIGHT, Continuous wave spectral profile of flow out of the LVOT; the profile is dagger shaped, consistent with a dynamic obstruction. The peak gradient is 90 to 100 mm Hg. MIDDLE LEFT, There is turbulence in the LVOT consistent with the obstruction, and there is also severe mitral insufficiency. MIDDLE RIGHT, Severe MR. BOTTOM LEFT, Pulmonary venous spectral flow profiles demonstrate systolic aliasing and flow reversal diagnostic of severe MR. BOTTOM RIGHT, LV inflow pattern reveals a summation of the E and A waves but A-wave dominance consistent with impaired relaxation. There is also IVRT flow consistent with a dynamic left ventricular cavity.

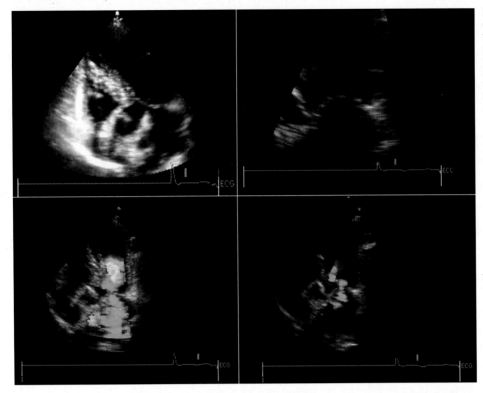

Figure 4-4. Transthoracic echocardiography. LEFT, Images before vasopressors and volume show severe SAM, prominent LVOT turbulence, and severe MR (due to the SAM). The distal LV has ballooned. RIGHT, Images taken after vasopressors and volume show much less SAM, less LVOT turbulence, and much less MR.

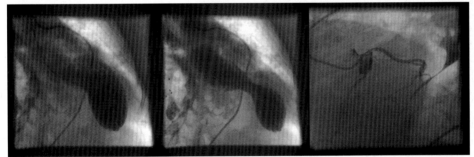

Figure 4-5. Contrast ventriculography demonstrates anteroapical (aneurysmal) ballooning and akinesis. Coronary angiography of left coronary artery shows no significant angiographic disease and marked distortion of anatomy: tortuous aorta, high kidney.

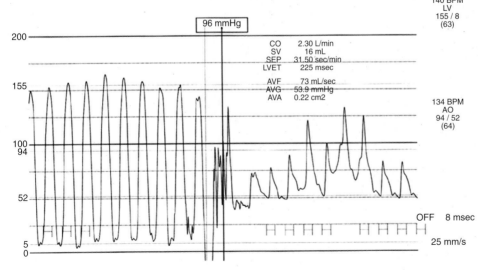

Figure 4-6. Cardiac catheterization. Left ventricle to aorta "pullback" gradient. Pullback (peak-to-peak) gradient 155 − 94 = 61 mm Hg.

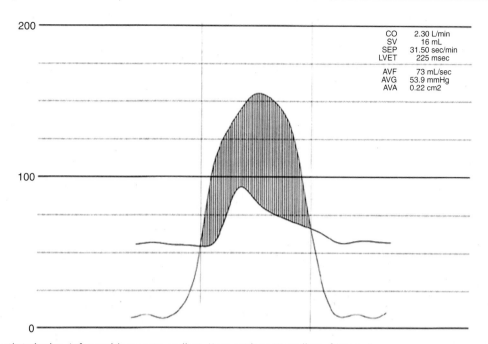

CO	2.30 L/min
SV	16 mL
SEP	31.50 sec/min
LVET	225 msec
AVF	73 mL/sec
AVG	53.9 mmHg
AVA	0.22 cm2

Figure 4-7. Cardiac catheterization. Left ventricle to aorta gradient. Mean aortic to LV gradient of 54 mm Hg.

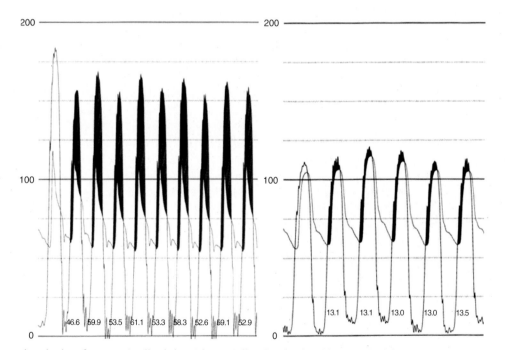

Figure 4-8. Cardiac catheterization after 500-mL saline bolus. A large gradient has developed between the left ventricle and the aorta. The 70 mm Hg gradient before volume infusion reduced to less than 5 mm Hg after volume infusion.

CASE 2

History

▸ 85-year-old woman presented with "indigestion" lasting for 4 hours and shortness of breath the day before; feeling "unwell" since
▸ Upper respiratory tract infection 3 weeks before, unremarkable
▸ Past medical history is significant for hypertension and hemodialysis for 3 years.
▸ On the day of presentation, hemodialysis was associated with an abrupt and severe blood pressure fall, which the patient said was unusual.

Physical Examination

▸ Elderly and frail appearing, no respiratory distress, severe kyphosis
▸ BP 105/60 mm Hg before dialysis, 50/– with ultrafiltration
▸ HR 110 bpm, RR 30/min
▸ Normal S_1, S_2; S_4 gallop
▸ No venous distention, normal carotid upstroke, no bruit or thrill
▸ SEM 3/6 at the base of the heart, no diastolic murmurs or rub
▸ Apex sustained and enlarged, mildly displaced
▸ No crepitations
▸ Troponin 15; CK 385, positive MB
▸ Because there had been no history of a murmur, an echocardiogram was obtained.

Clinical Impression

▸ Acute coronary syndrome–myocardial infarction
▸ Apical hypokinesis–ballooning and dynamic LVOT obstruction
▸ Hypotension and shock are due to acute infarction and LVOT obstruction (when the gradient rose above 80, the blood pressure fell below 80 mm Hg).

Management

▸ Avoidance of preload and afterload reduction
▸ Inotropic stimulation
▸ Brief infusion of phenylephrine (noninotropic vasopressor) to resuscitate blood pressure
▸ IV beta-blocker, followed by oral beta-blocker

Outcome

▸ Murmur was abolished and gradient eliminated
▸ BP rose to usual borderline hypertensive level and stabilized with hemodialysis
▸ The patient survived.

Comments

▸ LVOT obstruction and apical ballooning associated with an acute coronary syndrome
▸ Dynamic nature of LVOT was provoked by preload and afterload reduction (i.e., dialysis)
▸ Severe hypotension and pulmonary edema
▸ Murmurs of MR and outflow obstruction
▸ LVOT obstruction was corrected by increasing afterload and negative inotropy.
▸ Predisposing factors include chest deformity (severe kyphosis) angulating the ascending aorta and LVOT; left ventricular hypertrophy with a small and dynamic cavity; and apical wall motion abnormality with compensatory increase in contractility of the base of the left ventricle.
▸ Interestingly, her left ventricular systolic pressure (the sum of the systolic blood pressure and the LVOT gradient) was nearly always 160 mm Hg.

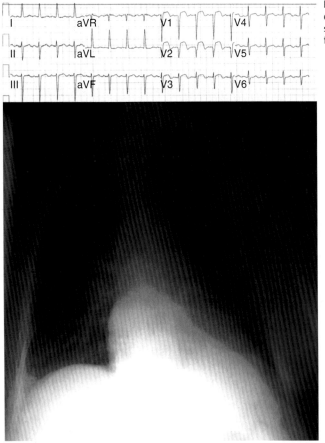

Figure 4-9. TOP, ECG shows sinus tachycardia, Q waves V_1 and V_2, and ST elevation V_1-V_4 consistent with anterior infarction. BOTTOM, Chest radiograph shows mildly enlarged CPS, bronchovascular markings in the left lower lung field, but no left-sided heart failure.

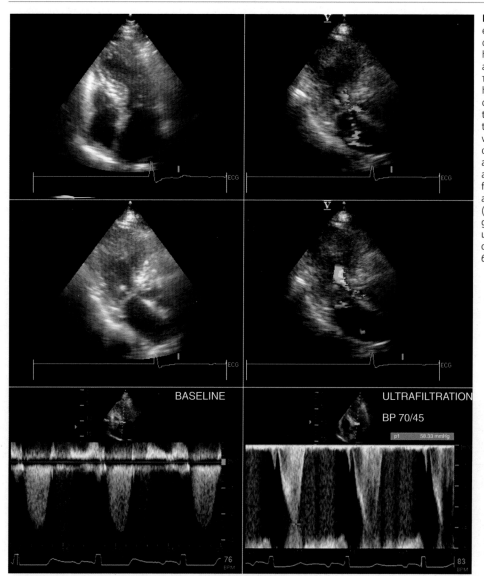

Figure 4-10. Transthoracic echocardiography. TOP LEFT, Apical 4-chamber view shows LV hypertrophy, hypokinesis or akinesis and dilation of the apex, and dynamic contraction elsewhere. TOP RIGHT, Apical 3-chamber view shows LV hypertrophy, apical dilation, and dynamic contraction of the base of the LV. There is turbulence (variance) in the LVOT, and there is MR. MIDDLE LEFT, Apical 3-chamber view shows LV hypertrophy, apical dilation, dynamic contraction at the base, and SAM at the LVOT level. MIDDLE RIGHT, Another apical 3-chamber view in addition shows flow acceleration at the base of the LVOT and MR. BOTTOM LEFT, In the resting state (before dialysis), there is a 25 mm Hg gradient in the LVOT. BOTTOM RIGHT, With ultrafiltration, there is provocation of the obstruction with development of a 60 mm Hg gradient.

CASE 3

History

▸ 50-year-old man with 3 hours of mild chest pressure and shortness of breath
▸ Past medical history is significant for chronic lung disease that the patient could not specify and for which he did not regularly take medications.

Physical Examination

▸ Fit and well appearing for age
▸ BP 80/50 mm Hg, HR 90 bpm, RR 13/min
▸ Marked pectus excavatum
▸ No venous distention, normal carotid upstroke, reduced volume
▸ Normal S_1, S_2; S_4 gallop
▸ Systolic ejection murmur 3/6 at the base of the heart, no associated diastolic murmurs or rub
▸ Systolic ejection murmur louder with post-PVC beat
▸ Pansystolic murmur 4/6 at the apex with axillary radiation
▸ Apex enlarged and sustained, not displaced
▸ Crepitations in the basal 25% of lung fields
▸ Troponin 20; CK 415, positive MB

Initial Clinical Impression

▸ Acute coronary syndrome–myocardial infarction
▸ Complex hemodynamics underlined by hypotension, pulmonary congestion, and two murmurs of undefined basis
▸ Possibilities include underlying aortic valve disease contributing to hypotension peri-infarct, early mitral disruption (mitral regurgitation murmur present), and apical myocardial infarction with LVOT obstruction and MR.
▸ Urgent echo was ordered to clarify basis of murmurs and to plan strategy.

Clinical Impression After Echocardiography

▸ Acute coronary syndrome–myocardial infarction
▸ Apical hypokinesis–ballooning and LVOT obstruction
▸ MR probably due to LVOT obstruction (because the mitral apparatus was itself normal)
▸ Pulmonary congestion from the myocardial infarction and the mitral regurgitation
▸ Hypotension due to acute infarction and LVOT obstruction
▸ Discordance between the size of the wall motion abnormality and the size of the CK rise

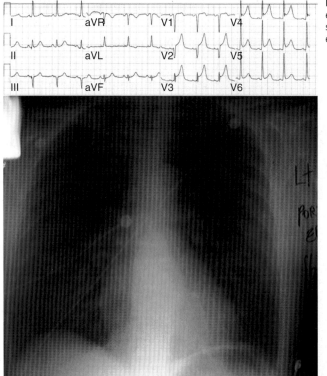

Figure 4-11. TOP, ECG shows sinus rhythm, Q waves V_1 and V_2, and ST elevation V_1-V_5 consistent with anterior infarction. BOTTOM, Chest radiograph shows borderline cardiomegaly (large lung fields) and interstitial pulmonary edema.

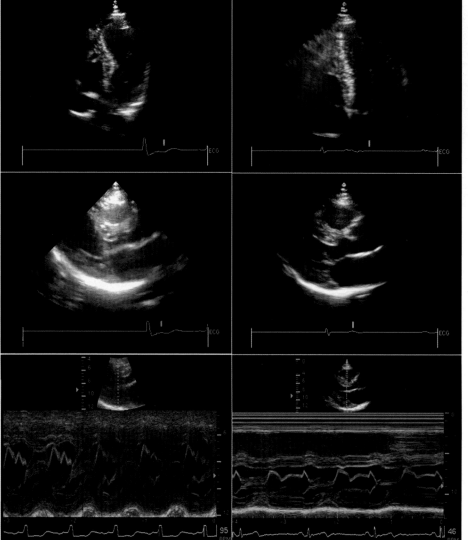

Figure 4-12. Images on the left were taken during initial admission, and images on the right were taken at 2-month follow-up. TOP LEFT, There is apical dilation (and akinesis). TOP RIGHT, At follow-up, the LV apex has normalized in size and systolic function. MIDDLE LEFT, At admission, there is severe SAM into the LVOT. MIDDLE RIGHT, At follow-up, there is only a "flick" of SAM. BOTTOM LEFT, At admission, there is severe SAM (prolonged apposition of the mitral valve leaflets against the septum). BOTTOM RIGHT, At follow-up, there is no SAM.

▸ Most of the wall motion abnormality was acute and due to stunning, not due to acute infarction.

▸ The wall motion abnormality represented a combination of prior infarction and a small acute infarction.

Management Plan

▸ Direct angiography with the view to urgent revascularization to improve anterior wall function and, it is hoped, to alleviate the LVOT obstruction

▸ Avoidance of preload reduction

▸ Afterload reduction

▸ Inotropic stimulation

▸ Small doses of IV pure vasopressors without inotropic effect (vasopressin)

▸ Concurrent small doses of IV beta-blocker, followed by oral beta-blocker

Outcome

▸ With increasing doses of beta-blocker, murmur was abolished, gradient was eliminated, BP returned to usual level, and heart failure cleared.

▸ The patient survived and was CCS class I, NYHA class I, and murmur free at follow-up.

Comments

▸ LVOT obstruction and apical ballooning associated with an acute coronary syndrome

▸ Murmurs of MR and outflow obstruction

▸ MR was secondary to the LVOT obstruction, mid and late systolic, and disappeared as the LVOT gradient was eliminated.

▸ Predisposing factors to the LVOT gradient include chest deformity (pectus excavatum) and aortic angulation, small and dynamic left ventricular cavity, and apical wall motion abnormality with compensatory increase in contractility of the base of the left ventricle.

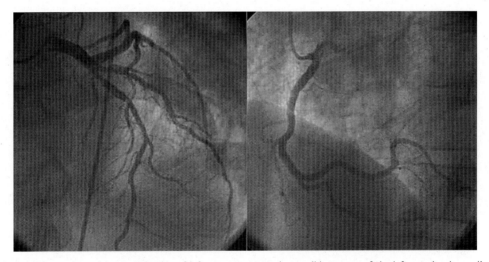

Figure 4-13. Selective coronary angiography. LEFT, Injection of left coronary artery shows mild stenoses of the left anterior descending coronary artery and first diagonal. RIGHT, Injection of right coronary artery shows mild stenoses of the left anterior descending coronary artery and first diagonal.

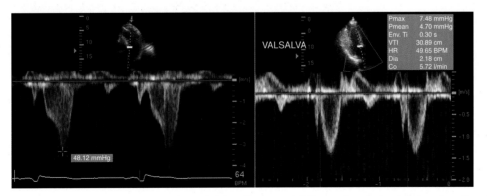

Figure 4-14. Continuous wave spectral profiles at initial admission (LEFT) and at 2-month follow-up (RIGHT). At admission, there is a 50 mm Hg peak gradient through the LVOT with atypical dagger shape of a dynamic obstruction. The gradient was at times 85 mm Hg. At follow-up, even with Valsalva preload reduction (strain phase), there is no provocation of a significant gradient. Low heart rate is due to beta-blockade.

References

1. Haley JH, Sinak LJ, Tajik AJ, et al: Dynamic left ventricular outflow tract obstruction in acute coronary syndromes: an important cause of new systolic murmur and cardiogenic shock. Mayo Clin Proc 1999;74:901-906.

2. Villareal RP, Achari A, Wilansky S, Wilson JM: Anteroapical stunning and left ventricular outflow tract obstruction. Mayo Clin Proc 2001;76:79-83.

3. Stollberger C, Finsterer J, Schneider B: Transient left ventricular dysfunction (tako-tsubo phenomenon): findings and potential pathophysiological mechanisms. Can J Cardiol 2006;22:1063-1068.

4. Abe Y, Kondo M, Matsuoka R, et al: Assessment of clinical features in transient left ventricular apical ballooning. J Am Coll Cardiol 2003;41:737-742.

5. Tsuchihashi K, Ueshima K, Uchida T, et al; Angina Pectoris–Myocardial Infarction Investigations in Japan: Transient left ventricular apical ballooning without coronary artery stenosis: a novel heart syndrome mimicking acute myocardial infarction. J Am Coll Cardiol 2001;38:11-18.

6. Hurst RT, Askew JW, Reuss CS, et al: Transient midventricular ballooning syndrome: a new variant. J Am Coll Cardiol 2006;48:579-583.

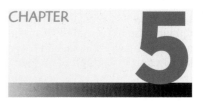

CHAPTER 5

Postinfarction Intracavitary Thrombi

KEY POINTS

▸ Postinfarction thrombi occur in larger infarctions, especially in non-anticoagulated cases.

▸ Thirty percent develop after discharge.

▸ Aneurysm, dyskinesis, and possibly akinesis are associated with thrombosis.

▸ CHF increases the risk of thrombus formation.

▸ Mobility and proximity to an infarct hinge point may suggest greater risk of embolization.

▸ Anticoagulation reduces the risk of thrombosis.

▸ Initiation of anticoagulation is based more on clinical judgment (size of infarction, severity of the wall motion abnormality, presence or absence of heart failure) than on merely whether thrombus was visualized on a single echo study.

▸ The optimal duration of anticoagulation therapy is unknown.

After myocardial infarction, intracavitary thrombi may form within any chamber of the heart. Although thrombi most commonly form within the left ventricle and are located at the apex, they may form as well over the left ventricular anterior wall, at the septum, and occasionally along the inferior wall. Left ventricular intracavitary thrombi may form as solitary or multiple lesions. Left atrial thrombi almost always occur in the context of atrial fibrillation, usually precipitated by left ventricular failure by the infarction. Rarely, right ventricular or right atrial thrombi may form after large right ventricular infarction. Hence, not all postinfarction thrombi are "apical."

The incidence of intracavitary thrombi has lessened in the current era because of the widespread use of anticoagulant therapy and is actually unknown. A scenario that continues to account for many thrombi is that of late presentation or delayed recognition of infarction, essentially replicating the natural history of infarction and allowing thrombi to form. From old postmortem series before the current era, approximately 20% of infarction cases, 30% to 40% of anterior infarction cases, and 60% of large anteroapical infarction cases developed thrombi. The incidence of thrombi among cases of inferior infarction is very low but is definitely not zero.

Thrombi may form within aneurysms and false aneurysms in any location. Aneurysms increase the risk of thrombus formation but engender some additional difficulties in recognizing thrombi. Aneurysms increase the area of endocardium to be assessed and the likelihood of missing small thrombi. Laminated thrombus along the wall of an aneurysm is difficult to appreciate

by echocardiography. Complete filling of an aneurysm by thrombus renders the aneurysm less readily appreciated.

The factors that cause intracavitary thrombi are not understood in detail, which explains why prevention and treatment are empirical. Local stagnation, such as low flow within aneurysms, is a factor, and impaired overall circulation (heart failure states) appears to compound local stagnation and further increase risk. Most thrombi are seen among ST elevation myocardial infarction (STEMI) or Q-wave infarction cases, presumably because of greater left ventricular regional and overall dysfunction.

Regional dyskinesis and aneurysmal deformation are associated with higher thrombus risk. Regional akinesia is not consistently associated with an increased risk of thrombus.[1,2]

DIAGNOSIS OF INTRACAVITARY THROMBI

The diagnostic test that bears the burden of identifying or predicting thrombi and thrombosis is echocardiography. And yet, echocardiography performed at 2 days after infarction identifies only half of the thrombi that will form. Several reasons are likely; the most likely is that patients at day 2 are still anticoagulated, and their findings do not predict non-anticoagulated outcomes. Some patients will experience progressive left ventricular dysfunction beyond day 2. As well, the sensitivity of echocardiography is not greater than 95%. Embolism occurs is 36% of those in whom a thrombus is imaged and in 7% of those in whom a thrombus is not imaged—which, although a lower rate, is not without embolism. Approximately 30% of thrombi develop after discharge as a result of discontinuation of anticoagulation or progression of left ventricular dysfunction. Postdischarge thrombi are most common if there is left ventricular aneurysm or dyskinesia, a predischarge ejection fraction of less than 35%, or a progressive deterioration of left ventricular systolic function.[1]

Few post-STEMI embolic episodes are seen because few patients at risk of thrombus formation are not anticoagulated (approximately 5%), only a minority develop thrombi (25% to 35%), and only a minority of cases with intracavitary thrombi evolve to recognizable embolism (10%). Therefore, the probability of embolism among all real-life STEMI cases is low, approximately 0.1% ($0.05 \times 0.05 \times 0.25$).

About half of all thrombi resolve, particularly if there is akinesia or use of warfarin.[1] Most thrombi that embolize do so early after infarction. Approximately 10% of non-anticoagulated thrombi embolize. The risk of embolization is greater if the thrombus is rounded or protuberant and particularly if there is hyperkinesis adjacent to the infarct territory (Fig. 5-1).[3] Mobile and protuberant thrombi have a high (80%) embolization rate. Thrombus location at a "hinge point" and readily visible thrombi also are at higher risk of embolization.[1,3]

Echocardiographic criteria of intracavitary thrombus include (1) delineation of the underlying endocardium : thrombus border, (2) specular echoes within the thrombus, and (3) the blood pool : thrombus border, all seen on more than a single view. Apical views are the most useful because most thrombi are apical. Transesophageal echocardiography (TEE) is probably more sensitive in detecting small apical thrombi,[4] but the relevance of such small thrombi is unknown, and TEE has not been well compared with cardiac magnetic resonance (MR) for the detection of small thrombi.

The left ventricular apex is prominently trabeculated, and small thrombi may rival the appearance of thrombi, and vice versa (Figs. 5-2 to 5-5).

Studies comparing detection rates of thrombi by echocardiography with another modality (e.g., indium In 111 scanning,

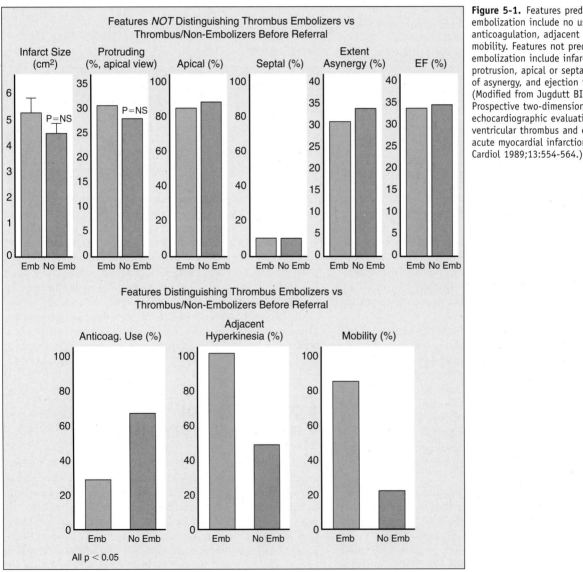

Figure 5-1. Features predictive of embolization include no use of anticoagulation, adjacent hyperkinesis, and mobility. Features not predictive of embolization include infarct size, protrusion, apical or septal location, extent of asynergy, and ejection fraction. (Modified from Jugdutt BI, Sivaram CA: Prospective two-dimensional echocardiographic evaluation of left ventricular thrombus and embolism after acute myocardial infarction. J Am Coll Cardiol 1989;13:554-564.)

5

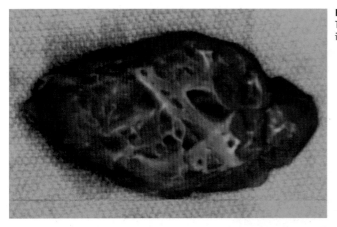

Figure 5-2. Normal left ventricular endocardial topography is complex. Trabeculations intersect and overlap and have differing size. Tomographic imaging struggles to discriminate small thrombi from trabeculations.

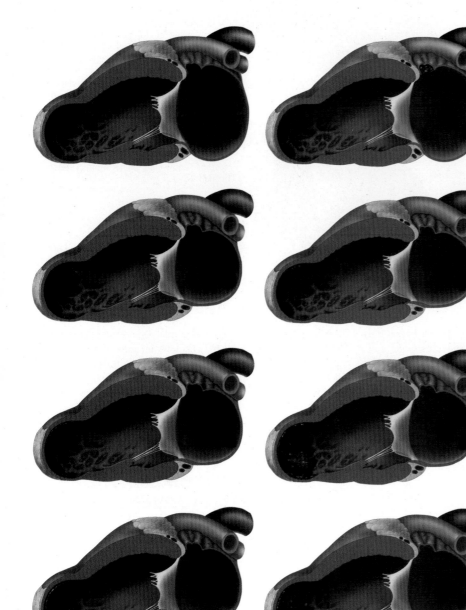

Figure 5-3. Left ventricular apical infarction, aneurysm, and thrombi. TOP ROW, LEFT, A well-formed, thin-walled (antero)apical aneurysm is present, typically the result of a mid-LAD occlusion. RIGHT, The apical aneurysm is without thrombus but is associated with left atrial enlargement, and a thrombus is present in the left atrial appendage as it may form in the presence of heart failure–associated atrial fibrillation. SECOND ROW, There are small, thin laminar thrombi scattered within the left ventricular apex. Such thrombi are readily missed by most imaging modalities because they are difficult to distinguish from trabeculations and may not obligingly fall onto the plane of imaging. THIRD ROW, LEFT, A laminar thrombus is present within the superior aspect of the aneurysm but again is readily missed by echocardiography because it may be interpreted as endocardium. RIGHT, Apical thrombus with some protrusion. The abnormal shape of the cavity within such an aneurysm-thrombus would strongly suggest the presence of a thrombus and should lead to its detection. BOTTOM ROW, LEFT, The apical aneurysm is largely filled with thrombus, and the shape of the thrombus confers only slight suggestion from the shape of the lumen of the presence of the thrombus. If the thrombus fills the aneurysm "flush" with the adjacent endocardium and restores the appearance of a normal cavity shape, the thrombus and aneurysm will not be detected by blood pool techniques but only by techniques that can image the thrombus and aneurysm directly. RIGHT, An obvious large protruding thrombus.

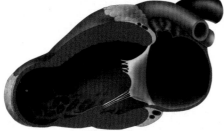 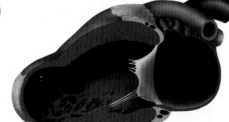

Figure 5-4. Protruding thrombi within an apical aneurysm. A narrow stalk is usually associated with motion of the thrombus, especially when the thrombus is located at the margin of an aneurysm, as in the right image, and if there is dyskinesis of the aneurysm. Dyskinesis of the aneurysm results in a simpler motion of thrombus in the central portion (LEFT IMAGE) and a more complex motion near the "hinge" with the normal myocardium (RIGHT IMAGE).

Figure 5-5. Although apical thrombi are the most numerous, and therefore the most often thought of, aneurysms (and false aneurysms) of the inferior wall (or lateral wall) may develop thrombi. LEFT UPPER IMAGE, Basal posterior wall aneurysm with a large amount of clot that is protruding. RIGHT UPPER IMAGE, Basal posterior wall aneurysm with an even larger amount of clot that is even more obviously protruding. Both of these thrombi should be apparent because they are large enough to be directly visualized and they distort the lumen, suggesting a thrombus. LEFT LOWER IMAGE, A thin laminar thrombus within the aneurysm is present and difficult to detect. RIGHT LOWER IMAGE, The thrombus has filled in the aneurysm, and if its top surface is flush with the adjacent endocardium, it would be difficult to detect by blood pool methods and would require a direct imaging modality.

autopsy, or surgical aneurysmectomy) are more than 10 years old and predate harmonic imaging. Although the sensitivity and negative predictive value of echocardiography are quite good (95% and 98%, respectively), the specificity and positive predictive value are less (72% and 86%, respectively). Interobserver agreement of transthoracic echocardiography is above 95%.

Common errors in the echocardiographic assessment of the apex include failure to systematically scan the entire apex, failure to recognize an aneurysm and a thrombus within it, and misdiagnosis of a false tendon or trabeculum as a thrombus (Figs. 5-6 and 5-7).

Other diagnostic modalities that may image intracavitary thrombi include contrast ventriculography (Fig. 5-8), which is best able to image protruding thrombi; blood pool scanning, which is also best able to image protruding thrombi; ^{111}In platelet scanning, which is not widely available; and cardiac MR. Cardiac MR is probably the most sensitive means by which to image thrombi (Figs. 5-9 to 5-11).[5] By SSFP sequences and inversion recovery sequences, thrombi are low signal (black) areas. Inversion recovery gadolinium delayed enhancement can corroborate infarction of the underlying myocardium.

There have been few (six) trials randomizing postinfarction patients to anticoagulation, totaling only 560 patients, and they

are obviously underpowered to tabulate the effect of anticoagulation on thromboembolism. The few data that exist suggest an approximately 50% reduction in thrombus formation. Clearly, despite full anticoagulation, thrombi can form, as has been demonstrated by serial echocardiographic imaging.[6]

ACC/AHA RECOMMENDATIONS FOR THE MANAGEMENT OF PATIENTS WITH ACUTE MYOCARDIAL INFARCTION: ANTICOAGULATION[7]

Class I

- Patients with LV thrombus
- Secondary prevention in patients unable to take aspirin
- Persistent atrial fibrillation

5

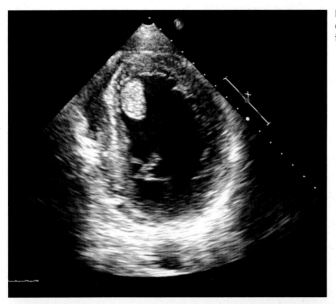

Figure 5-6. Transthoracic echocardiography—off-axis view of the apex to optimally image the thrombus. There is aneurysmal deformation of the inferior apex. Note the demarcation of the endocardium under the thrombus.

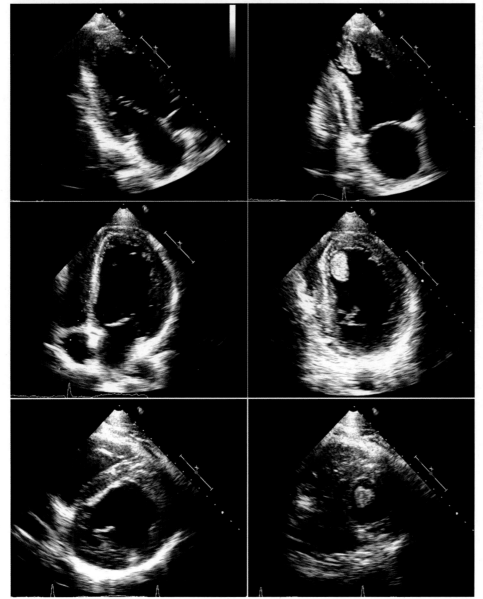

Figure 5-7. Transthoracic echocardiography reveals a large and protruding apical thrombus. The images on the left are obtained along a plane in which the thrombus does not fall. The images on the right have been optimized to view the thrombus. The thrombus resides in an inferior apical aneurysm; given the tendency of apical views to foreshorten the apex, the area of disease is less apparent on standard views.

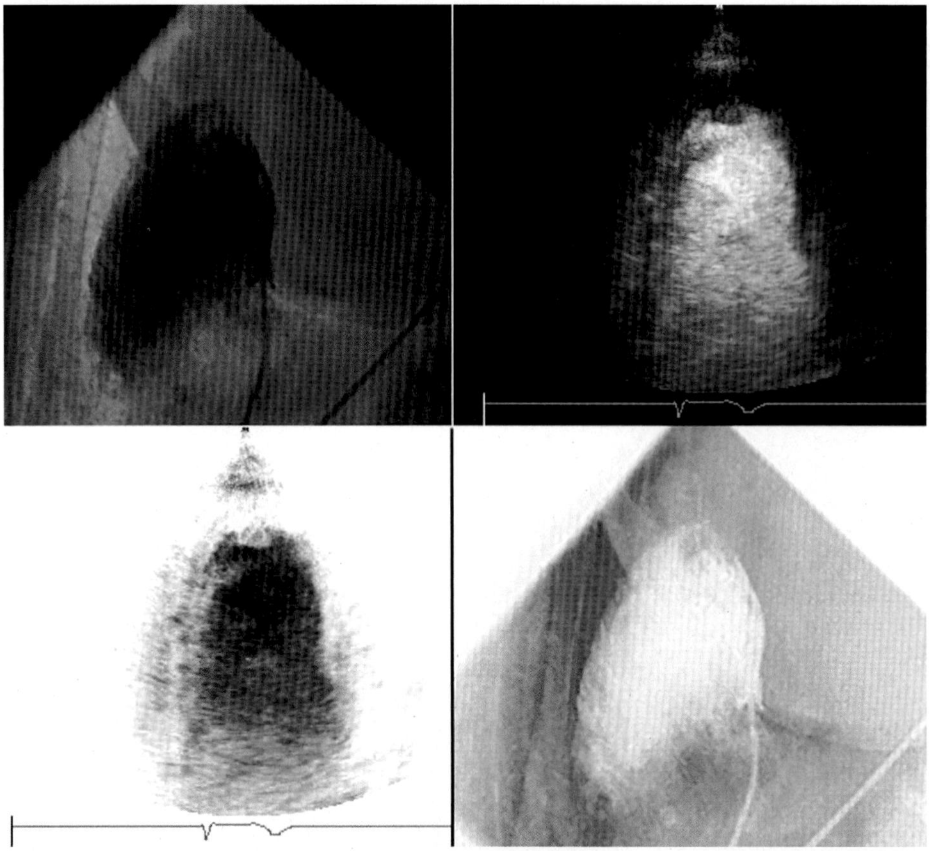

Figure 5-8. TOP, Contrast ventriculography (LEFT) and contrast echocardiography (RIGHT) images of the same case. BOTTOM, Black and white inverted contrast echocardiography (LEFT) and black and white inverted contrast ventriculography (RIGHT).

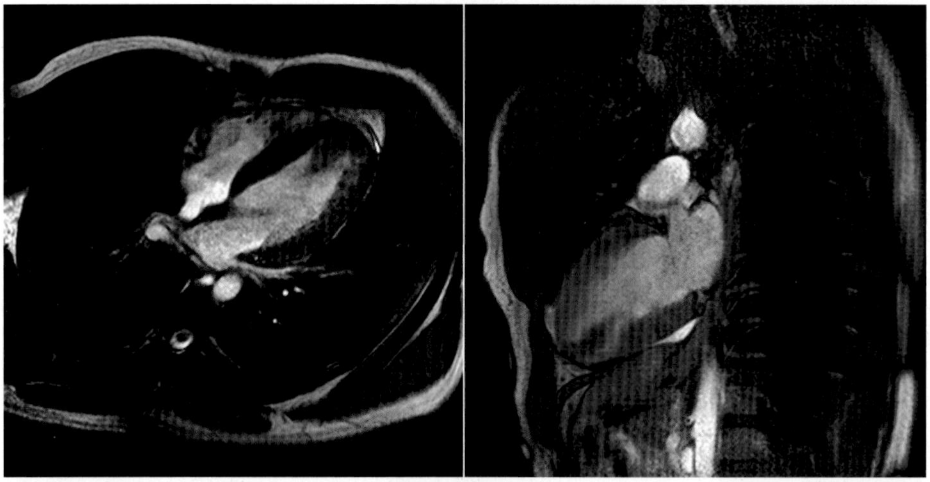

Figure 5-9. MRI SSFP sequences. The apical thrombus is apparent as a region of low signal within an inferior apical aneurysm that is akinetic.

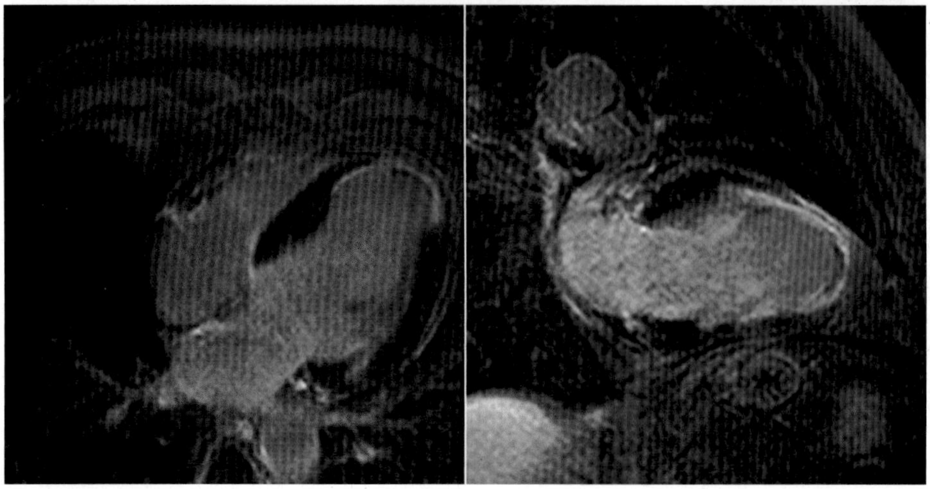

Figure 5-10. Inversion recovery sequences revealing delayed gadolinium enhancement of the distal anterior wall, distal septum, and apex consistent with prior infarction and a laminated thrombus (low signal layer). (Courtesy of Andrew Yan, MD, Toronto, Canada.)

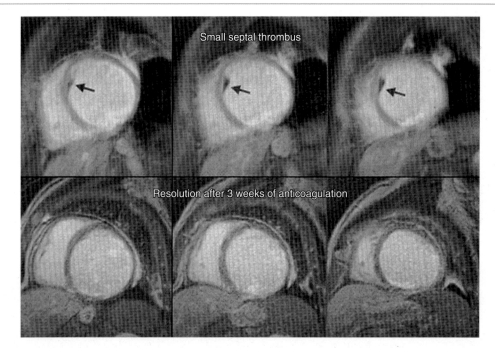

Small septal thrombus

Resolution after 3 weeks of anticoagulation

Figure 5-11. By SSFP cardiac MRI, thrombi are apparent as low signal areas, typically against wall motion abnormalities. (From Mollet NR, Dymarkowski S, Volders W, et al: Visualization of ventricular thrombi with contrast-enhanced magnetic resonance imaging in patients with ischemic heart disease. Circulation 2002;106:2873-2876.)

Class IIa

- Extensive wall motion abnormalities
- Paroxysmal atrial fibrillation

Class IIb

- Severe LV systolic dysfunction with or without congestive heart failure (CHF)

The contribution of thrombolysis to the management of intracavitary thrombosis appears negligible; the risk of fragmentation of thrombus and embolization has been established as prominent. In a small series of four patients with mobile apical thrombus at predischarge echocardiographic evaluation who were given thrombolysis, lysis occurred without complications in two patients; in the other two, systemic embolism occurred, of which one was fatal.

CASE 1

History

▸ 77-year-old man suffered a postdischarge cardiac arrest
▸ Past medical history is significant for previous myocardial infarctions.
▸ Previous VT and ICD implantation 6 years before for secondary prevention
▸ CCS class II angina, NYHA class III dyspnea

Physical Examination

▸ Normal blood pressure, heart rate; appears well perfused
▸ Enlarged and displaced apex

▸ S_3 and S_4
▸ No murmurs

Comments

▸ Chronic apical thrombus in a large apical aneurysm in the background of heart failure
▸ Significant for association of heart failure, aneurysm, and thrombus
▸ On receiving warfarin, the patient experienced two GI bleeds.
▸ Anticoagulation could not be continued because the source of bleeding could not be found.
▸ The clot has not enlarged over time.

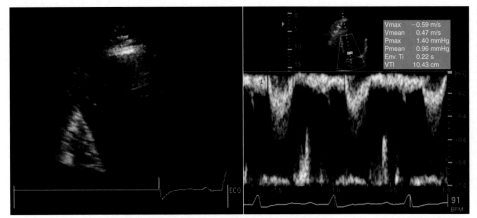

Figure 5-12. Transthoracic echocardiography. LEFT, Shallow apical 2-chamber view. There is an apical aneurysm, which was also dyskinetic. There are both a false tendon linearly traversing the dilated apex (blood pool–linear interface–blood pool) and an elliptical soft tissue mass within the most apical portion of the apex, largely filling it, with the typical features of thrombus (blood pool interface—specular echoes from the interface to the endocardium = thrombus). RIGHT, Spectral flow profile of LVOT flow (VTI 10 cm; normal range is 18 to 23 cm), revealing a severely reduced stroke volume, consistent with severe left ventricular systolic dysfunction.

CASE 2

History

- 67-year-old man
- Late-presentation anterior STEMI (hour 17)
- Did not receive fibrinolytics
- Heart failure present at the onset and persistent in the hospital

Physical Examination

- BP 100/60 mm Hg, HR 90 bpm, tachypneic
- Rales over 50% of the lung fields
- Quiet heart sounds
- S₃ gallop
- No murmurs

Comments

- Large anterior and apical infarction and thrombus
- The greatest bulk of the thrombus is along the anterior wall, not the apex.
- The "jelly-like" wobbling is consistent with fresh, nonorganized thrombus.
- No (recognized) embolic events occurred.
- Heart failure and thrombus developed early.
- Heart failure was refractory, and the patient died 4 weeks later.
- Early thrombus formation may be a marker of low output (CHF) and therefore high early mortality.

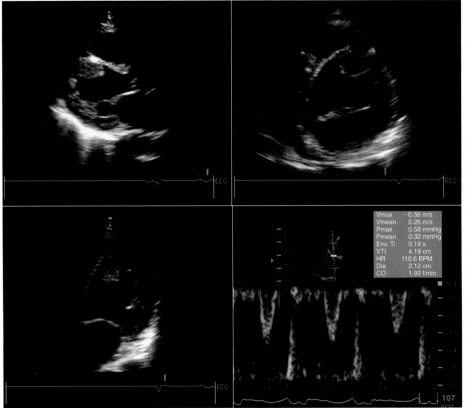

Figure 5-13. Transthoracic echocardiography. TOP LEFT, Parasternal long-axis view. There is a large, round soft tissue mass within the left ventricular cavity attached to the anterior septum. The cavities are dilated. TOP RIGHT, Parasternal short-axis view. Dilated left ventricular cavity with akinesis (and thinning) of the septum. Soft tissue mass in the anteroseptal cavity of the left ventricle with motion independent of the adjacent wall. Low-output motion of the mitral and aortic valves. BOTTOM LEFT, Off-axis apical view. Thinned, noncontractile septum and bright—suggestive of prior, chronic infarction. Thrombus extending into the cavity from the anteroseptal wall. BOTTOM RIGHT, Spectral profile of left ventricular outflow velocity. In this case, flow is extremely reduced (VTI 5 cm; stroke volume only 17 mL). Elevated heart rate is alone responsible for the borderline cardiac output.

CASE 3

History

▸ 69-year-old man admitted in advanced heart failure
▸ Anterior infarction 3 months before, received fibrinolytics
▸ There was little heart failure during the initial hospitalization.
▸ He was not discharged on warfarin.

Physical Examination

▸ BP 110/65 mm Hg, HR 90 bpm, tachypneic
▸ Enlarged apical impulse and mesoapical impulse

▸ S_3
▸ No murmurs

Comments

▸ Large anterior and anteroseptal thrombus developed after discharge within an anteroapical aneurysm.
▸ "Remodeling" of the left ventricle after discharge furthered the development of heart failure and thrombosis.
▸ Although the thrombus is well layered and apparent, it is not obvious.

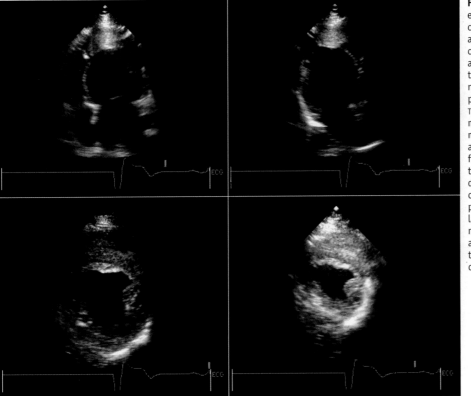

Figure 5-14. Transthoracic echocardiography. TOP LEFT, Apical 4-chamber view. The left cavities of the heart are enlarged compared with the right heart chambers. Although there is near-field artifact over the apex, it can also be seen that the left ventricular apex is filled in nearly entirely with thrombus, leaving a peculiarly round left ventricular cavity. TOP RIGHT, Apical 2-chamber view. The magnitude of the near-field artifact would make it easy to dismiss that there is an abnormality at the apex. BOTTOM LEFT, At first glance, the geometry of the heart on this plane appears normal. However, dyskinesis of the anterior wall prompts consideration of an aneurysm, which is present and is filled by 1.5 cm of laminated thrombus—thicker than the myocardium. BOTTOM RIGHT, A bulging anterior aneurysm is best defined between the 12-o'clock and 2-o'clock positions, completely filled in by thrombus.

CASE 4

History

▸ 79-year-old man, admitted with a hip fracture from a mechanical fall
▸ Late-presentation anterior STEMI 3 months ago (few details); discharged on beta-blocker, ASA, statin, ACE-I (not receiving warfarin)

Physical Examination

▸ Enlarged, displaced, and sustained apex
▸ S_3
▸ Echocardiography performed preoperatively

Comments

▸ Small, rounded thrombus at the left ventricular apex within a mobile, adversely remodeled dyskinetic segment

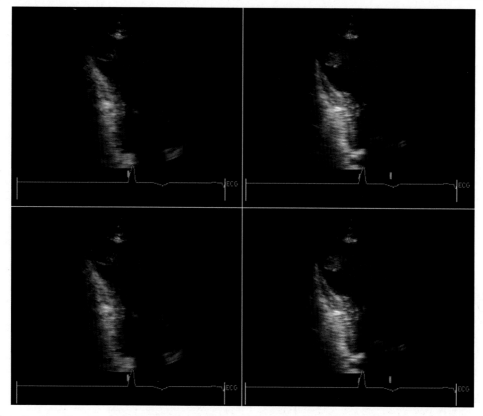

Figure 5-15. Transthoracic echocardiography—apical 2-chamber views. An apical aneurysm is present; depending on the frame, there is either a ghostly appearing or a more obvious appearing round marble-sized apical thrombus within the aneurysm.

CASE 5

History

▸ 63-year-old woman 7 days after inferior myocardial infarction, with associated large clinical right ventricular myocardial infarction causing protracted cardiogenic shock
▸ Recurrent GI bleeds requiring 7 transfusions

Physical Examination

▸ Venous distention
▸ No murmurs or rubs

Comments

▸ Large right ventricular myocardial infarction with associated right ventricle failure, low output, and right ventricular thrombosis
▸ Early heart failure after MI, early thrombosis, and in-hospital death

5

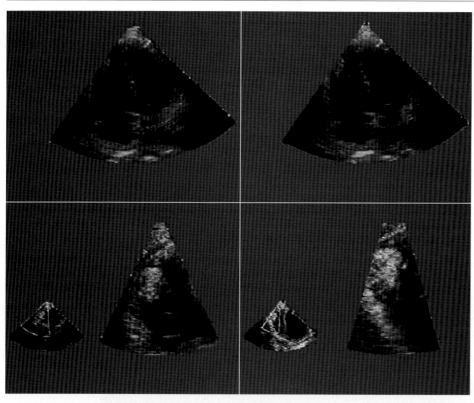

Figure 5-16. Transthoracic echocardiography. TOP IMAGES, Apical 4-chamber views. BOTTOM IMAGES, Zoom apical 4-chamber views. The right ventricle is severely dilated. The left atrium is small, consistent with severe right ventricular failure. The non-zoom views suggest an abnormality along the distal lateral wall of the right ventricle, which was akinetic. The zoom views are strongly suggestive of a rounded thrombus attached to the right ventricular free wall, attached to the underlying akinetic segment of the right ventricle.

CASE 6

History

▸ 76-year-old man admitted with heart failure
▸ Q-wave myocardial infarction 10 months previously, few details
▸ Slow insidious development of heart failure since discharge (not receiving warfarin)

Physical Examination

▸ Large displaced and sustained apex
▸ S_3, S_4

Comments

▸ Large mural thrombus filling an anteroapical aneurysm
▸ Progressive heart failure, and thrombosis, incited by adverse remodeling

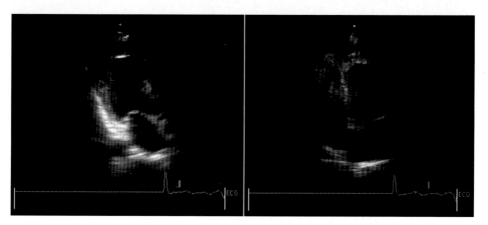

Figure 5-17. Transthoracic echocardiography. LEFT, Apical 2-chamber view. The left ventricular apex appears abnormal (flat apical surface), but it is not well enough seen to be assessed. RIGHT, Apical 4-chamber view. A kidney-shaped thrombus is present within the dilated left ventricular apex. The blood : clot interface, the bright specular echoes of the clot, and the distinct clot : endocardium interface of the thrombus are far more obvious on this plane of imaging.

CASE 7

History

- ▸ 29-year-old woman
- ▸ Late-presentation anterior STEMI (hour 17)
  - ▸ Hypotension without shock
  - ▸ Hemodynamic improvement during 3 days
  - ▸ Left anterior descending coronary artery: proximal irregularities, no stenosis, TIMI III flow
  - ▸ Discharged angina and heart failure free and prescribed warfarin for 6 months because of a large apical akinesis and in-hospital heart failure
- ▸ Risk factors: hypertension, dyslipidemia, smoking
- ▸ Thrombophilia work-up negative

Physical Examination

- ▸ Normotensive, normal heart rate
- ▸ No signs of heart failure
- ▸ No murmurs
- ▸ Enlarged and sustained apex

Evolution and Management

- ▸ Warfarin was stopped after 6 months of empirical treatment.
- ▸ There was no heart failure or definite apical thrombus.
- ▸ Routine echocardiography was performed 3 weeks later.

Comments

- ▸ Rapid formation of a thrombus after cessation of anticoagulation
- ▸ Mobile and pedunculated apical thrombus (high embolic potential) formed in a localized dyskinetic apical aneurysm.
- ▸ No thrombus had been seen before in this area of the heart, but the patient had been receiving anticoagulation at the time.
- ▸ In retrospect, the patient admitted to amaurosis fugax the morning of admission for repeated anticoagulation.
- ▸ Apparent need for long-term anticoagulation

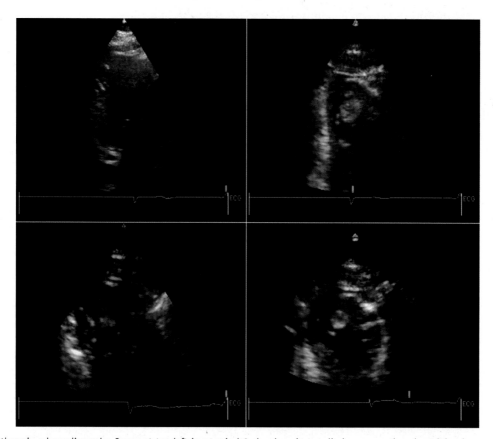

Figure 5-18. Transthoracic echocardiography. Image at top left is an apical 2-chamber view at discharge—no thrombus. Other images were taken once warfarin had been stopped. There is a round, mobile, marble-sized thrombus in the apex that formed after discontinuation of the warfarin.

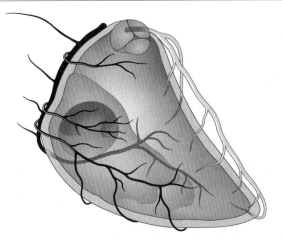

Figure 6-3. The right coronary artery and blood supply to the right ventricle and other structures. The walls of the right ventricle are depicted in pale brown and represent the complex shape of the right ventricle—convex on the free wall, concave on the septal side, tubular out the RVOT, and flat at the tricuspid valve orifice base. The normal vascular anatomy that supplies the right ventricle is composed of the conus branch that perfuses the RVOT region and that may evolve to collateralize to the LAD; acute marginal branches, of which there are usually two or three angiographically apparent branches that runover and perfuse the mid–free wall of the right ventricle and that may supply collaterals to the LAD; small anterior diagonal branches that arise from the LAD anteriorly to supply the medial anterior wall of the right ventricle and often its apex; and small posterior diagonal branches that arise from the posterior descending coronary artery that supply the medial posterior aspect of the right ventricle. The inferior septum, which contributes to right ventricular systolic and diastolic function, is supplied by inferior septal branches of the posterior descending coronary artery (not shown), and the anterior superior septum is similarly supplied by septal perforator branches by the LAD, which also contribute to right ventricular function or dysfunction. Septal function contributes to both right ventricular systolic and diastolic function. Inferior septal rupture may occur with occlusion of a dominant right coronary artery; hence, importantly, right ventricular infarction and septal rupture may be concurrent. Atrial branches also arise from the right coronary artery and sustain the atrial systolic function to deliver preload to the right ventricle, which is its principle means of compensation during infarction. The artery to the sinoatrial node usually (in 60% of cases) arises as the first branch of the right coronary artery. The artery to the atrioventricular node arises in most patients about 1 cm distal to the "crux" of the right coronary/ posterior descending artery. The posteromedial papillary muscle is perfused by branches of the right coronary from the posterior descending coronary artery or posteroventricluar branches off the ongoing distal right coronary artery and right coronary occlusion may lead to mitral insufficiency and papillary muscle rupture. The right coronary artery supplies blood flow to a large number of structures within the heart (contractile, valvular, and electrical), and thus permutations of cardiac dysfunction and the clinical complications are greater in right coronary infarction than in infarction caused by either other coronary artery.

marginal branches to the lateral and inferior walls of the right ventricle—resulting in right ventricular dysfunction of a sufficient extent to be recognized in most cases. Interestingly, only half of proximal right coronary occlusions produce right ventricular infarction, suggesting resistance of the (nonhypertrophied) right ventricle to ischemia and potentially of collateralization from the left coronary artery in an important proportion of cases. The relevance of right ventricular thebesian veins to right ventricular oxygen supply is controversial.[2]

Although the most prominent right ventricular infarctions are the consequence of right coronary artery occlusions, 10% of LAD-generated infarctions have pathologically and clinically apparent right ventricular infarction.[11]

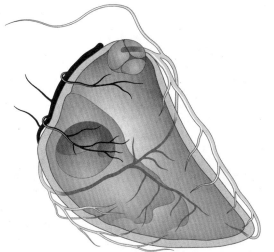

Figure 6-4. In ≤10% of patients, the left circumflex coronary artery supplies perfusion to a significant proportion of the right ventricle (whereas it normally does not), through posterior diagonal branches off the posterior descending coronary artery and from acute marginal branches of an ongoing circumflex after the crux. In 40% of cases, the artery to the sino-atrial node arises off the circumflex artery, not the right coronary artery.

DIFFERENCES OF RIGHT VENTRICULAR INFARCTION AND LEFT VENTRICULAR INFARCTION

- Right-sided heart failure versus left-sided heart failure
- Prominent need for adequate right ventricular preload
- Pericardium-mediated ventricular interdependence is an active phenomenon in right ventricular infarction because the right ventricle is more prone to rapid dilation.
- Recoverability of the right ventricle is greater and faster than that of the left ventricle.
- Preinfarction angina protects against right ventricular infarction.
- Right atrial pressure mechanical function is important and may be lost in atrial fibrillation, heart block, and atrial infarction.
- Right ventricular hypertrophy increases right ventricular ischemia.

COMPLICATIONS OF RIGHT VENTRICULAR INFARCTION

- Low output
- Shock (usually with little pulmonary congestion)
- Right ventricular papillary muscle rupture ($^1/_{20}$ of papillary muscle ruptures)
- Right ventricular free wall rupture ($^1/_7$ of myocardial ruptures)
- Patency of a foramen ovale with right-to-left shunting (hypoxemia unresponsive to supplemental oxygen) (Fig. 6-5)
- Pulmonary embolism of a right ventricular apical thrombus
- Pacer perforations
- Pericarditis

THE NORMAL RIGHT VENTRICLE

The stroke volume of the right ventricle is the same as that of the left ventricle, but the right ventricle pumps against a lesser arterial pressure (one fifth of systemic) and resistance (one tenth of systemic); hence, the right ventricle in its usual state is a less forceful

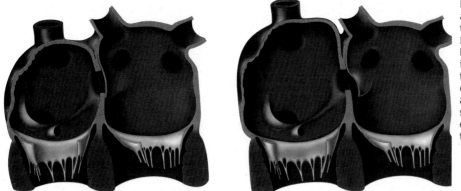

Figure 6-5. LEFT IMAGE, Normal atrial size and anatomy. In about one quarter of individuals, there is patency of the foramen ovale. RIGHT IMAGE, Enlargement of the right side of the heart as a consequence of right ventricular infarction. The right atrium is dilated, and a foramen ovale is both stretched open by the chamber dilation and pushed open by a right atrial to left atrial gradient due to the right-sided heart failure and general absence of equally prominent left-sided heart failure in the context of right ventricular infarction.

pump, having one sixth of the muscle mass, having one third of the wall thickness, and performing one fourth of the stroke work of the systemic ventricle. The right ventricle receives systemic venous blood at lower diastolic filling pressures than does the left ventricle and also with greater respiratory fluctuations in filling pressure. The normal right ventricle functions despite variations in preload. In contradistinction, the ischemic right ventricle is highly sensitive to variations in preload. The pattern of contraction of the right ventricle differs from that of the left ventricle, which contracts radially and longitudinally. The right ventricular free wall contracts toward the interventricular septum, with also some longitudinal shortening. The interventricular septum normally pushes into the right ventricle, contributing to right ventricular function.

THE INFARCTED RIGHT VENTRICLE

Smaller infarctions of the right ventricle, such as those due to LAD occlusion, result in little hemodynamic disturbance. Infarctions of the right ventricular lateral wall and posterior wall, as occur with an occlusion of the right ventricle proximal to most of the acute marginal branches, would usually result in disturbed hemodynamics. The ischemic right ventricle is prominently dependent on preload as a means to maintain filling of the chamber that has less compliant walls from the ischemia. To achieve adequate filling, right atrial contraction augments to adapt to right ventricular ischemic noncompliance. This is apparent by an increase in the right atrial A-wave magnitude and x descent prominence.[12] As stroke volume falls from right ventricular systolic failure, heart rate rises to maintain cardiac output. A larger proportion of right ventricular ejection is effected by septal contraction, as free wall contraction fails because of ischemia.

Right-sided heart failure, when it is due to right ventricular infarction, results in a low-output, hypotension syndrome. There is rarely a prominent concurrent amount of left-sided heart failure because the right ventricular infarction reduces filling of the left side of the heart. The transmural distending pressure of the left ventricle (diastolic pressure minus the intrapericardial pressure) is profoundly influenced by right-sided heart failure and dilation. The intrapericardial pressure and the right-sided heart diastolic pressures are nearly identical and very low. Left ventricular filling (transmural distending pressure) is normally approximately 10 mm Hg minus 0 mm Hg; whereas in right ventricular infarction, the left ventricular filling (transmural distending pressure) is markedly reduced (approximately 10 mm Hg minus 10 mm Hg).

Hypotension, due to underfilling of the left side of the heart, is the most obvious manifestation of right ventricular infarction.

The thin-walled right ventricle and atrium are prone to early dilation. Significant dilation will challenge the acute pericardial (volume) reserve. Excessive right-sided heart dilation will achieve a compressive phenomenon within the pericardial space, elevating diastolic pressures. The dilated right-sided chambers will compete for space with the left-sided chambers. Maneuvers that further augment right-sided heart filling, such as volume loading, will actually compromise left-sided heart filling within the finite intrapericardial space.[13]

Factors that impair right atrial systolic function may lead to a prominent fall in right ventricular function. The development of atrial fibrillation and complete heart block typically result in prompt hypotension. Right atrial infarction, which is difficult to diagnose, has the same detrimental effect as atrial fibrillation.[14] The more proximal the occlusion of the right coronary artery, the greater the likelihood of right atrial branch loss and right atrial infarction, which is apparent as a lack of an increase in the right atrial A wave and x descent and an M pattern of the right atrial waveform, whereas a mid right coronary occlusion without extensive right atrial branch loss and without significant right atrial infarction is associated with an augmented right atrial A wave and x descent and a W pattern of the right atrial waveform.[12]

Septal contraction is an important component of right-sided heart function in right ventricular infarction because the right ventricular free wall is not contributing to contraction and may be dyskinetic, detracting from systolic function. In most individuals, the extent of concurrent septal infarction is small because the posterior septal perforators from the posterior descending coronary artery supply normally only the basal posterior septum and some proportion of the mid posterior septum. In individuals in whom the coronary anatomy generates a larger septal infarction, the compromising effect on right-sided heart systolic function will be larger.

Right ventricular ischemic or infarcting myocardium exhibits a steeper pressure : volume (length : tension) relationship and is therefore more sensitive to variation in filling.[12] Use of venodilators, such as nitroglycerin, or diuretics will deprive the right ventricle of venous return and preload, and nitroglycerin intolerance is a common occurrence in right ventricular infarction.

Elevation of right atrial pressure (from right ventricular infarction) will enable right-to-left shunting in those with patency of the foramen ovale. Dilation of the right atrium from right ventricular failure will enlarge the foramen ovale, augmenting shunt flow.

Table 6-2. Preinfarction Angina Decreases the Risk of Right Ventricular Infarction and Complications

	With Angina (N = 62)	Without Angina (N = 51)	
ST elevation V₄R	27%	71%	<.001
Complete AV block	11%	33%	.004
Hypotension or shock	8%	53%	<.001
In-hospital death	5%	10%	.26

The systolic function of the right ventricular free wall recovers faster and more completely than does that of the left ventricular inferior wall,[3] although not all cases recover enough or fast enough to elude shock and death. The reasons that the right ventricle demonstrates greater recoverability are not well understood. The lesser right ventricular myocardial demand (less mass, pressure), the presence of collaterals from the left coronary system, the balanced pattern (systolic and diastolic) of right coronary blood flow versus left coronary blood flow (diastolic predominant), and potentially the oxygen supply through right ventricular thebesian veins may contribute to the fact that the right ventricle is more likely to stun than to infarct. Preinfarction angina reduces the risk of right ventricular infarction and its complications, presumably because of ischemic preconditioning and collateral recruitment (Table 6-2).[8] Less than half of proximal dominant occlusions produce recognized right ventricular infarction. The extent of recovery of the right ventricle has prompted some to propose that the right ventricle experiences ischemia rather than infarction.

CLINICAL PRESENTATIONS OF RIGHT VENTRICULAR INFARCTION

- Hypotensive inferior infarction
- Inferior infarction, cardiogenic shock
- Inferior infarction with venous distention, Kussmaul sign
- Inferior infarction, blood pressure intolerant of nitroglycerin
- Larger biomarker rise than anticipated from inferior infarction
- Greater amount of hypotension than expected from a first infarct with a small or moderate creatine kinase rise

Differential diagnosis of myocardial infarction with prominent hypotension but without proportionally as much pulmonary edema:

- Underfilling of the left ventricle
  - Hypovolemia, may be from medications
  - Right ventricular infarction
- Vasodepression
  - Excessive effect of medications
  - Medication-induced anaphylaxis
  - Vagal vasodepressant state
- Tamponade
- Ventricular septal rupture

DIAGNOSIS OF RIGHT VENTRICULAR INFARCTION

Physical Diagnosis

Right ventricular infarction can be diagnosed at the bedside. The combination of jugular venous pressure higher than 8 cm and a Kussmaul sign is 88% sensitive and 76% specific for right ventricular infarction. The triad of hypotension, venous distention, and clear lung fields in the setting of inferior infarction is 96% specific for right ventricular infarction but only 25% sensitive.[15] Hypovolemia and hypervolemia obscure jugular venous findings of right ventricular infarction.

Electrocardiography

Electrocardiography (ECG) is useful for the diagnosis of right ventricular infarction, as long as the baseline ECG recording is normal and if ECG is performed very early in the infarction. Several ECG patterns have been advanced. Right-sided chest leads (V₄R) demonstrating more than 0.5 mV or more than 1 mV of ST elevation suggest right ventricular infarction. Use of 0.5 mV or mm is more sensitive but less specific; 1 mm of ST elevation 0.08 second after the J point is seen in most (>80%) cases and has a high pathologic correlation with right ventricular infarction (100%).[16] A significant caveat is that the finding of ST elevation in V₄R is evanescent, lasting only 24 to 48 hours and normalizing in half of cases within 10 hours. False-positives are also common and may be generated by pulmonary embolism, pericarditis, acute anteroseptal ST elevation myocardial infarction (STEMI), and anteroseptal aneurysm. ST elevation in V₁ through V₄ is associated with pure right ventricular infarction.[17] ST elevation in standard limb lead III more than in standard limb lead II is 97% sensitive and 70% specific.[18]

Other common, clinically important but not diagnostic ECG findings in right ventricular infarction include sinus bradycardia, sinus tachycardia, atrial fibrillation (seen in up to one third of cases),[19] atrioventricular block and third-degree block, and right bundle branch block. Right bundle branch block has been noted in up to 48% of cases of right ventricular infarction and is associated with a poor prognosis.[20,21]

Echocardiography

Echocardiography is useful to corroborate findings of right ventricular systolic dysfunction and to identify or to exclude associations and complications of inferior infarction or of the right ventricular infarction itself. Older echocardiographic and nuclear signs of right ventricular infarction were simply right ventricular dilation and overall systolic dysfunction. With improved imaging, assessment of regional right ventricular systolic function is now possible and useful because it correlates with the right coronary anatomy and the location of occlusion. The posterior wall of the right ventricle is most commonly affected by right ventricular infarction because it is the most distal right coronary territory.[22] Combined right ventricular lateral and posterior wall motion abnormalities are produced by more proximal right coronary artery occlusions and are the typical findings of hemodynamically

Table 6-3. Echocardiographic Views That Assist with Right Ventricular Regional Wall Motion Assessment

	Segment of the Right Ventricle	Vascular Supply	If Wall Motion Assessment Suggests Site of Occlusion
Echocardiographic view			
Parasternal long-axis view	RVOT	Conus branch	Very proximal RCA
Parasternal short-axis view	Anterior RV	Diagonal branches off the LAD	LAD
	Lateral wall	Acute marginal branches	Before one (mid RCA) or all acute marginal (proximal RCA) branches
	Posterior wall	Diagonal branches off the PDA/PIV	PDA/PIV or anywhere proximal to PDA/PIV, including dominant left circumflex artery
RV inflow view			
Apical 4-chamber view	Lateral wall	Acute marginal branches	Before one (mid RCA) or all acute marginal (proximal RCA) branches
Subcostal long-axis view	Lateral wall	Acute marginal branches	Before one (mid RCA) or all acute marginal (proximal RCA) branches
Subcostal long-axis view	Posterior wall	Diagonal branches off the PDA/PIV	PDA/PIV or anywhere proximal to PDA/PIV, including dominant left circumflex artery
	Lateral wall	Acute marginal branches	Before one (mid RCA) or all acute marginal (proximal RCA) branches
	Anterior RV	Diagonal branches off the LAD	LAD

LAD, left anterior descending coronary artery; PDA/PIV, posterior descending (interventricular) artery; RCA, right coronary artery; RV, right ventricle; RVOT, right ventricular outflow tract.

significant right ventricular infarction. In the context of inferior infarction, right ventricular akinesis or hypokinesis (segmental) is 83% sensitive and 93% specific for right ventricular infarction.[23]

Right ventricular wall motion abnormalities do occur in other disease states, such as pulmonary hypertension, pulmonary embolism, and trauma, and after poor pump protection. Views that assist with right ventricular regional wall motion assessment are listed in Table 6-3. Echocardiographic findings in right ventricular infarction are summarized in Table 6-4.

Radionuclide Angiography

The diagnosis of right ventricular infarction by radionuclide technique is possible by use of the combination of overall depression of right ventricular systolic function (<40%; normal range is 45% to 75%) and regional right ventricular systolic dysfunction.[2] Technetium pyrophosphate scanning is specific but not sensitive.[2]

Cardiac Magnetic Resonance

Cardiac magnetic resonance (MR) is able to image the increased myocardial water (edema) by T2 weighting and by gadolinium contrast enhancement.[26] Cardiac MR SSFP sequences elegantly depict right and left ventricular regional wall motion.

Hemodynamics, Cardiac Catheterization, and Angiography

Right-sided heart catheterization is seldom necessary for diagnosis of right ventricular infarction, but waveforms are revealing of the physiology. As described before, as long as right atrial infarction has not occurred, right atrial systolic function (Starling forces) is recruited to enable filling of a noncompliant right ventricle, resulting in an augmented A wave and x descent of the right atrial pressure and a W pattern. When significant right atrial infarction has occurred, the right atrial A wave is therefore diminished, as is the x descent, and the right atrial waveform has an M pattern.[13] Pericardial restraint will also contribute to the M pattern ("square root" or "dip-and-plateau" pattern) typical of severe and larger right ventricular infarction with impaired right ventricular compliance and pericardial restraint.[22] The x descent predominance can also be seen. The right ventricular systolic waveform becomes broad and sometimes bifid, reflecting lesser dP/dt (upslope from systolic failure), impaired relaxation (reduced −dP/dt), and septal bulge into the right ventricle.

The most prominent pressure waveform of right ventricular infarction is the combination of diastolic failure (elevated right atrial and right ventricular diastolic pressure) and systolic failure (lower right ventricular systolic pressure). Thus, a right atrial pressure:pulmonary capillary wedge pressure (RAP:PCWP) above 0.86 (normal <0.6) is 82% sensitive and 97% specific for right ventricular infarction in the setting of inferior infarction.[27]

MANAGEMENT

Management principles are based on the following:

- Optimize right ventricular preload
  - Optimize volume status (central venous pressure [CVP] of 15 mm Hg)
  - Maintain atrioventricular synchrony by maintaining or restoring sinus rhythm (if in atrial fibrillation) or sequential pacing for complete heart block

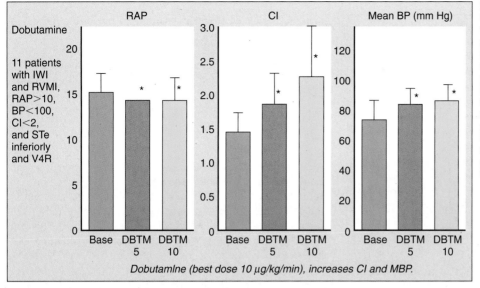

Figure 6-9. In patients with right ventricular infarction and inferior left ventricular infarction optimized with right atrial pressure above 10 mm Hg but still hypotensive and with low output, inotropic doses of dobutamine lower right atrial pressure (RAP) and increase cardiac index (CI) and arterial blood pressure. The asterisks indicate significance. IWI, inferior wall infarction; RVMI, right ventricular myocardial infarction. (Data from Ferrario M, Poli A, Previtali M, et al: Hemodynamics of volume loading compared with dobutamine in severe right ventricular infarction. Am J Cardiol 1994;74:329-333.)

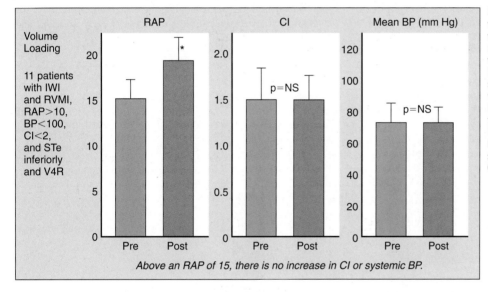

Figure 6-10. In patients with right ventricular infarction and inferior left ventricular infarction already with optimal right ventricular filling pressures, further volume loading does not improve arterial hemodynamics. The asterisks indicate significance. CI, cardiac index; IWI, inferior wall infarction; RAP, right atrial pressure; RVMI, right ventricular myocardial infarction. (Data from Ferrario M, Poli A, Previtali M, et al: Hemodynamics of volume loading compared with dobutamine in severe right ventricular infarction. Am J Cardiol 1994 1994;74:329-333.)

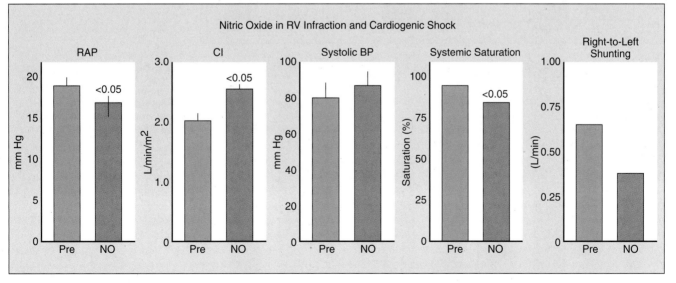

Figure 6-11. LEFT THREE IMAGES, The effect of inhalation of 80 ppm of nitric oxide (NO) on the hemodynamics of patients with right ventricular (RV) infarction and cardiogenic shock. Inhaled nitric oxide reduces right atrial pressure (RAP), increases cardiac index (CI), and systemic arterial pressure. RIGHT TWO IMAGES, The effect of inhalation of 80 ppm of nitric oxide on right-to-left shunting in 3 patients with right ventricular infarction and cardiogenic shock. A significant volume of right-to-left shunting occurred at baseline, particularly when considering the low overall cardiac indices. Inhalation of nitric oxide reduced right-to-left shunting and increased systemic arterial saturation. (From Inglessis I, Shin JT, Lepore JJ, et al: Hemodynamic effects of inhaled nitric oxide in right ventricular myocardial infarction and cardiogenic shock. J Am Coll Cardiol 44:793-798, 2004, with permission from Elsevier.)

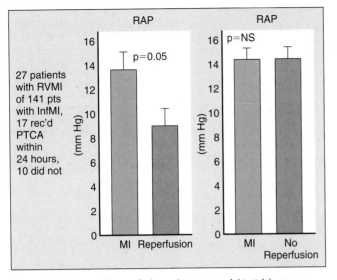

Figure 6-12. Successful reperfusion reduces mean right atrial pressure (RAP). PTCA, percutaneous transluminal coronary angioplasty; RVMI, right ventricular myocardial infarction. (Data from Kinn JW, Ajluni SC, Samyn JG, et al: Rapid hemodynamic improvement after reperfusion during right ventricular infarction. J Am Coll Cardiol 1995;26:1230-1234.)

maintaining atrioventricular synchrony; atrial pacing at the same rate increased the stroke volume by a mean of 42%.[32]

Observational data suggest that when reperfusion can be established, the mean right atrial pressure nearly normalizes (Fig. 6-12),[33] and right ventricular systolic function (ejection fraction) may also nearly normalize.[34] Unsuccessful percutaneous coronary intervention (PCI) is associated with absence of improvement of right ventricular systolic function, persistence of hypotension and low cardiac index, and significantly higher mortality (Fig. 6-13).[3] Among patients in whom PCI was successful, the percentage with persistent hypotension and low cardiac output is significantly less, as is mortality.[3] The effect of successful PCI on right ventricular systolic function, right atrial pressure, and cardiac index is demonstrable at 1 hour after the procedure and there is further benefit at 1 and 3 days (Figs. 6-14 to 6-16).[3] The percentage of cases in which right ventricular systolic function has normalized at 1 month is significantly greater after successful reperfusion (Fig. 6-17).[3]

Although PCI has not been shown in large prospective trials to reduce mortality in right ventricular infarction, the available evidence favors its use, particularly early use, and suggests that it is underused.

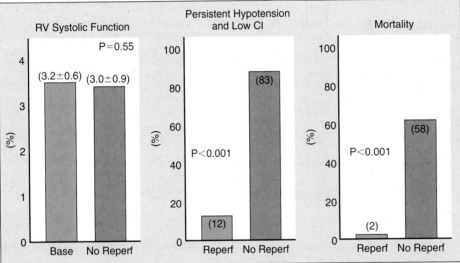

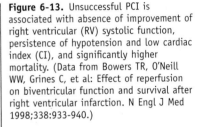

Figure 6-13. Unsuccessful PCI is associated with absence of improvement of right ventricular (RV) systolic function, persistence of hypotension and low cardiac index (CI), and significantly higher mortality. (Data from Bowers TR, O'Neill WW, Grines C, et al: Effect of reperfusion on biventricular function and survival after right ventricular infarction. N Engl J Med 1998;338:933-940.)

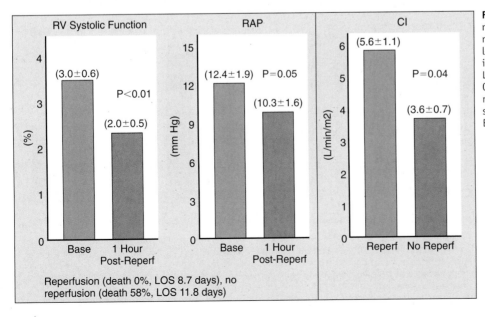

Reperfusion (death 0%, LOS 8.7 days), no reperfusion (death 58%, LOS 11.8 days)

Figure 6-14. PCI, effective in establishing reperfusion, is associated with improved right ventricular (RV) systolic function, lower right atrial pressure (RAP), and improved cardiac output and index (CI). LOS, length of stay. (Data from Bowers TR, O'Neill WW, Grines C, et al: Effect of reperfusion on biventricular function and survival after right ventricular infarction. N Engl J Med 1998;338:933-940.)

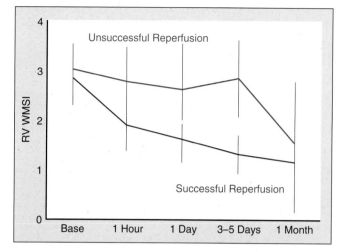

Figure 6-15. Successful PCI leads to early improvement (fall in right ventricular wall motion score index [RV WMSI]) in right ventricular function, whereas PCI unsuccessful in achieving reperfusion is associated with delayed recovery. (Data from Bowers TR, O'Neill WW, Grines C, et al: Effect of reperfusion on biventricular function and survival after right ventricular infarction. N Engl J Med 1998;338:933-940.)

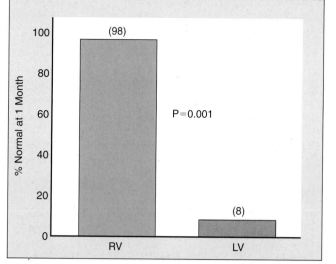

Figure 6-17. At 1 month after infarction, almost all survivors have normal right ventricular (RV) systolic function, but few have normalized left ventricular (LV) systolic function. (Data from Bowers TR, O'Neill WW, Grines C, et al: Effect of reperfusion on biventricular function and survival after right ventricular infarction. N Engl J Med 1998 1998;338:933-940.)

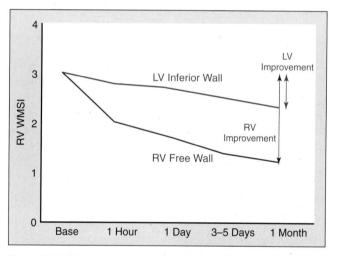

Figure 6-16. The right ventricle (RV) recovers more and faster than does the inferior wall of the left ventricle (LV). RV WMSI, right ventricular wall motion score index. (From Bowers TR, O'Neill WW, Grines C, et al: Effect of reperfusion on biventricular function and survival after right ventricular infarction. N Engl J Med 1998;338:933-940. Copyright © [2001] Massachusetts Medical Society. All rights reserved.)

Therapy for right ventricular infarction cases should be individualized. General principles of therapy are summarized in Table 6-6.[35]

Table 6-6. General Principles of Therapy for Right Ventricular Infarction Cases

Type of Case	Therapy
Asymptomatic	Avoid diuretics and vasodilators that may precipitate low output and hypotension.
Symptomatic low-output state and normotensive with right atrial pressure or pulmonary capillary wedge pressure <15 mm Hg	Add fluid to increase the pulmonary capillary wedge pressure to 15-18 mm Hg. If cardiac output does not increase adequately, add a vasodilator. If the cardiac output still does not increase adequately, add dobutamine or amrinone. Reperfusion therapy should be considered.
Symptomatic low-output state and normotensive with right atrial pressure or pulmonary capillary wedge pressure >15 mm Hg	Add intravenous dobutamine or amrinone. Additional vasodilator with fluid therapy support may be added. Reperfusion therapy should be considered.
Cardiogenic shock	Sustain blood pressure with dopamine; additional dobutamine may increase cardiac output. Consider right ventricular assist or pulmonary artery counterpulsation for select cases. Reperfusion therapy should be strongly considered.

OUTCOMES

The in-hospital mortality of right ventricular infarction is, as expected, graded according to the severity of the hemodynamic disturbances (Killip I: 5% mortality; Killip IV, cardiogenic shock: 55% mortality) and the occurrence of complications or associated lesions. The in-hospital mortality of inferior infarction without right ventricular infarction is 6%; with right ventricular infarction, 31%; and with right ventricular infarction and cardiogenic shock, 50% to 60%.[36]

The long-term survival of patients discharged from the hospital is good. Most do recover a large proportion of right ventricular systolic function and therefore have their prognosis determined by the degree of postinfarction left ventricular function and the extent and severity of coronary artery disease. However, postinfarction persistence of right ventricular dysfunction is an independent predictor of the development of heart failure and of death.[37]

CASE 1

History

▸ 83-year-old man with chronic renal insufficiency, presenting with 9 hours of ischemic chest pain

Physical Examination

▸ BP 110/60 mm Hg, HR 48 bpm, RR 12/min
▸ Venous distention to the angle of the jaw
▸ Normal S_1, S_2; S_4 present
▸ No murmurs or rubs
▸ Extremities warm, mentation normal

Management

▸ Avoidance of preload-reducing maneuvers
▸ As the neck veins were indicative of adequate preload, no volume was given.
▸ As the output was clinically adequate, no inotropes were given.

Evolution and Outcome

▸ Right-sided heart failure resolved after 3 hours.
▸ The remainder of the hospital course was uneventful: no recurrent pains, no reversible defect on perfusion scanning.
▸ Well at follow-up

Comments

▸ Right ventricular myocardial infarction diagnosed by elevated neck veins in the context of an acute inferior STEMI; echocardiography corroborative
▸ No major hemodynamic disturbances other than mild hypotension
▸ Early spontaneous recovery of right ventricular systolic function

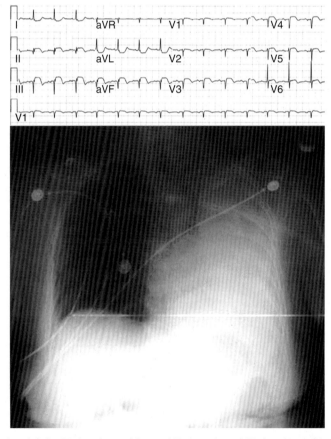

Figure 6-18. TOP, ECG shows sinus rhythm, inferior ST elevation, and inverted T waves. Lateral ST elevation and inverted T waves suggest acute inferolateral infarction. BOTTOM, Chest radiograph shows no pulmonary edema within the right lung field and a large left pleural effusion.

6

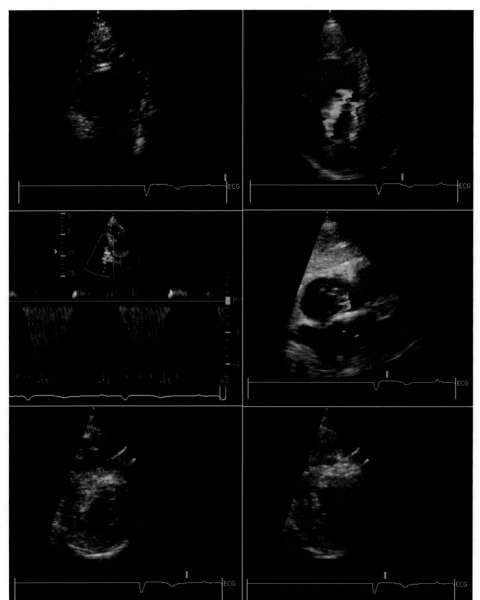

Figure 6-19. Transthoracic echocardiography. TOP ROW, Apical 4-chamber views oriented to the right. There is dilation and "sphericalization" of the right ventricle, consistent with infarction and systolic dysfunction. There is moderate tricuspid insufficiency due to the right ventricular systolic dysfunction. MIDDLE LEFT, Tricuspid regurgitation spectral profile. Right ventricular systolic pressure: $4 \times V^2 +$ RAP = 13 + 15 = 28 mm Hg. The right ventricular systolic pressure is low for a typical myocardial infarction case with shock, and the diastolic pressure (the right atrial pressure) is disproportionately high (50% of the systolic pressure). The delayed velocity rise (slope) of the tricuspid regurgitation is consistent with impaired right ventricle dP/dt. MIDDLE RIGHT, Right atrial and right ventricular dilation. There is marked systolic bulging of the right atrium due to right atrial pressure exceeding that of the left atrium. BOTTOM ROW, Diastolic (LEFT) and systolic (RIGHT) views. There is diastolic flattening of the interventricular septum due to elevation of the right ventricular diastolic pressure from the right ventricular infarction.

CASE 2

History

- 75-year-old man presenting with 3 syncopal episodes; no chest pain
- Found by EMS to be in third-degree aortic valve block, BP 55/– mm Hg
- Mechanical ventilation and vasopressors started at community hospital
- Transferred for a pacer

Physical Examination

- BP 90/60 mm Hg, HR 55 bpm
- Cool extremities
- Head trauma from syncope, 5-cm laceration across the forehead

- Venous distention to the angle of the jaw
- Quiet heart sounds
- No gallops, rubs, or murmurs
- CK 3000, creatinine 300

Management

- Temporary pacer inserted, with poor capture
- High-dose vasopressors and inotropes used
- IABP inserted

Outcome

- Arrived in shock, remained in shock
- Died within an hour of arrival, within 4 hours of presentation to the community hospital

▸ Died despite the preceding measures and before angiography could be obtained

Comments

▸ Massive right ventricular infarction associated with inferior infarction
▸ Cardiogenic shock in the context of an inferior STEMI is usually due to right ventricular infarction, as it was here.
▸ Acute right-sided heart failure (venous distention and hypotension) is usually due to tamponade, pulmonary embolism, or right ventricular myocardial infarction.
▸ The difficulty in achieving capture with the pacer was likely due to the right ventricle's infarction.
▸ Pulseless electrical activity likely resulted from progression of the right ventricle's failure, worsened by acidosis; right ventricle perforation, after infarction or due to the pacer.
▸ An unfortunate example of the real risk that some right ventricular infarctions confer

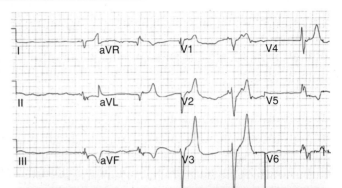

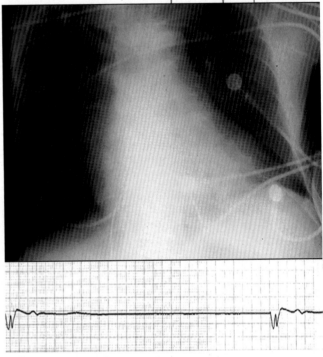

Figure 6-20. TOP, ECG shows complete heart block with an irregular wide complex ventricular rhythm. There is no pacemaker capture due to right ventricular infarction. MIDDLE, Chest radiograph shows normal-sized cardiopericardial silhouette, no pulmonary edema. BOTTOM, ECG on arrival shows asystole with ventricular escape beats.

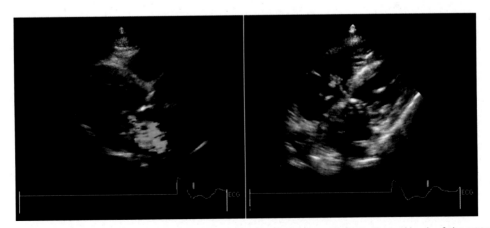

Figure 6-21. Transthoracic echocardiography. LEFT IMAGE, Parasternal long-axis view. Contracting anterior septum, akinesis of the posterior wall. Prominent jet of mitral regurgitation. RIGHT IMAGE, Subcostal view (right ventricle free wall akinesis). Right ventricular and atrial dilation and tricuspid insufficiency.

CASE 3

History

- 79-year-old man collapsed at home
- Recent prolonged air travel
- Various chest pains the day before

Physical Examination

- Awake, intubated, very weak, cool extremities
- BP 80/50 mm Hg, HR 110 bpm, tachypneic
- Venous distention to the angle of the jaw, S_3
- No murmurs or rubs
- CK 500
- Oliguric

Clinical Impression

- Although there was a high index of suspicion of pulmonary embolism, CT scanning was normal, as were leg Doppler studies.
- The patient was ventilated for airway management.
- Transesophageal echocardiography was performed because transthoracic images were poor.

Management

- Avoidance of preload reduction
- With pulmonary artery catheter guidance, the CVP was kept at 15 to 18 mm Hg.
- Dobutamine was given to increase cardiac output.
- Hemodynamics were acceptable with this regimen, and his hemodynamics spontaneously normalized on day 5.

Outcome

- Discharged angina and heart failure free

Comments

- Initial confusion over the cause of the right heart failure
- Large submassive right ventricular infarction
- Late presentation
- Volume optimizing and inotropes corrected the hypotension and low output.
- Spontaneous recovery
- Postdischarge echo showed normalized right ventricular systolic function.

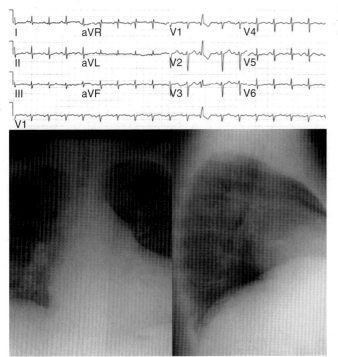

Figure 6-22. TOP, ECG shows sinus tachycardia with one premature ventricular contraction and nonspecific repolarization abnormalities. BOTTOM, Chest radiograph shows cardiomegaly and mild pulmonary edema.

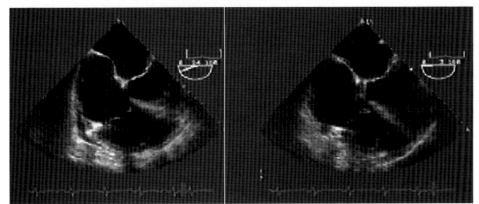

Figure 6-23. Transesophageal echocardiography images show marked right atrial and right ventricular dilation. The left-sided heart chambers are small because of underloading. Interatrial septal bulging to the left side suggests that right atrial pressure is greater than left atrial pressure. The right ventricular free wall is severely hypokinetic or akinetic, despite inotropic support. There is no pericardial effusion.

CASE 4

History

- 54-year-old man developed indigestion at 5 PM
- At 7 PM, experienced a cardiac arrest on the street
- 20 minutes of bystander CPR, defibrillation by EMS

Physical Examination

- Deeply comatose, basal skull laceration
- BP 80/50 mm Hg, HR 100 bpm, ventilated
- Marked venous distention
- S_1, S_2 normal
- S_4
- No murmurs or rubs

Impression and Evolution

- Although there was a high index of suspicion of pulmonary embolism, CT scanning and leg Doppler studies were normal.
- The patient was ventilated for airway management.
- Transesophageal echocardiography was performed because transthoracic images were poor.

Management

- Avoidance of preload reduction
- With pulmonary artery catheter guidance, the CVP was kept at 15 to 18 mm Hg.

- Dobutamine was given to increase cardiac output.
- Hemodynamics were acceptable with this regimen, and his hemodynamics spontaneously normalized on day 5.

Outcome

- Arrived in shock, remained in shock
- After 5 days, hemodynamic therapy was no longer needed, but ventilatory support was continued because of persistent neurologic impairment.
- Eventually (60 days later), he died of sepsis while still on a ventilator.

Comments

- Large right ventricular infarction complicating inferior STEMI
- Initial hypotension due to right ventricular myocardial infarction and recent cardiac arrest
- Hemodynamic resuscitation was straightforward.
- Clinical outcome was determined by neurologic sequelae of the out-of-hospital cardiac arrest, not cardiac performance.

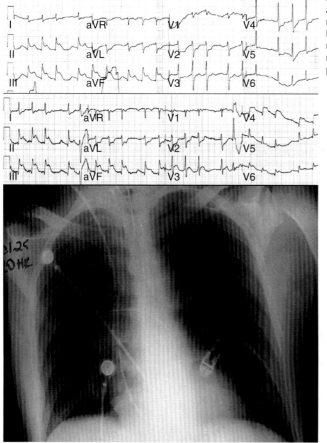

Figure 6-24. TOP, ECG shows atrial fibrillation, inferior ST elevation (II, II, aVF), and septal and lateral ST depression, suggesting acute inferior myocardial infarction with septal ischemia or "reciprocal" pattern. MIDDLE, Right-sided ECG shows atrial fibrillation with inferior ST elevation. There is more than 1 mm of ST elevation in V_4R. BOTTOM, Chest radiograph shows normal cardiopericardial silhouette and clear lung fields. There is no pulmonary edema because of the underloading of the left side of the heart.

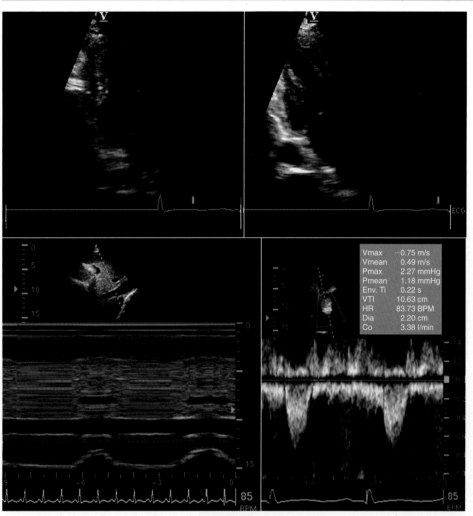

Figure 6-25. Transthoracic echocardiography. TOP ROW, Apical 3-chamber views in systole (LEFT) and diastole (RIGHT). There is dyskinesis of the basal inferior wall. The two bodies of the posterior papillary muscle are intact. BOTTOM LEFT, Subcostal M-mode study of the inferior vena cava. Caval (inferior vena cava) dilation without respiratory collapse = elevated central venous pressure. BOTTOM RIGHT, Left ventricular outflow tract pulsed wave Doppler sampling: reduced VTI (10.6 cm; normal, 18 to 22 cm) consistent with severely reduced stroke volume.

Vmax	−0.75 m/s
Vmean	0.49 m/s
Pmax	2.27 mmHg
Pmean	1.18 mmHg
Env. Ti	0.22 s
VTI	10.63 cm
HR	83.73 BPM
Dia	2.20 cm
Co	3.38 l/min

CASE 5

History

▸ 62-year-old man presented to a community hospital with 9 hours of chest pain
▸ Received tPA at hour 10, but pain continues, as do ST elevations

Physical Examination

▸ Ventilated, BP 85/50 mm Hg, HR 110 bpm
▸ Prominent venous distention
▸ S_1, S_2 normal
▸ No gallops, rubs, or murmurs
▸ Chest clear

Impression and Evolution

▸ Inferior myocardial infarction with large right ventricular myocardial infarction
▸ Hypoxemia due to large amount of shunting through a patent foramen ovale (PFO)

▸ The ventilator time became protracted because of persistent elevation of the CVP (18 mm Hg) and shunting through the PFO. Maintenance of adequate oxygenation was difficult.
▸ There was no significant left ventricular failure (PCWP 13 mm Hg).
▸ PFO closure with a device was considered, but first it was thought worth exploring whether occlusion of the PFO would really increase the oxygenation.

Comments

▸ Right ventricular infarction complicating inferior STEMI
▸ Right-to-left shunting through a PFO contributing to arterial hypoxemia
▸ Consideration of percutaneous closure of the PFO was given because the time course on the ventilator was becoming prolonged, but fevers precluded.
▸ Eventual recovery of right ventricular systolic function; concurrent with this was recovery of diastolic function as seen by spontaneous closure of the PFO and hypoxemia resolving.
▸ Postdischarge echo showed only mild left ventricular and right ventricular systolic function.

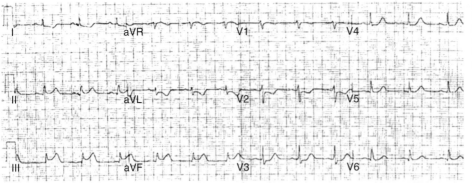

Figure 6-26. ECG shows sinus rhythm, ST elevation in II and aVF consistent with acute inferior infarction, and ST depression in V₂ and early R-wave transition, suggestive of acute infarction of the contiguous posterior wall.

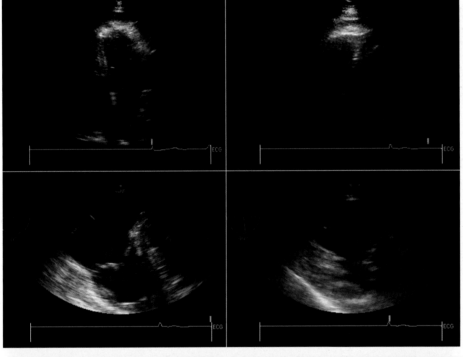

Figure 6-27. TOP IMAGES, Transthoracic echocardiography. BOTTOM IMAGES, Transesophageal echocardiography. TOP LEFT, The left ventricle on this plane appears normal. TOP RIGHT, The right ventricle is substantially dilated and "sphericalized." BOTTOM LEFT, The right atrium is prominently dilated, as is the coronary sinus, because of the elevation of the right atrial pressure. BOTTOM RIGHT, The anterolateral papillary muscle is intact.

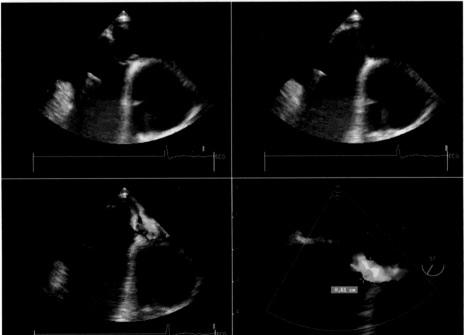

Figure 6-28. Transesophageal echocardiography. TOP LEFT, The interatrial septum is mobile, and there is flow across it because of the elevation of the right atrial pressure, above that of the left atrial pressure, and the presence of a patent foramen ovale. TOP RIGHT, A catheter is being advanced across the interatrial septum. BOTTOM LEFT, A wire has been advanced across the interatrial septum. BOTTOM RIGHT, A balloon has been inflated across the interatrial septum, resulting in prominent reverberations.

6

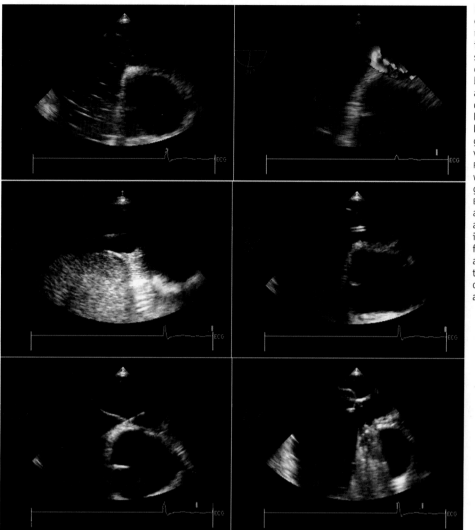

Figure 6-29. Transesophageal echocardiography. TOP LEFT, View of the right and left atria. The interatrial septum is revealing a patent foramen ovale. A saline injection has resulted in marginal contrast effect in the right atrium. Two bubbles have crossed the PFO into the left atrium. TOP RIGHT, Color flow mapping depicts the right-to-left flow at the atrial level. MIDDLE LEFT, Inferior vena cava in long axis as it enters the right atrium. A guide wire is seen extending to the inferior vena cava : right atrial junction. MIDDLE RIGHT, A catheter (note the near and far wall echoes) has been advanced over the guide wire and has just traversed the PFO. BOTTOM LEFT, The guide wire has been advanced through the PFO into the left atrium. BOTTOM RIGHT, A balloon has been inflated within the left atrium and has filled the PFO. There are near and far wall artifacts from the balloon. With inflation of the balloon within the left atrium and occlusion of the PFO by the balloon, the arterial oxygenation increased.

References

1. Sanders AO: Coronary thrombosis with complete heart-block and relative ventricular tachycardia: a case report. Am Heart J 1930;6:820-823.

2. Kinch JW, Ryan TJ: Right ventricular infarction. N Engl J Med 1994;330: 1211-1217.

3. Bowers TR, O'Neill WW, Grines C, et al: Effect of reperfusion on biventricular function and survival after right ventricular infarction. N Engl J Med 1998;338:933-940.

4. López-Sendón J, López de Sá E, Roldán I, et al: Inversion of the normal interatrial septum convexity in acute myocardial infarction: incidence, clinical relevance and prognostic significance. J Am Coll Cardiol 1990;15: 801-805.

5. Mehta SR, Eikelboom JW, Natarajan MK, et al: Impact of right ventricular involvement on mortality and morbidity in patients with inferior myocardial infarction. J Am Coll Cardiol 2001;37:37-43.

6. Hochman JS, Buller CE, Sleeper LA, et al: Cardiogenic shock complicating acute myocardial infarction—etiologies, management and outcome: a report from the SHOCK Trial Registry. SHould we emergently revascularize Occluded Coronaries for cardiogenic shocK? J Am Coll Cardiol 2000;36(Suppl A):1063-1070.

7. Jacobs AK, Leopold JA, Bates E, et al: Cardiogenic shock caused by right ventricular infarction: a report from the SHOCK registry. J Am Coll Cardiol 2003;41:1273-1279.

8. Shiraki H, Yoshikawa T, Anzai T, et al: Association between preinfarction angina and a lower risk of right ventricular infarction. N Engl J Med 1998; 338:941-947.

9. Isner JM, Roberts WC: Right ventricular infarction complicating left ventricular infarction secondary to coronary heart disease. Frequency, location, associated findings and significance from analysis of 236 necropsy patients with acute or healed myocardial infarction. Am J Cardiol 1978; 42:885-894.

10. Ratliff NB, Hackel DB: Combined right and left ventricular infarction: pathogenesis and clinicopathologic correlations. Am J Cardiol 1980;45:217-221.

11. Tahirkheli NK, Edwards WD, Nishimura RA, Holmes DR Jr: Right ventricular infarction associated with anteroseptal myocardial infarction: a clinicopathologic study of nine cases. Cardiovasc Pathol 2000;9:175-179.

12. Goldstein JA: Pathophysiology and management of right heart ischemia. J Am Coll Cardiol 2002;40:841-853.

13. Goldstein JA, Vlahakes GJ, Verrier ED, et al: The role of right ventricular systolic dysfunction and elevated intrapericardial pressure in the genesis of low output in experimental right ventricular infarction. Circulation 1982;65:513-522.

14. Goldstein JA, Tweddell JS, Barzilai B, et al: Right atrial ischemia exacerbates hemodynamic compromise associated with experimental right ventricular dysfunction. J Am Coll Cardiol 1991;18:1564-1572.

15. Dell'Italia LJ, Starling MR, O'Rourke RA: Physical examination for exclusion of hemodynamically important right ventricular infarction. Ann Intern Med 1983;99:608-611.

16. Erhardt LR, Sjogren A, Wahlberg I: Single right-sided precordial lead in the diagnosis of right ventricular involvement in inferior myocardial infarction. Am Heart J 1976;91:571-576.

17. Logeart D, Himbert D, Cohen-Solal A: ST-segment elevation in precordial leads: anterior or right ventricular myocardial infarction? Chest 2001;119: 290-292.

18. Saw J, Davies C, Fung A, et al: Value of ST elevation in lead III greater than lead II in inferior wall acute myocardial infarction for predicting in-hospital mortality and diagnosing right ventricular infarction. Am J Cardiol 2001;87:448-450, A6.

19. Sugiura T, Iwasaka T, Takahashi N, et al: Atrial fibrillation in inferior wall Q-wave acute myocardial infarction. Am J Cardiol 1991;67:1135-1136.

20. Berger PB, Ryan TJ: Inferior myocardial infarction. High-risk subgroups. Circulation 1990;81:401-411.

21. Braat SH, de Zwaan C, Brugada P, et al: Right ventricular involvement with acute inferior wall myocardial infarction identifies high risk of developing atrioventricular nodal conduction disturbances. Am Heart J 1984;107: 1183-1187.

22. López-Sendón J, Garcia-Fernandez MA, Coma-Canella I, et al: Segmental right ventricular function after acute myocardial infarction: two-dimensional echocardiographic study in 63 patients. Am J Cardiol 1983;51: 390-396.

23. Bellamy GR, Rasmussen HH, Nasser FN, et al: Value of two-dimensional echocardiography, electrocardiography, and clinical signs in detecting right ventricular infarction. Am Heart J 1986;112:304-309.

24. López-Sendón J, Gonzalez Garcia A, Sotillo Marti J, Roldán I: Complete pulmonic valve opening during atrial contraction after right ventricular infarction. Am J Cardiol 1985;56:486-487.

25. Come PC: Transient right atrial thrombus during acute myocardial infarction: diagnosis by echocardiography. Am J Cardiol 1983;51:1228-1229.

26. Kumar A, Abdel-Aty H, Kriedemann I, et al: Contrast-enhanced cardiovascular magnetic resonance imaging of right ventricular infarction. J Am Coll Cardiol 2006;48:1969-1976.

27. Shah PK, Maddahi J, Berman DS, et al: Scintigraphically detected predominant right ventricular dysfunction in acute myocardial infarction: clinical and hemodynamic correlates and implications for therapy and prognosis. J Am Coll Cardiol 1985;6:1264-1272.

28. Goldstein JA, Vlahakes GJ, Verrier ED, et al: Volume loading improves low cardiac output in experimental right ventricular infarction. J Am Coll Cardiol 1983;2:270-278.

29. Johnston WE, Lin CY, Feerick AE, et al: Volume expansion increases right ventricular infarct size in dogs by reducing collateral perfusion. Chest 1996;109:494-503.

30. Ferrario M, Poli A, Previtali M, et al: Hemodynamics of volume loading compared with dobutamine in severe right ventricular infarction. Am J Cardiol 1994;74:329-333.

31. Inglessis I, Shin JT, Lepore JJ, et al: Hemodynamic effects of inhaled nitric oxide in right ventricular myocardial infarction and cardiogenic shock. J Am Coll Cardiol 2004;44:793-798.

32. Topol EJ, Goldschlager N, Ports TA, et al: Hemodynamic benefit of atrial pacing in right ventricular myocardial infarction. Ann Intern Med 1982;96: 594-597.

33. Kinn JW, Ajluni SC, Samyn JG, et al: Rapid hemodynamic improvement after reperfusion during right ventricular infarction. J Am Coll Cardiol 1995;26:1230-1234.

34. Schuler G, Hofmann M, Schwarz F, et al: Effect of successful thrombolytic therapy on right ventricular function in acute inferior wall myocardial infarction. Am J Cardiol 1984;54:951-957.

35. Chatterjee K: Pathogenesis of low output in right ventricular myocardial infarction. Chest 1992;102(Suppl 2):590S-595S.

36. Zehender M, Kasper W, Kauder E, et al: Right ventricular infarction as an independent predictor of prognosis after acute inferior myocardial infarction. N Engl J Med 1993;328:981-988.

37. Zornoff LA, Skali H, Pfeffer MA, et al: Right ventricular dysfunction and risk of heart failure and mortality after myocardial infarction. J Am Coll Cardiol 2002;39:1450-1455.

Acute and Subacute Free Wall Rupture

Of the different forms of postinfarction myocardial rupture, rupture through a free wall is the most calamitous and unfortunately also the most common form of myocardial rupture (2 to 9 times as common as septal rupture).[1] Free wall rupture occurs as an acute massive and usually immediately definitive event, or it may stutter for a period lasting days with a subacute course. Most patients with free wall rupture will succumb, but a few will survive by undergoing surgical repair, which was first performed successfully in 1970 by Hatcher.

The incidence of postinfarction free wall rupture is approximately 3% to 4%, accounting for 10% to 20% of deaths from ST elevation myocardial infarction (STEMI). Approximately 25,000 cases of free wall rupture per year occur in the United States. Free wall rupture usually occurs as a solitary lesion or event; but in a few percent of cases, it may be associated with other forms of postinfarction rupture, such as ventricular septal defect or papillary muscle rupture.[1,2]

Postinfarction myocardial rupture occurs before the necrotic myocardium has fibrosed and is therefore an early postinfarction occurrence (Fig. 7-1).

Acute free wall rupture results in sudden, generally unsuspected, catastrophic and almost always fatal tamponade from which only a few cases can be salvaged. Two thirds of patients with acute free wall rupture die in minutes and only one third survive a matter of hours, leaving little time to salvage most cases. The presentations of acute free wall rupture are chest pain, acute severe tamponade, electromechanical dissociation, and sudden death.

The subset of *subacute* free wall rupture experiences premonitory symptoms and has a higher salvage rate; the majority die in days, not minutes or hours. There usually are premonitory symptoms that may arouse alert. The median time until death in subacute free wall cases is 4 days; 87% of patients die within the first week.[3] A rupture may occur with a subacute course because thrombus partially "plugs" the tear, a serpiginous tear does not allow free flow through the tear, a false aneurysm restrains the rupture transiently, or intrapericardial pressure equilibrates with left ventricular pressure, stopping leakage. Presentations of subacute postinfarction rupture include nausea, vomiting, unexplained nonischemic pains, pericarditis, abnormal postinfarction repolarization patterns, unexpected finding on imaging, tamponade, and electromechanical dissociation. Maintenance of an index of suspicion and evaluation of atypical postinfarction symptoms as potentially being due to subacute rupture will enable salvage of some cases.[4]

The location of free wall rupture is usually the mid left ventricle along the anterolateral or posterolateral wall; but it may be elsewhere over the left ventricular free wall or, on occasion, the right ventricle or an atrium (Table 7-1). The majority of free wall rupture cases have underlying single- or two-vessel coronary artery disease (Table 7-2), but angiographic three-vessel coronary artery disease is present in about 25% of cases.

Clinical risk factors for free wall rupture are similar to those for septal rupture: female patient, older, first infarction.[1,10,11] Lack of prior chronic coronary artery disease facilitates transmural infarction through lack of collaterals. Absence of prior

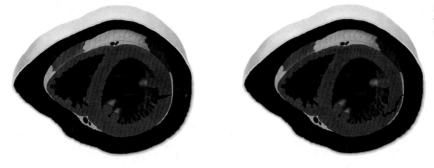

Figure 7-1. Rupture of the free wall may occur through a straight rent (LEFT), through necrotic myocardium, or through a serpiginous tear (RIGHT).

Table 7-1. Sites of Postinfarction Rupture in 70 Patients[5]

Base-Apex Location		Segmental Location		Infarct-Related Artery	
Basal	14%	Anterior	36%	LAD	42%
Middle	76%	Lateral	38%	Circumflex	35%
Apical	10%	Inferior	26%	RCA	23%

LAD, left anterior descending coronary artery; RCA, right coronary artery.

infarction confers high residual left ventricular systolic function after acute infarction—sufficient to generate the physical forces necessary to rupture the infarcted segment. Hypertension, concurrent aortic stenosis, undue physical activity early after infarction, and straining all increase intracavitary pressure and the chance of rupture.[8]

Undue effort before rupture has been noted in 26% of cases of myocardial rupture (agitation, repeated vomiting, protracted coughing requiring specific medications): 33% of free wall rupture, 18% of ventricular septal rupture, and 30% of papillary muscle rupture.[8] Similar observations of higher than expected rupture rates have been made in psychiatric patients, in whom usual postinfarction bed rest was infrequently achieved.

It has not been conclusively proved, but beta-blocker use appears to reduce myocardial rupture after STEMI (Table 7-3).[12]

The effect of reperfusion on myocardial rupture is complex and appears to depend on the timing of reperfusion and the type of reperfusion treatment (fibrinolytic use or percutaneous coronary intervention [PCI]), resulting in a bidirectional effect of reperfusion and fibrinolytics on myocardial rupture according to time of administration. Unsuccessful or late reperfusion appears to lead to transmural infarction and necrosis.[1] Hemorrhagic conversion of a late infarction may lead to hemorrhagic dissection of the infarct segment and to rupture.[13] Fibrinolytic administration within the first 7 hours probably reduces the risk of rupture (22% versus 46%, TIMI data). Fibrinolytic administration past the 7-hour mark probably increases the risk of rupture (Fig. 7-2; Table 7-4).[13] Because of bidirectional effects, overall, fibrinolytics do not influence the rate of rupture, but they may influence the timing of rupture, rendering it earlier.[14] Although there is an overall clinical benefit to administration of fibrinolytics, they appear to increase the risk of myocardial rupture in the first 48 hours (Fig. 7-3).[15]

Primary angioplasty (versus fibrinolytic use) may be associated with less septal rupture and myocardial rupture. If this is true, it is another implication that myocardial hemorrhage from fibrinolytics is deleterious.[10,16,17]

In a series of 1247 patients (33 subacute free wall ruptures, 1214 without), there was significantly more syncope, recurrent chest pain, tamponade, effusion, intrapericardial echoes, right atrial collapse, right ventricular collapse, and hemopericardium on pericardiocentesis.[18]

A review of the clinical courses of 70 cases of postinfarction myocardial rupture versus 100 nonrupture transmural infarction cases observed that free wall rupture is often clinically unsuspected but, pathologically, appears stuttering (Figs. 7-4, 7-5, 7-6).[5] It was noted that 80% of rupture cases had two or more of the following: pericarditis, repetitive emesis, restlessness, agitation; whereas only 3% of nonrupture cases did (P < .002). Deviation from expected T-wave pattern was seen in 94% of rupture cases and 34% of controls (Table 7-5). The usual site of rupture in this series was the mid lateral wall, following left circumflex artery occlusion and inferoposterolateral infarction; 21% of ruptures had an initial hypotensive or bradycardic episode before arrest (Table 7-6).[5]

Free wall rupture is a challenging clinical diagnosis based on (1) a plausible (postinfarction) clinical scenario establishing a pretest probability and (2) test results indicating the presence of a significant effusion with compressive or tamponade-like physiology and some evidence that the effusion is blood or blood clot. Echocardiography is a helpful test but is only one aspect of building the overall clinical case of free wall rupture. The combination of a pericardial effusion of more than 5 mm, hypotension, and central venous pressure above 10 mm Hg after infarction has been suggested as highly specific (>99%) for free wall rupture.[18] The utility of echocardiography is to identify a large (>5 mm thick) effusion (the mean thickness in one series was 24 mm)[19] that is usually circumferential but may be localized, to identify signs of chamber collapse to support compressive physiology, and to enable detection of intrapericardial echoes that are consistent with intrapericardial blood or clot.[19] Although imaging of the rupture tract is possible, particularly by transesophageal echocardiography,[20,21] it is difficult to achieve, but imaging of some forms of disruption of the myocardium is useful and more possible. Flow out of a cardiac chamber through a disruption into the pericardium is not likely to be imaged or still ongoing,[21] and even if it is found, it will be short-lived, as will be the patient.[20]

The management of free wall rupture is to obtain emergent surgical inspection and repair[18] (patch repair ± "glue," ± cardiopulmonary bypass, ± aortocoronary bypass)[3] in reasonable candidates. Hence, consideration of a probable diagnosis of postinfarction rupture entails a surgical decision.[18,22]

Table 7-2. Angiographic Findings in Postinfarction Rupture

Angiographic Disease	Septal Rupture			Papillary Muscle Rupture		Postinfarction MR, No Papillary Muscle Rupture	Free Wall Rupture
Reference	6	7	8	7	8	9	8
Single-vessel	50%	36%	57%	30%	46%	16%	58%
Two-vessel	40%	27%	33%	35%	29%	24%	38%
Three-vessel	11%	36%	10%	35%	25%	60%	4%

MR, mitral regurgitation.

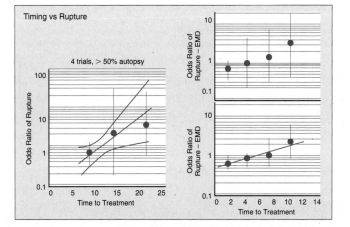

Figure 7-2. Among four fibrinolytic trials, an influence of timing of administration of fibrinolytic on myocardial rupture and electromechanical dissociation (EMD) was seen. (From Honan MB, Harrell FE Jr, Reimer KA, et al: Cardiac rupture, mortality and the timing of thrombolytic therapy: a meta-analysis. J Am Coll Cardiol 1990;16:359-367.)

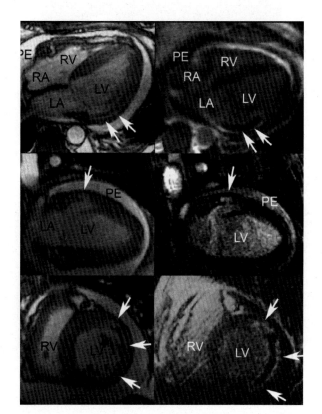

Figure 7-4. Cardiovascular MR in a patient with left ventricular free wall rupture. LEFT COLUMN, Systolic cine images. RIGHT COLUMN, Myocardial late gadolinium enhancement images. (From Shiozaki AA, Filho RA, Dallan LA, et al: Left ventricular free-wall rupture after acute myocardial infarction imaged by cardiovascular magnetic resonance. J Cardiovasc Magn Reson 2007;9:719-721, with permission.)

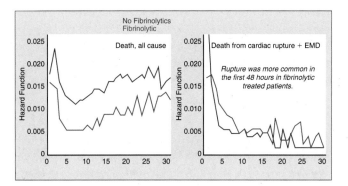

Figure 7-3. Fibrinolytics increase the risk of rupture in the first 48 hours; but overall, there are clinical benefits to their use. In the National Registry of Myocardial Infarction, 350,755 patients were analyzed by multivariate analysis. Use of fibrinolytics, female gender, hypertension, and intravenous beta-blocker use were associated with rupture. EMD, electromechanical dissociation. (From Becker RC, Gore JM, Lambrew C, et al: A composite view of cardiac rupture in the United States National Registry of Myocardial Infarction. J Am Coll Cardiol 1996;27:1321-1326, with permission from Elsevier.)

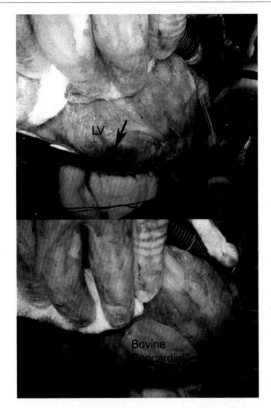

Figure 7-5. Surgical views. TOP, The location of the ventricular wall rupture. BOTTOM, Surgical repair with a bovine pericardial patch. (From Shiozaki AA, Filho RA, Dallan LA, et al: Left ventricular free-wall rupture after acute myocardial infarction imaged by cardiovascular magnetic resonance. J Cardiovasc Magn Reson 2007;9:719-721, with permission.)

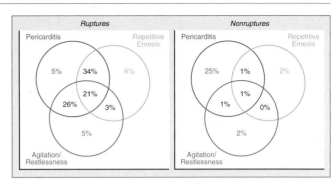

Figure 7-6. Postinfarction myocardial rupture cases commonly experience pericarditis, repetitive emesis, or agitation or restlessness. One fifth experience all three symptoms. One quarter of non–myocardial rupture infarction cases experience pericarditis, but only a few experience repetitive emesis or agitation or restlessness. Almost none (1%) experience all three symptoms. (From Oliva PB, Hammill SC, Edwards WD: Cardiac rupture, a clinically predictable complication of acute myocardial infarction: report of 70 cases with clinicopathologic correlations. J Am Coll Cardiol 1993;22:720-726.)

Table 7-3. Effect of Beta-Blocker Use on Myocardial Rupture After STEMI

Cause of Death	Atenolol	Control
Cardiac rupture (confirmed at autopsy)	5	17
Electromechanical dissociation	15	37
Ventricular fibrillation	5	13
Bradycardia or asystole	10	3

STEMI, ST elevation myocardial infarction.

Table 7-4. Rupture by Timing of Fibrinolytic Administration[13]

Study	Agent	Mean Time to Treatment (hours)	Odds Ratio
European Cooperative Study Group (ECSG)	SK	9	0.63
European Working Party (EWP)	SK	9	0.67
Heikinheimo	SK	14	2.4
Amery	SK	21	3.8

SK, streptokinase.

Table 7-5. Clinical Features of Postinfarction Myocardial Rupture

	Sensitivity	Specificity	PPV
Pericarditis	86%	72%	68%
Repetitive emesis	64%	95%	90%
Restlessness, agitation	55%	95%	86%
≥2 symptoms	84%	97%	95%
ST deviation	61%	72%	58%
T-wave deviations	94%	66%	66%
ST-T wave deviations	61%	68%	64%

PPV, positive predictive value.
From Oliva PB, Hammill SC, Edwards WD: Cardiac rupture, a clinically predictable complication of acute myocardial infarction: report of 70 cases with clinicopathologic correlations. J Am Coll Cardiol 1993;22:720-726.

Table 7-6. Predictors of Cardiac Rupture[17]

Variable	OR	CI	P Value
Age (years)	1.68*	1.26-2.28	.0006
Female	2.13	1.14-4.02	.02
Killip > I	2.42	1.25-4.72	.009
Thrombolytic	3.32	1.75-6.54	.0003
Heart rate > 100 bpm	1.19†	1.04-1.35	.009
Systolic blood pressure < 100 mm Hg	1.83‡	0.74-0.93	.001

*OR for an increase of 10 years.
†OR for an increase of 10 beats.
‡OR for a decrease of 10 mm Hg.
CI, confidence interval; OR, odds ratio.

Supportive measures (ventilation, volume loading or inotropes, intra-aortic balloon counterpulsation [IABP][23]) are to be undertaken while definitive surgical repair is arranged. The performance of pericardiocentesis is controversial because it is not a definitive treatment and its effect may be unpredictable and is often unsuccessful. Pericardiocentesis with autotransfusion has been successful.[24] A tap may be useful to establish the presence of hemopericardium supportive of diagnosis of rupture, and drainage may improve hemodynamics; but drainage may also worsen hemodynamics (by reducing intrapericardial pressure, leading to complete blowout of the rupture), and ongoing drainage will lead to further blood loss, causing hypovolemic shock. Also, if the blood within the pericardial space has begun to clot, it cannot be evacuated by a needle.

DIAGNOSIS OF FREE WALL RUPTURE

- Surgical inspection is definitive.[25]
- Clinical probable diagnosis can be made on the basis of the following:
  - Background of recent transmural infarction, often with prodromal features (subacute cases mainly)
  - Evidence of cardiac compression (usually severe), including hypotension, venous distention, and pulseless electrical activity (PEA)
  - Evidence of blood in the pericardial space. On echocardiography, pericardial blood appears as fine specular echoes within fluid or fine specular echoes within gelatinous material; also, pericardial tap will return blood.
  - Some imaging evidence of disruption of the myocardium is reassuring toward the diagnosis. However, a straight-through rupture will not readily reveal endocardial or myocardial disruption.

Acute free wall rupture cases can be successfully salvaged with surgical repair, with good long-term results.[3,4,19,26] Subacute rupture cases have better surgical salvage rates because they are less likely to be in shock and also have good long-term results.[18]

Somewhat surprisingly, about one third of patients with subacute rupture will survive for months or years without surgical repair. An important series of 81 consecutive subacute rupture cases after a first transmural myocardial infarction that presented with hypotension (tamponade) or electromechanical dissociation observed 47 deaths within 2 hours, with 15 patients undergoing surgery and 2 surviving, leaving 19 patients (10 electromechanical dissociation, 9 tamponade) resuscitated by fluid and inotropes; 15 patients underwent pericardiocentesis. All were managed with bed rest, blood pressure control, and beta-blockers. Four patients died, and 13 patients survived a mean of 52 ± 35 months.[19]

CASE 1

History

- 73-year-old man presented with inferior STEMI 5 days before and received fibrinolytic therapy at hour 5
- Recurrent pains of several qualities
- Past medical history is significant for hypertension and type 2 diabetes.

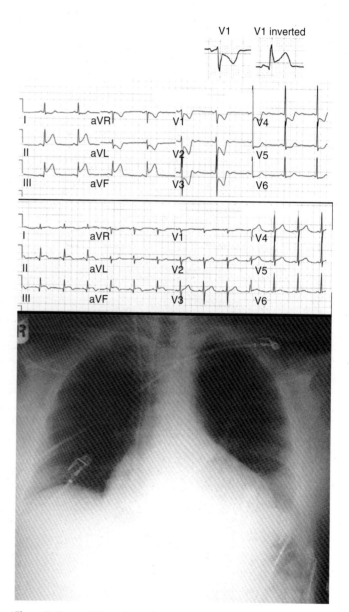

Figure 7-7. TOP, ECG on day 1 shows sinus rhythm, inferior (II, II aVF) ST elevation, inferior Q waves, T-wave inversions, and ST depression V_1-V_4: reciprocal versus posterior myocardial infarction, indicative of acute inferior infarction ± posterior infarction. MIDDLE, ECG on day 2 shows sinus tachycardia, inferior Q waves and ST elevation, early precordial R-wave transition ("posterior" Q waves?), ST elevation also in V_5-V_6, suggesting possible infarction or pericarditis. BOTTOM, Chest radiograph shows normal cardiopericardial silhouette and no signs of pulmonary edema.

Physical Examination

▸ BP 150/60 mm Hg, HR 75 bpm, RR 12/min
▸ Good color, extremities warm, alert
▸ No jugular venous distention, no edema
▸ S_1, S_2 normal; S_4 present
▸ Initially, no rubs or murmurs. Pericardial rub developed on day 3 and subsided on day 4.
▸ CK 2690

Evolution and Outcome

▸ During the resuscitation, hanging fluids off the ceiling was the only means to overcome the elevated pericardial pressure and to infuse the fluid.

▸ The resuscitation was initially unusually successful but was not enduring enough to get the patient to surgery, and he died.

Comments

▸ Variable chest pains before rupture were probably herald pains before the complete rupture.
▸ The anterior pericardial fluid and small posterior clot (near the inferoposterior infarction) were the key signs.

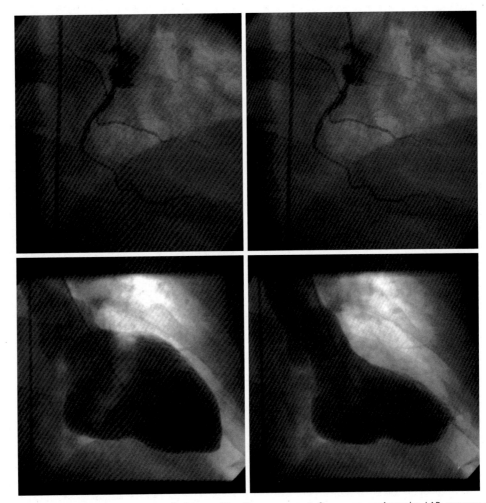

Figure 7-8. TOP LEFT, Right coronary angiography shows occlusion at midportion. TOP RIGHT, Left coronary angiography. LAD coronary artery: 70% and 80% stenoses. LCx: 70% OM1 stenosis. BOTTOM, Contrast ventriculography (RAO): diastole (LEFT), systole (RIGHT). There is akinesis of the inferior wall, with some aneurysmal (wide neck and base) development at the basal portion.

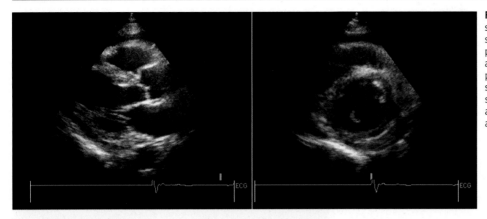

Figure 7-9. LEFT, Parasternal long-axis view shows normal RVOT and normal anterior septal contraction as well as basal posterior dyskinesis and mid posterior akinesis, suggesting possible anterior pericardial effusion. RIGHT, Parasternal short-axis view shows normal anterior septal contraction and basal inferior septal and inferior dyskinesis, suggesting possible anterior pericardial effusion.

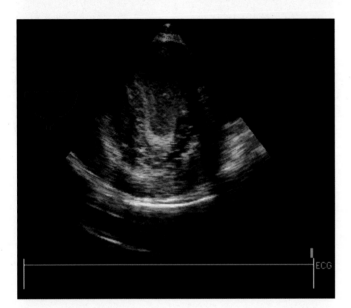

Figure 7-10. Echocardiogram shows normal anterior septal contraction as well as basal inferior septal and inferior dyskinesis, suggesting possible anterior pericardial effusion.

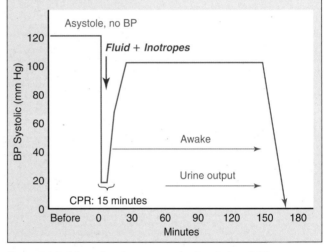
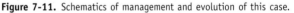

Figure 7-11. Schematics of management and evolution of this case.

CASE 2

History

▶ 86-year-old woman, frail
▶ Late-presentation inferior STEMI (8 hours), but received fibrinolytic at hour 9 because of ongoing pain
▶ No heart failure symptoms
▶ Past medical history is significant for hypertension, type 2 diabetes, and chronic renal insufficiency.

Physical Examination

▶ BP 85/50 mm Hg, HR 55 bpm, RR 13/min
▶ Venous distention and Kussmaul sign
▶ S_1, S_2 normal
▶ 2/6 pansystolic murmur at the LLSB, S_3 at LLSB
▶ No pericardial rub

Clinical Impression and Evolution

▶ Inferolateral myocardial infarction with right ventricle involvement (elevated neck veins) and tricuspid regurgitation (pansystolic murmur at the LLSB)

▶ Well for 2 days
▶ Developed recurrent chest pains of typical ischemic quality, without ECG changes
▶ Coronary angiography arranged

Evolution

▶ More pains developed, with increasingly atypical components, but with some typical ones
▶ Prolonged minor pains without ECG changes, nitroglycerin relief, or pericardial rub
▶ One episode of vomiting

Impression, Management, and Outcome

▶ Inferior infarction complicated by right ventricular infarction
▶ Probable subacute rupture (from the infarcted left ventricle or right ventricle)
▶ 30 minutes after echocardiography was performed, the patient experienced cardiovascular collapse (PEA). Volume resuscitation, inotropes, and pericardiocentesis achieved 20 minutes of partial recovery, before recurrent and refractory PEA. Surgical exploration

was considered, but given the cardiac arrest status and advanced age, it was declined.
▸ Death

Comments

▸ Herald symptoms before complete rupture
▸ Evanescent success with volume and inotropes
▸ Either the left ventricle or the right ventricle may have been the site of rupture.
▸ The right ventricular infarction and elevated right-sided pressures altered the findings of tamponade (in this patient, the left ventricle and left atrium collapsed more than the right ventricle and right atrium).

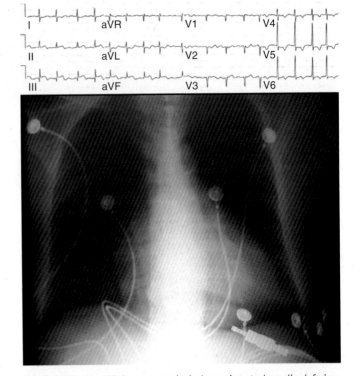

Figure 7-12. TOP, ECG (at presentation) shows sinus tachycardia, inferior (II, II, aVF) ST elevation suggesting acute inferior infarction, and nonspecific anterolateral repolarization abnormalities. BOTTOM, Chest radiograph shows normal cardiopericardial silhouette, no signs of pulmonary edema, and marked intimal calcification of the aortic arch.

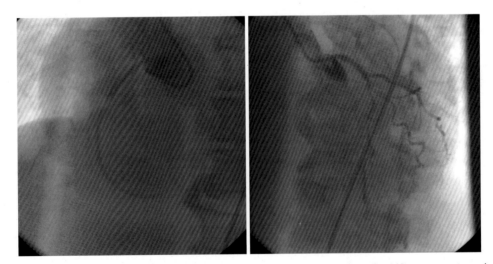

Figure 7-13. LEFT, Right coronary angiography. RCA: 90% proximal stenosis. RIGHT, Left coronary angiography. LAD coronary artery: significant disease. LCx: 80% OM1 stenosis.

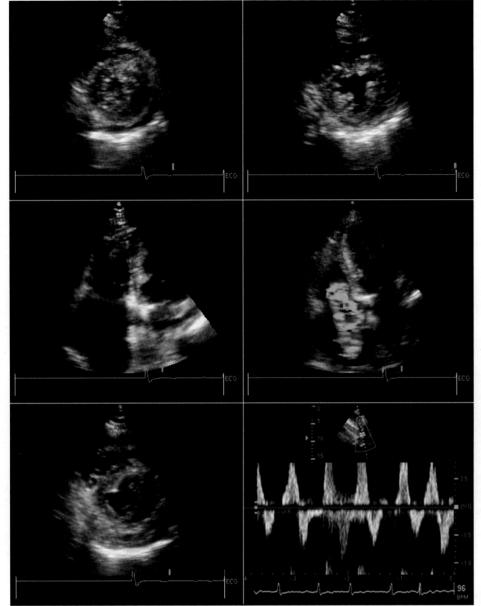

Figure 7-14. Transthoracic echocardiography. TOP ROW, Parasternal short-axis views in systole (LEFT) and diastole (RIGHT). There is diastolic septal flattening and a small pericardial effusion. MIDDLE ROW, Apical 4-chamber views. The right ventricle is dilated, as is the right atrium. There is severe tricuspid regurgitation. BOTTOM LEFT, There is material within the pericardial space posterior to the LV that has a specular appearance. BOTTOM RIGHT, Spectral display of hepatic venous flow. Severe tricuspid regurgitation: systolic flow reversal (up) in the superior hepatic veins. The severe tricuspid regurgitation may be opposing right heart compression signs from the effusion.

CASE 3

History

▸ 75-year-old man received in transfer with post–myocardial infarction rupture
▸ Had presented to a community hospital 6 hours earlier with an inferoposterior STEMI, markedly hypertensive, Killip class I
  ▸ Received tPA 4 hours before
  ▸ Developed pleuritic chest pains 3 hours before, and falling blood pressure despite volume and inotropes
  ▸ Several abrupt PEA episodes at the other hospital
  ▸ Echocardiography showed pericardial fluid (pericardial drain had been inserted, draining frank blood).
  ▸ Repeated PEA arrests in transfer
  ▸ Acidotic before transfer (pH 7.2; lactate 15 mmol)
▸ Past medical history is significant for hypertension and smoking.

Physical Examination

▸ BP 50/– mm Hg, HR 30 bpm, ventilated
▸ Cold, blue
▸ Marked jugular venous distention, no edema
▸ Heart sounds not audible
▸ No rubs or murmurs

Impression

▸ Early post–myocardial infarction rupture
▸ Hypertension at presentation may have been a contributing factor.
▸ Large amount of clotted blood, advanced cardiac arrest state

Management and Outcome

▸ Insertion of a larger bore catheter to increase drainage and connection of this to the femoral vein = autotransfusion
▸ Transvenous pacer at 100 bpm
▸ Bicarbonate boluses and infusion

▸ Consideration of surgery (but the total elapsed cardiac arrest time was 75 minutes already)
▸ The patient died because the resuscitative measures did not restore the circulation.

Comments

▸ Autopsy found a 1-cm blowout hole in the posterolateral wall, confirming an inferoposterior hemorrhagic infarction.
▸ The hypertension at presentation may have contributed to early rupture.

▸ Diagnosis by echocardiography (clot and blood)
▸ The blood clot never evacuated through drainage catheters, as would be expected, and the heart remained nonviably compressed. The patient's best chance would have been surgical evacuation very early on, had it been available.

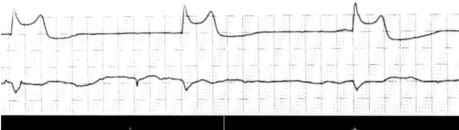

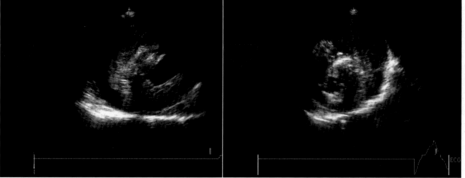

Figure 7-15. TOP, ECG on arrival shows marked junctional bradycardia and inferior ST elevation (lead II). BOTTOM, Transesophageal echocardiography during PEA arrest. Large amount of blood or clot (gelatinous intrapericardial echoes) in the pericardial space has a layered appearance, suggesting successive episodes of bleeding (strata). Heart cavities are very small because of compression by clot.

CASE 4

History

▸ 48-year-old man, very physically active (manual laborer)
▸ Initially admitted for evaluation of severe abdominal pains and abnormal liver enzymes. Abdominal ultrasound examination had serendipitously identified a 65-mm abdominal aortic aneurysm.
▸ No history of angina or heart failure; no prior transient ischemic attacks or strokes or peripheral vascular disease symptoms
▸ Past medical history is significant for hypertension and smoking.
▸ Preoperative stress testing was scintigraphically normal. Nifedipine was changed to metoprolol.

Physical Examination

▸ BP 85/50 mm Hg, HR 55 bpm, RR 13/min
▸ No venous distention or edema; no vascular bruits
▸ Palpable abdominal aortic aneurysm
▸ S_1, S_2 normal
▸ No pericardial rub or murmur
▸ Underwent abdominal aortic aneurysm repair—more adhesions than usual, but operation was otherwise unremarkable

Impression and Management

▸ Acute inferior STEMI without right ventricle involvement
▸ Normal hemodynamics: Killip class I, no RV infarction
▸ Reperfusion therapy (fibrinolytic) was out of the question.
▸ Primary PCI was discussed. Given the small size of the infarction, the lack of hemodynamic problems, and the higher than usual concern for bleeding if clopidogrel ± IIb/IIIa antagonists were used, the decision was made to manage the infarction conservatively with ASA, beta-blockers, and nitrates.

Evolution

▸ For the next 4 days, the patient was stable without heart failure, hypotension, or chest pains. The peak CK was 1100. There were no arrhythmias. There was mild to moderate surgical bleeding, requiring transfusion.
▸ On fifth postoperative day, he developed sudden band-like chest pain of an atypical quality, associated with shortness of breath.
▸ BP 130/90 mm Hg, HR 70 bpm; clear chest; venous distention; new pansystolic murmur at the apex; no rub
▸ No ECG changes; no relief to nitroglycerin

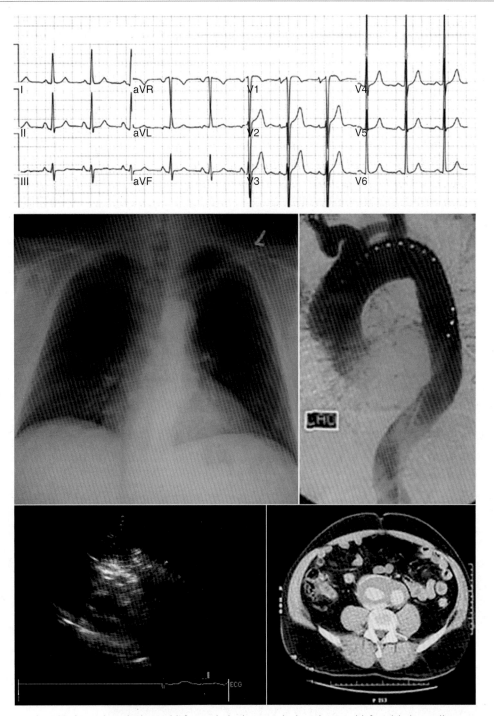

Figure 7-16. TOP, Preoperative ECG shows sinus rhythm and left ventricular hypertrophy by voltage and left atrial abnormality. MIDDLE LEFT, Preoperative chest radiograph shows normal cardiopericardial silhouette, normal lung fields, and tortuous thoracic aorta. MIDDLE RIGHT, Preoperative aortogram shows mildly enlarged ascending aorta and tortuous thoracic aorta. BOTTOM LEFT, Preoperative transthoracic echocardiography, parasternal short-axis view, shows mildly dilated ascending aorta, mild left ventricular hypertrophy, and normal left atrial size (and systolic function). BOTTOM RIGHT, Preoperative contrast-enhanced CT scan shows abdominal aortic aneurysm extending into common iliacs. Lumen with contrast material (white). Large amount of clot (speckled gray) in the anterior portion of the abdominal aortic aneurysm and circumferentially in the iliac aneurysms.

▸ The patient rapidly became distressed, his BP rose to 180/100, then he seized and collapsed. He had no pulse despite electrical activity to the heart.

Impression and Management

▸ Post–myocardial infarction acute rupture, compression of the heart from clot
▸ Infusion of volume, epinephrine
▸ No improvement with pericardiocentesis
▸ Bedside surgical evacuation of clot through subcostal incision and immediate transfer to surgery for emergent exploration and repair
▸ Time between collapse and arrival in the operating room was less than 30 minutes, but no circulation during that time

Outcome

▸ Surgery revealed a 4-cm blowout rupture of the basal inferior wall and infarcted posterior papillary muscle.

▸ Patch repair of the tear was performed and held.
▸ Tremendous difficulty in getting the heart to start up once coming off pump
▸ Death despite repair

Comments

▸ Myocardial rupture occurring in a non-reperfused STEMI
▸ Infarction was well tolerated to that point, and the infarction was neither enzymatically nor hemodynamically large. This underscores that preserved residual systolic function and elevated intracavitary pressures are important determinants of rupture.
▸ Large rupture consistent with fulminant tamponade
▸ The pansystolic murmur heard immediately before rupture may have been myocardial regurgitation, or potentially the rupture itself.
▸ Unfortunate and discouraging outcome, given that the rupture was diagnosed within 5 minutes of occurrence and the surgical response was within minutes

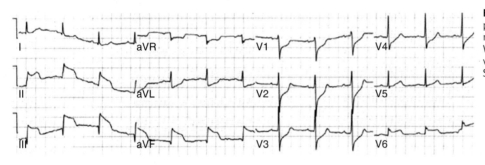

Figure 7-17. ECG taken 4 hours postoperatively shows sinus rhythm, marked inferior ST elevation (II, III, aVF, V$_6$), ST depression V$_1$-V$_4$—septal ischemia, versus reciprocal changes, versus posterior ST elevation.

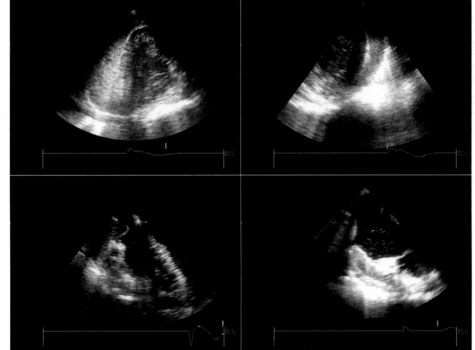

Figure 7-18. Transesophageal echocardiography during arrest shows clot in pericardial space, under the posterior wall (TOP LEFT), beside the lateral wall of the LV (TOP RIGHT) and severely collapsing the RA wall (BOTTOM LEFT). The bottom right image was taken after surgical suction extraction of a large amount of fresh intrapericardial clot at the beside, allowing better RA filling. Bubbles in the right side of the heart are from intravenous infusions. Asystolic heart.

CASE 5

History

▸ 79-year-old woman, very frail
▸ Late-presentation inferior STEMI (11 hours)
▸ No heart failure symptoms
▸ Past medical history is significant for hypertension and type 2 diabetes.

Physical Examination

▸ Well appearing, BP 180/90 mm Hg, HR 95 bpm, RR 13/min
▸ Clear chest
▸ No venous distention, no edema
▸ S_1, S_2 normal; S_4 present
▸ No rubs or murmurs
▸ Not given fibrinolytics at hour 12 because pain had subsided and late time
▸ CK at arrival 800, peaked at 2400
▸ No heart failure; occasional mild atypical chest discomforts
▸ Dipyridamole (Persantine), sestamibi; fixed inferior defect

Impression and Evolution

▸ Late-presentation inferoposterior STEMI with mild peri-infarct heart failure
▸ The patient was well for 4 days, then experienced sudden severe weakness and mild chest pain

▸ BP 60/−, HR 120 bpm, dyspneic
▸ Chest clear
▸ Venous distention, no edema
▸ Heart sounds distant; no rub or murmurs

Impression, Management, and Outcome

▸ Acute postinfarction rupture with severe tamponade and cardiac compression
▸ Pericardiocentesis performed, as the patient had become cold and overtly shocky within 5 minutes. Frank blood returned, as did some blood pressure, but clinically, cardiac output did not return.
▸ Deemed too elderly and frail to undergo surgical exploration and repair
▸ Lasted 2 hours, then became asystolic and died

Comments

▸ Herald symptoms before complete rupture
▸ Evanescent success with pericardiocentesis, volume, and inotropes
▸ The aneurysmal mid inferior left ventricle was the presumed site of rupture
▸ The volume of blood return from the pericardial space (3 L in 2 hours, with the catheter verified to be in the pericardial space) inferred massive ongoing bleeding into the pericardial space.

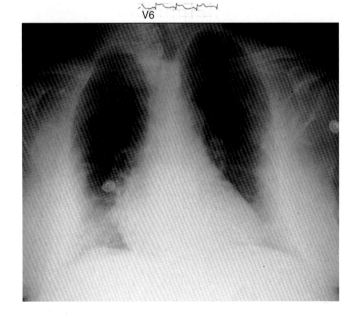

Figure 7-19. ECG at presentation shows sinus rhythm, inferior and lateral ST elevation and Q waves, early precordial R-wave evolution, and ST depression, suggesting acute inferolateral and posterior infarction. Chest radiograph shows normal cardiopericardial silhouette and mild left-sided heart failure.

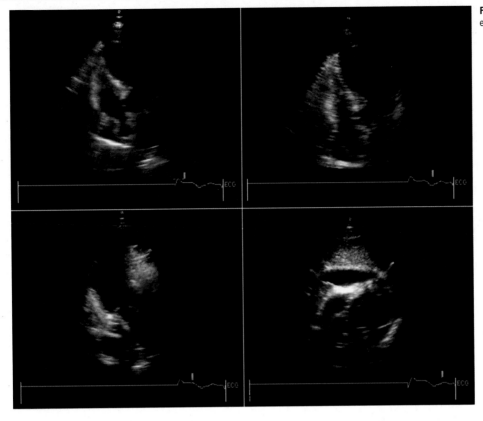

Figure 7-20. Transthoracic echocardiography views.

CASE 6

History and Physical Examination

▶ 58-year-old man transferred for rescue PCI after presumed failed fibrinolytic therapy for anterior STEMI
▶ Had presented at hour 12 with ongoing chest pains, Killip II, and anterior ST elevation, but Q waves had already formed
▶ Fibrinolytics had been given at hour 12:45; received at hour 16 for rescue PCI
▶ Dyspneic and severely hypotensive on arrival
▶ Dopamine started for vasopressor support; presumed progression to Killip class IV
▶ Intubated for airway and ventilatory support during PCI and because of shock
▶ Venous pressures appeared elevated, but the patient was lying supine and on PEEP
▶ No murmurs or rub

Management

▶ Angiography revealed occlusion of the LAD proximally, which was readily dilated and stented. Only TIMI I-II flow after, and no improvement in blood pressure, which was still prominently dependent on vasopressor and inotropic support.
▶ To assess for other causes of cardiogenic shock, right- and left-sided heart catheterization was proceeded with and urgent echocardiography requested.
▶ It was unknown if the tamponade represented a PCI complication or an early rupture. Rapidly, his pressure and output fell.

Evolution and Outcome

▶ With emergency drainage of 75 mL of blood, no hemodynamic improvement occurred.
▶ IABP was inserted, and the patient emergently underwent surgical inspection and repair.
▶ The patient had frankly arrested by the time the chest was opened.
▶ A 4-cm tear through the aneurysmal (expanded) apex was found and patched. The apex was severely hemorrhagic in appearance. The ventricle did not start up.

Comments

▶ Early acute free wall rupture through the apex
▶ Large tear, severe compression
▶ Neither transthoracic echocardiography (TTE) nor transesophageal echocardiography (TEE) established that the pericardial fluid was blood, but pericardial tap did.
▶ Confusing, rapidly evolving case that initially appeared to be early cardiogenic shock or pump failure from a large anterior STEMI with early infarct expansion
▶ In this case, PCI did not precipitate tamponade.
▶ Rupture through the area of infarct expansion (aneurysm). Chronic aneurysms are unlikely to rupture, but acute early ones may.
▶ Late presentation, later use of fibrinolytics; hemorrhagic transformation of the infarct observed

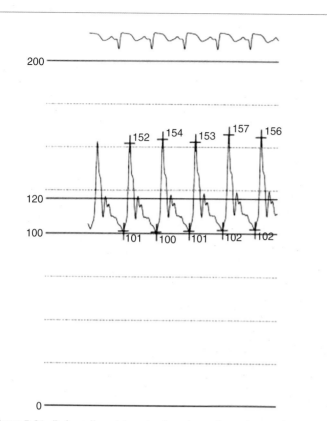

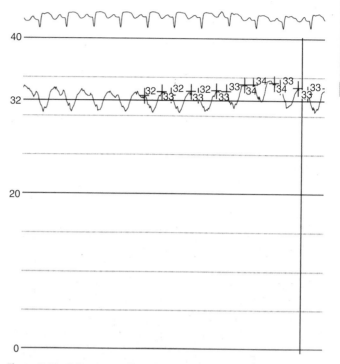

Figure 7-21. Tachycardia and hypertension—hyperadrenergic state from the dopamine. The contour of the systolic waveform is incomplete, consistent with a small stroke volume.

Figure 7-22. Pulmonary capillary wedge pressure (PCWP) tracing. The mean pressure is severely elevated and the contour is grossly abnormal with a diminutive y descent and a prominent x descent, consistent with tamponade. The PCWP is greater than the right atrial pressure because of the effect of the large acute anterior LV infarction.

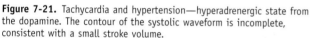

Figure 7-23. Transthoracic echocardiography. TOP LEFT, Parasternal short-axis view. There is left ventricular hypertrophy, and the LV cavity is very small at the mid ventricle level. There is a pericardial effusion that is not small. The right ventricular cavity is very small and probably compressed by the effusion. TOP RIGHT, Apical 4-chamber view. The apex prominently is aneurysmal—early infarct expansion. The right atrium is collapsed, as is the distal half of the right ventricle. BOTTOM LEFT, Subcostal long-axis view. Moderate-sized effusion with specular echos and severe right ventricular collapse along its length. BOTTOM RIGHT, Transesophageal echocardiography view of the right atrium, which is collapsed by pericardial fluid.

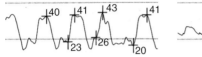

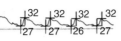

Figure 7-24. Right ventricular pressure tracings. LEFT, Initial recording notable for a prominent elevation of the diastolic pressure. RIGHT, Recording at the moment of PEA. There is almost no pulse pressure generated by the right ventricle, which is presumably too compressed to fill.

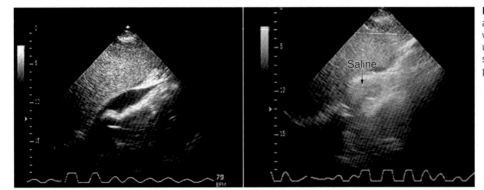

Figure 7-25. The near cardiac arrest–attempted pericardial aspiration, which withdrew blood of uncertain origin and under some pressure. Injection of agitated saline confirms the needle tip in the pericardial effusion *(arrow).*

CASE 7

History

▸ 78-year-old woman admitted with a late-presentation (hour 18) inferior STEMI
▸ Past medical history of hypertension; BP 165/97 mm Hg at admission

Physical Examination

▸ No right ventricular infarction findings
▸ No murmurs or rubs and normal venous pressures

Evolution

▸ Pain free until day 3, when distress, agitation, and vomiting occurred abruptly

▸ BP 100/60 mm Hg, HR 80 bpm (with beta-blockers)
▸ Searing severe chest pain occurred, distress then asystole
▸ Bedside echocardiography was performed during attempted resuscitation.

Outcome

▸ All resuscitation efforts were unsuccessful, and the patient died.

Comments

▸ Probable acute posterior free wall rupture
▸ Associated severe bradyarrhythmia, asystole
▸ Brief prodrome of distress, agitation, vomiting, pain
▸ History of hypertension

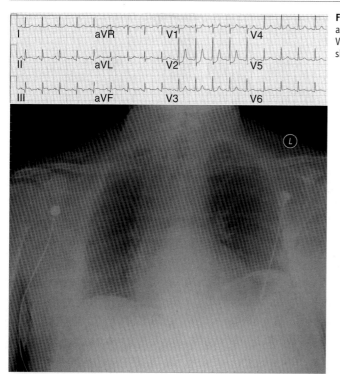

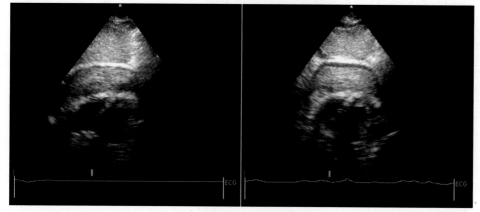

Figure 7-26. TOP, ECG at presentation shows sinus rhythm, inferior Q waves, and ST elevation. Early precordial R-wave transition and ST depression also in V_1 and V_2, suggesting associated posterior infarction. BOTTOM, Chest radiograph shows clear lung fields, normal-sized heart shadow.

Figure 7-27. Transesophageal echocardiography subcostal views. There is a large amount of clot-like material within the pericardial space; the heart cavities are small. Note the asystole on the ECG.

CASE 8

History

▸ 76-year-old woman 2 days after inferolateral STEMI; had received fibrinolytics at hour 10 because of ongoing chest pain and ST elevation; peak troponin 80, CK 2200

▸ Past medical history is significant for hypertension.

▸ Initial physical examination: BP 175/100 mm Hg, HR 85 bpm, Killip I, no murmurs or rubs

▸ Initial echocardiography showed only a moderate-sized inferolateral akinetic area.

▸ Restlessness developed late at night; distress and burning chest pain different from her initial infarction-like pain

Physical Examination

▸ Appeared unwell and pale

▸ Cool extremities

▸ BP 100/60 mm Hg; pulsus paradoxus of 15 mm Hg, HR 95 bpm

▸ Venous distention

▸ No murmur or pericardial rub, clear chest

▸ Repeated echocardiography performed

Clinical Impression

▸ Probable postinfarction rupture—a large amount of blood (clot) in the pericardial space and severe cardiac compression

▸ Plan: urgent angiography and surgical inspection and repair

Outcome

▸ Slow postoperative course, but survived

▸ No angina

▸ NYHA class II heart failure symptoms

Comments

▸ Acute-subacute lateral wall rupture (the most common site)

▸ Early rupture; had received fibrinolytics at hour 10

▸ Because the rupture was small, the cardiac compression, although severe, was not unsupportable.

▸ Restlessness, agitation, and chest pains were indicative symptoms.

▸ The site of rupture (distal lateral wall) approximately corresponded to the persistent ST elevation on the ECG and to the peculiar thickened wall seen on TTE.

▸ TTE demonstrated a small effusion but did not well represent the clot, which was readily appreciated by TEE.

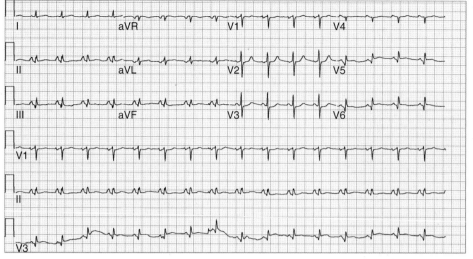

Figure 7-28. Repeated ECG shows sinus rhythm, Q waves in the inferior and lateral leads. The standard limb lead voltages are low (<5 mm). There is ST elevation in V_5 and V_6.

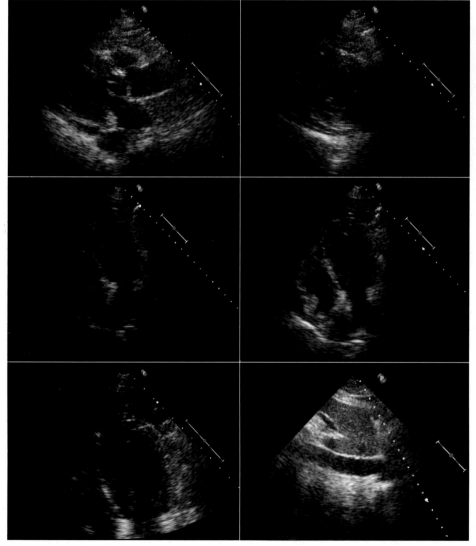

Figure 7-29. Transthoracic echocardiography. TOP ROW, Parasternal long- and short-axis views. Mild left ventricular hypertrophy. There is a small posterior pericardial effusion. MIDDLE ROW, Apical 4-chamber views. There is a small pericardial effusion at the apex. BOTTOM LEFT, The apicolateral wall has a peculiar thickening to it. BOTTOM RIGHT, The inferior vena cava is dilated, consistent with elevated pressure.

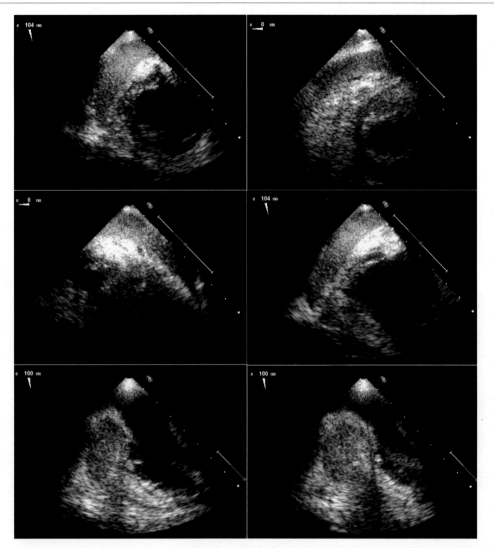

Figure 7-30. Transesophageal echocardiography. TOP AND MIDDLE ROWS, Transgastric views demonstrate a 2-cm clot within the pericardial space that appears as fine specular material with the appearance of liver. The ventricular cavities are small. BOTTOM ROW, There is clot also lateral to the right atrium, which is prominently compressed. No disruption to the endocardium or myocardium could be seen.

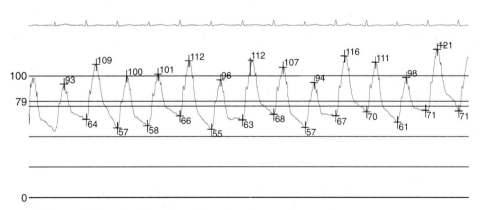

Figure 7-31. Aortic pressure tracing, with dopamine. There is an 18 mm Hg pulsus paradoxus.

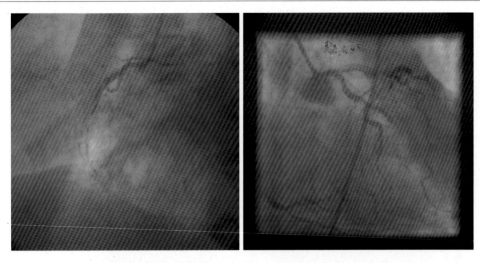

Figure 7-32. Selective coronary angiography. LEFT, Right coronary injection. The right coronary is completely occluded. RIGHT, Left coronary injection. There is prominent collateralization from the distal left circumflex artery to the distal right coronary artery and the posterior descending. A large first obtuse marginal branch is occluded.

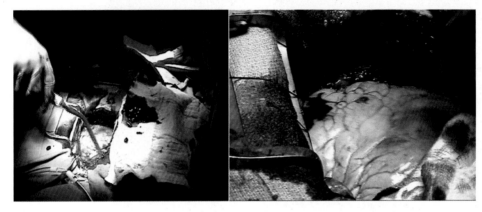

Figure 7-33. Intraoperative photographs. LEFT, With the chest opened, a large amount of gelatinous blood clot is evacuated from the pericardial space. RIGHT, Blood seeps into the pericardial space from the lateral aspect of the left ventricle, the source of which was a small distal lateral wall rupture that underwent patch repair. Aortocoronary bypass grafting was performed to the distal right coronary and obtuse marginal branch.

References

1. Reddy SG, Roberts WC: Frequency of rupture of the left ventricular free wall or ventricular septum among necropsy cases of fatal acute myocardial infarction since introduction of coronary care units. Am J Cardiol 1989;63:906-911.
2. Aravot DJ, Dhalla N, Banner NR, et al: Combined septal perforation and cardiac rupture after myocardial infarction. Clinical features and surgical considerations of a correctable condition. J Thorac Cardiovasc Surg 1989;97:815-820.
3. Núñez L, de la Llana R, López-Sendón J, et al: Diagnosis and treatment of subacute free wall ventricular rupture after infarction. Ann Thorac Surg 1983;35:525-529.
4. Roberts JD, Mong KW, Sussex B: Successful management of left ventricular free wall rupture. Can J Cardiol 2007;23:672-674.
5. Oliva PB, Hammill SC, Edwards WD: Cardiac rupture, a clinically predictable complication of acute myocardial infarction: report of 70 cases with clinicopathologic correlations. J Am Coll Cardiol 1993;22:720-726.
6. Crenshaw BS, Granger CB, Birnbaum Y, et al: Risk factors, angiographic patterns, and outcomes in patients with ventricular septal defect complicating acute myocardial infarction. GUSTO-I (Global Utilization of Streptokinase and TPA for Occluded Coronary Arteries) Trial Investigators. Circulation 2000;101:27-32.
7. Kishon Y, Iqbal A, Oh JK, et al: Evolution of echocardiographic modalities in detection of postmyocardial infarction ventricular septal defect and papillary muscle rupture: study of 62 patients. Am Heart J 1993;126 (pt 1):667-675.
8. Figueras J, Cortadellas J, Calvo F, Soler-Soler J: Relevance of delayed hospital admission on development of cardiac rupture during acute myocardial infarction: study in 225 patients with free wall, septal or papillary muscle rupture. J Am Coll Cardiol 1998;32:135-139.
9. Edwards BS, Edwards WD, Edwards JE: Ventricular septal rupture complicating acute myocardial infarction: identification of simple and complex types in 53 autopsied hearts. Am J Cardiol 1984;54:1201-1205.
10. Moreno R, López-Sendón J, Garcia E, et al: Primary angioplasty reduces the risk of left ventricular free wall rupture compared with thrombolysis in patients with acute myocardial infarction. J Am Coll Cardiol 2002;39:598-603.
11. Mann JM, Roberts WC: Rupture of the left ventricular free wall during acute myocardial infarction: analysis of 138 necropsy patients and comparison with 50 necropsy patients with acute myocardial infarction without rupture. Am J Cardiol 1988;62:847-859.
12. Mechanisms for the early mortality reduction produced by beta-blockade started early in acute myocardial infarction: ISIS-1. ISIS-1 (First International Study of Infarct Survival) Collaborative Group. Lancet 1988;1:921-923.
13. Honan MB, Harrell FE Jr, Reimer KA, et al: Cardiac rupture, mortality and the timing of thrombolytic therapy: a meta-analysis. J Am Coll Cardiol 1990;16:359-367.
14. Gertz SD, Kragel AH, Kalan JM, et al: Comparison of coronary and myocardial morphologic findings in patients with and without thrombolytic therapy during fatal first acute myocardial infarction. The TIMI Investigators. Am J Cardiol 1990;66:904-909.
15. Becker RC, Gore JM, Lambrew C, et al: A composite view of cardiac rupture in the United States National Registry of Myocardial Infarction. J Am Coll Cardiol 1996;27:1321-1326.

16. Kinn JW, O'Neill WW, Benzuly KH, et al: Primary angioplasty reduces risk of myocardial rupture compared to thrombolysis for acute myocardial infarction. Cathet Cardiovasc Diagn 1997;42:151-157.

17. Solodky A, Behar S, Herz I, et al: Comparison of incidence of cardiac rupture among patients with acute myocardial infarction treated by thrombolysis versus percutaneous transluminal coronary angioplasty. Am J Cardiol 2001;87:1105-1108, A9.

18. López-Sendón J, González A, López de Sá E, et al: Diagnosis of subacute ventricular wall rupture after acute myocardial infarction: sensitivity and specificity of clinical, hemodynamic and echocardiographic criteria. J Am Coll Cardiol 1992;19:1145-1153.

19. Figueras J, Cortadellas J, Evangelista A, Soler-Soler J: Medical management of selected patients with left ventricular free wall rupture during acute myocardial infarction. J Am Coll Cardiol 1997;29:512-518.

20. Fein SA, Vargas M: Transesophageal echocardiographic diagnosis of cardiac rupture. J Am Soc Echocardiogr 1991;4:415-416.

21. Deshmukh HG, Khosla S, Jefferson KK: Direct visualization of left ventricular free wall rupture by transesophageal echocardiography in acute myocardial infarction. Am Heart J 1993;126:475-477.

22. Stiegel M, Zimmern SH, Robicsek F: Left ventricular rupture following coronary occlusion treated by streptokinase infusion: successful surgical repair. Ann Thorac Surg 1987;44:413-415.

23. Hochreiter C, Goldstein J, Borer JS, et al: Myocardial free-wall rupture after acute infarction: survival aided by percutaneous intraaortic balloon counterpulsation. Circulation 1982;65:1279-1282.

24. Proli J, Laufer N: Left ventricular rupture following myocardial infarction treated with streptokinase: successful resuscitation in the cardiac catheterization laboratory using pericardiocentesis and autotransfusion. Cathet Cardiovasc Diagn 1993;29:257-260.

25. Raitt MH, Kraft CD, Gardner CJ, et al: Subacute ventricular free wall rupture complicating myocardial infarction. Am Heart J 1993;126: 946-955.

26. Padro JM, Mesa JM, Silvestre J, et al: Subacute cardiac rupture: repair with a sutureless technique. Ann Thorac Surg 1993;55:20-23.

7

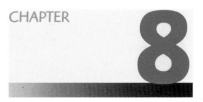

False Aneurysms of the Left Ventricle

▸ Adhesions within the pericardial space from prior peri- carditis avert immediate tamponade in some cases of myocardial rupture and lead to formation of false aneu- rysms, which allow some chance of recognition and surgical intervention.

▸ Presentations are subtle. Basic clinical evaluation (physical examination, chest radiography) will be sug- gestive in some cases.

▸ Echocardiography and contrast ventriculography are the most commonly performed tests, but cardiac MR (SSFP) and gated cardiac CT may be superior.

▸ Because no imaging modality can compare with histol- ogy for determining that the wall of the false aneurysm

is not composed of all the usual layers of myocardium, the gross morphologic findings are used to distinguish false from true aneurysms of the left ventricle.

▸ The gross morphologic findings of a narrow neck and wide body are generally useful to distinguish false aneu- rysms and true aneurysms, except for lesions located between the posterior papillary muscle and the mitral annulus.

▸ Obtain angiography and surgical repair.

▸ Most patients do well with reparative surgery, but surgi- cal mortality is affected by the extent of left ventricular dysfunction, and surgical failures occur.

False aneurysms, also known as pseudoaneurysms, have several important features that distinguish them from true aneurysms (Table 8-1). The incidence of postinfarction false aneurysms of the left ventricle is unknown, as is the overall natural history. The natural history of symptomatic unrepaired false aneurysms is likely to progress to death. The natural history of asymptomatic false aneurysms is almost entirely unknown; few are ever identi- fied. It is known that even small (2 cm) false aneurysms may rupture, resulting in fatal hemopericardium,[1] but survival up to 6 years without surgical repair has been reported.[2]

A postinfarction false aneurysm is an incomplete rupture of the heart. The usual false aneurysm represents a tear through the ventricular myocardium due to transmural necrosis from infarction. The tear is complete, leaving no myocardium lining part of the outside wall of the false aneurysm,[3] but preexisting pericardial (parietal to visceral) adhesions limit the distribution to a portion of the pericardial cavity, avoiding generalized distri- bution of the blood and tamponade. If the false aneurysm is large, it commonly contains a large amount of mural thrombus. The limitation imparted by adhesions is impermanent. The size of the intrapericardial cavity is variable, from a few centimeters to a dimension as large as the heart itself. The outside wall of the cavity is composed of parietal pericardium and is often lined with mural thrombus, but it always lacks myocardium (Fig. 8-1). The neck (of the tear) that affords communication of the left ventricular cavity

with the "body" of the false aneurysm is typically narrow (<50% of the dimension of the body of the intrapericardial cavity). In some cases, the neck is prominently narrow, virtually a tract. In other cases in which the false aneurysm body has grown to an advanced size, the neck may become very wide. Rarely, a false aneurysm may develop from a true aneurysm.[4,5] The reported locations and sizes of false aneurysms are summarized in Table 8-2.[6,7]

CLINICAL PRESENTATIONS OF POSTINFARCTION FALSE ANEURYSMS

The most common presenting signs of left ventricular false aneurysms include the following:

- A murmur (in approximately 70%)[6] that may be a systolic murmur or a to-and-fro murmur. The common proximity of false aneurysms to papillary muscles often engenders mitral insufficiency from distortion of ventricular geometry, and the murmur of mitral insufficiency may dominate that of the false aneurysm (Fig. 8-2A,B).

Table 8-1. Differences between False and True Aneurysms

False Aneurysm	True Aneurysm
Tearing of myocardium	Stretching of myocardium
Narrow neck	Wide neck
No myocardial wall or partial-thickness wall, tentatively restrained by adherent pericardium	Full-thickness wall
Likely to rupture	Unlikely to rupture. Few *chronic* myocardial aneurysms rupture, but ruptures have been reported. *Acute* infarct expansion or *early* aneurysm rupture accounts for a proportion of free wall rupture.
	May rarely develop into a false aneurysm

Table 8-2. Location and Size of Left Ventricular False Aneurysms

	Frances et al[6]	Gueron et al[7]
Location		
Posterior	43	45
Lateral	28	14
Apical	24	18
Inferior	19	5
Anterior	18	18
Basal	14	
PA diameter (cm)	1.5, 20.1	
Orifice diameter (cm)	0.1, 9.0	
Orifice/PA diameter ratio	0.02, 1.0	

PA, pseudoaneurysm.

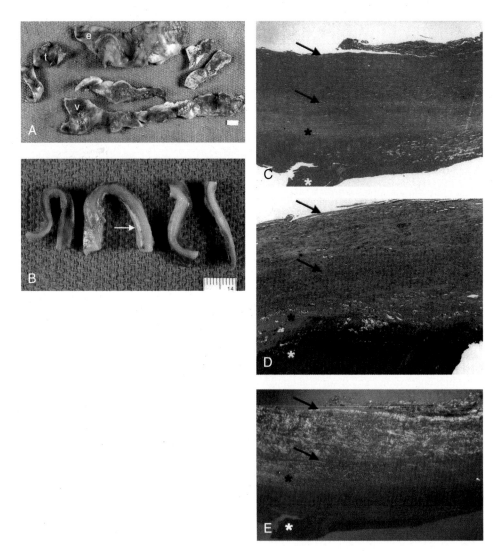

Figure 8-1. A, Strips of ventricular aneurysmal tissue showing the endocardial surface with overlying red-brown thrombus. v, endocardial surface; e, epicardial surface; t, thrombus. **B,** Longitudinal strips of gray-white tissue from the resected ventricular wall. The endocardial surface is indicated by the arrow. The wall thickness ranges from 2 to 4 mm. **C** and **D,** Histologic sections of the wall show no residual myocardium. The parietal pericardium is seen *(arrows)* and is thickened by fibrosis and overlying organizing thrombus *(asterisks)*. **E,** A photomicrograph with polarized light showing the birefringent pericardial collagen *(arrows)* with overlying fibrous tissue and thrombus *(asterisks)*. (From Butany J, Dias B, Grapa J, et al: Left ventricular pseudoaneurysm. Can J Cardiol 2002;18:1122-1123.)

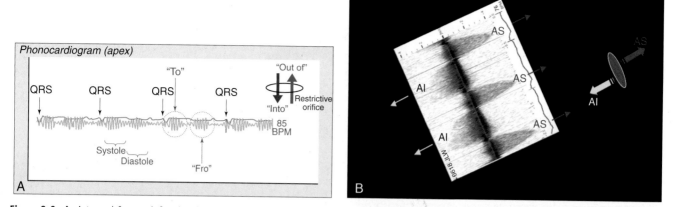

Figure 8-2. A, A to-and-fro postinfarction false aneurysm murmur phonocardiogram, recorded on an echo system. The systolic and diastolic components can be appreciated, representing turbulent flow into (systole) and out of (diastole) the body of the false aneurysm. **B,** The reciprocating murmur of aortic stenosis (AS) or aortic insufficiency (AI) is similar to that of the to-and-fro murmur of a false aneurysm. Both are due to turbulent flow that alternates direction with each phase of the cardiac cycle.

- Congestive heart failure due to postinfarction left ventricular dysfunction and loss of stroke volume into the false aneurysm (the cavity, which may be as large as the left ventricular cavity, may accommodate a large proportion of the stroke volume) (Fig. 8-4)
- Basal septal rupture. Most postinfarction inferobasal septal ruptures have complex anatomy and often a frank false aneurysm into the floor of the inferior wall or septum.[8,9]
- Chest pains due to pericardial distention, irritation
- Unexplained pericardial effusion due to leakage from the cavity into the pericardial space
- Abnormal bulge on chest radiography (in more than half)[6]; mass of the false aneurysm (Fig. 8-3)
- Tamponade due to rupture or fistulization into the pericardial space
- Systemic embolism of thrombus within the cavity

DIAGNOSIS OF POSTINFARCTION LEFT VENTRICULAR FALSE ANEURYSM

Echocardiography

Echocardiography is a good test and has the advantage of being readily portable; it is able to image the myocardial disruption (neck) and, by use of Doppler study, the flows through it (Fig. 8-5). The cavity of the false aneurysm is generally visible, but often incompletely if it extends deeply into the chest.[10,11] One of the advantages of transesophageal echocardiography is greater ability to visualize posterior false aneurysms.[12,13] Color Doppler and pulsed wave Doppler study assist in characterizing the pathologic flow pattern into and out of the false aneurysm.[14]

Contrast Ventriculography

Contrast ventriculography is a very useful test to depict the abnormal contour, location, and systolic expansion of the body of

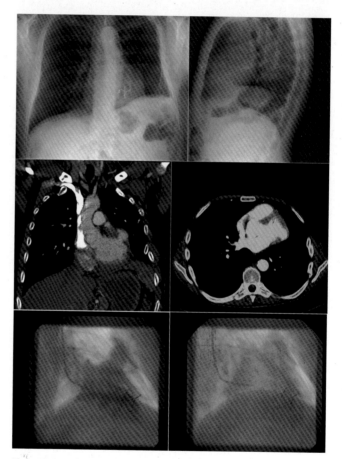

Figure 8-3. False aneurysm of the left ventricle. TOP, PA and lateral chest radiographs show a prominent bulge along the left heart border. On the PA view the lesion projects away from the LV chamber and is more apparent. MIDDLE LEFT, Contrast-enhanced coronal CT scan shows a contrast-enhancing cavity outside the LV cavity along its anterolateral wall and connected to the LV cavity via a narrow neck, where the bulge was seen on the PA radiograph. MIDDLE RIGHT, Contrast-enhanced axial CT scan shows the cavity beside the anterolateral wall of the LV. BOTTOM, Contrast ventriculography in systole (LEFT) and diastole (RIGHT). On these RAO views, the lesion projects away from the LV cavity and is well seen, especially in systole.

Diastole   Systole

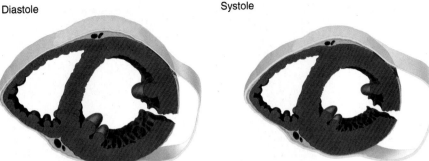

Figure 8-4. Systolic contraction of the left ventricle typically results in bulging of the cavity of the false aneurysm. The pulsatility of the body of the false aneurysm may be prominent. Stroke volume is reduced by the underlying infarction, by loss into the body of the false aneurysm, and by any infarction-associated mitral insufficiency.

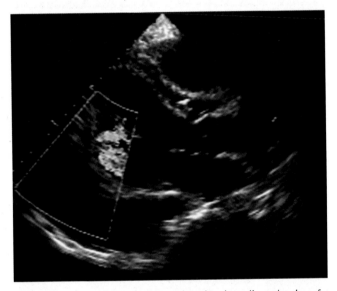

Figure 8-5. Parasternal long-axis transthoracic echocardiography view of a leaking postinfarction posterior false aneurysm. There is turbulent flow through a very narrow neck in the mid-distal posterior wall, into a large saccular cavity behind the posterior wall. The right ventricular outflow tract is severely compressed by fluid.

the false aneurysm and its neck.[6] The view must have the correct projection to depict the false aneurysm body away from the left ventricle. Neither the myocardium nor the actual plane of parietal pericardium is as clearly depicted by contrast ventriculography as by computed tomography (CT) or magnetic resonance (MR). Coronary angiography has an important role in the evaluation of postinfarction false aneurysms, as the anticipated treatment is surgical repair of the defect and coronary artery bypass grafting. Coronary angiography usually reveals the myocardial wall by achieving a "blush." Furthermore, the coronary arteries lie on the epicardium, assisting with localizing the myocardial wall. In the presence of a true aneurysm, the coronary arteries "drape" over the aneurysm, whereas in the presence of a false aneurysm, the coronary arteries do not drape over the false aneurysm.[15]

Cardiac Computed Tomography

Electrocardiography (ECG)–gated cardiac CT offers an excellent means to delineate the anatomic details of the false lumen, mural thrombus, and myocardial and pericardial layers, but even older non–ECG-gated CT was able to show large false aneurysms in detail.[16]

Cardiac Magnetic Resonance

Cardiac MR also affords an excellent means to depict the blood pool, the myocardium and pericardium, the systolic motion, and the presence of mural thrombus, making it the best overall test to image false aneurysms. SSFP sequences will demonstrate the anatomy, the motion, and the flow into and out of a false aneurysm (Fig. 8-6). T1-weighted black blood sequences will depict anatomic findings, and cine SSFP will depict pulsatility and flow.[17-20] Inversion recovery gradient echo sequences will depict delayed enhancement in the territory with myocardial infarction.

Gross Imaging Features Differentiating False from True Aneurysms

Because no imaging modality currently has the spatial resolution to accurately determine the nature of the tissue that composes the outer wall of the suspected false aneurysm, gross morphologic findings that can be identified with available imaging modalities are used to distinguish false aneurysms from true aneurysms.

The most useful gross imaging feature is that the width of the neck is far smaller than the diameter of the body; this proportion appears to be maintained irrespective of the size of the false aneurysm (Fig. 8-7). True aneurysms, with one exception, have wide necks. The mean ratio of neck width is 0.37 ± 0.07 for false aneurysms and 1.00 ± 0.08 for true aneurysms.[21] The exception to this rule involves true aneurysms at the base of the posterior wall, between the mitral annulus and the base of the posteromedial papillary muscle. Most true aneurysms in this location have a narrow-appearing neck, as the tension of the mitral valve on the papillary muscle prevents the neck from widening to the extent that it does elsewhere in the heart. In this location, true and false aneurysm necks may be similar.[22] A very narrow neck or other findings, such as obvious tissue disruption and excessive myocardial (free) motion at the neck, would be needed to build a case for a false aneurysm. Aneurysms, including giant ones, do occur along the inferior wall of the left ventricle.[23]

Other imaging features are that the cavity that appears extrinsic to the myocardium has a saccular or globular contour. The appearance of a sharp discontinuity at the neck or site of communication is useful to establish that myocardial disruption occurred. A severe regional wall motion abnormality around the neck is an important finding to infer location (transmural infarction as the substrate for the contained rupture).

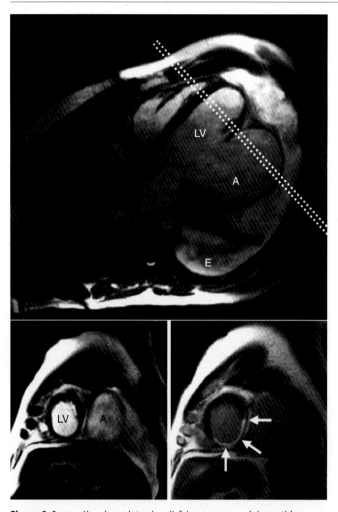

Figure 8-6. TOP, Very large lateral wall false aneurysm. A large thin-walled cavity, arising from a narrow neck, extends off the internal wall of the left ventricle (LV) and appears to be at least as large as the left ventricular cavity is. A, false aneurysm. E, large left pleural effusion. BOTTOM, Inversion recovery gradient echo delayed enhancement sequences. There is transmural delayed enhancement of the myocardium adjacent to the false aneurysm cavity, indicative of prior transmural infarction, the substrate of the false aneurysm.

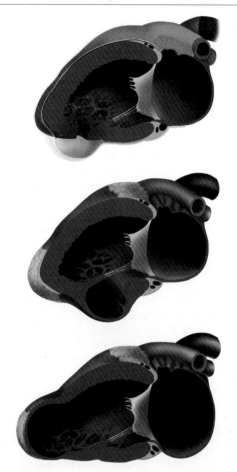

Figure 8-7. TOP, Depiction of a postinfarction false aneurysm of the distal inferior wall. There is a narrow neck through the disrupted myocardium that has allowed the blood pool to communicate with the pericardial space. Pericardial adhesions, though, have limited the spread of the cavity, at least for an interval. The neck of a false aneurysm is usually about a third of the width of the body. MIDDLE, Depiction of a true aneurysm of the base of the posterior wall. There is some similarity of appearance of this true aneurysm to a false aneurysm, as assessment of the neck is confounded by the overarching papillary muscle, but there is no irregularity of the margins to suggest myocardial disruption. Tension exerted by chordae on nearby myocardium will influence the remodeling of an aneurysm. BOTTOM, Depiction of a typical apical aneurysm with a wide neck.

Notably, current imaging modalities, such as gated cardiac CT and SSFP MR sequences, are not well represented in the literature. Most postinfarction complication series are older and representative of older technology (Table 8-3).[6]

Angiography, Catheterization, and Hemodynamics

Angiography should be performed in all cases to establish the severity and extent of underlying infarction (Table 8-4). Surgical repair is the intended treatment, and aortocoronary bypass grafting should be performed concurrently.

Catheterization reveals hemodynamic findings due to loss of stroke volume into the false aneurysm, loss of contractile function due to the underlying infarction, and occasionally a pericardial restraint effect that may occur if the false aneurysm enlarges rapidly.

Table 8-3. Diagnostic Accuracy of Imaging Modalities in Patients with Left Ventricular False Aneurysms (in 1988)[6]

Modality	Diagnostic (%)	Helpful (%)	Inadequate (%)	N
Ventriculography	87	11	2	197
Echocardiography				
Two-dimensional	26	65	9	115
Color Doppler	29	56	15	41
Pulsed wave Doppler	35	55	13	23
Transesophageal	75	25	0	16
Multiple gaited acquisition	12	74	14	43
Computed tomography	7	93	0	15
Magnetic resonance	53	47	0	17

Table 8-4. Angiographic Findings in Postinfarction Rupture

Angiographic Disease	Septal Rupture			Papillary Muscle Rupture		Postinfarction MR, No Papillary Muscle Rupture	Free Wall Rupture
Reference	24	25	26	25	26	27	26
Single-vessel	50%	36%	57%	30%	46%	16%	58%
Two-vessel	40%	27%	33%	35%	29%	24%	38%
Three-vessel	11%	36%	10%	35%	25%	60%	4%

MR, mitral regurgitation.

MANAGEMENT OF LEFT VENTRICULAR FALSE ANEURYSMS

The management of symptomatic left ventricular false aneurysms consists of obtaining prompt surgical repair (closure, patch repair) and aortocoronary bypass grafting. Asymptomatic cases should also undergo repair because the natural history is believed to eventuate in rupture. The proximity of a false aneurysm to the mitral valve and underlying prior infarction may render the mitral valve incompetent, necessitating concurrent mitral valve repair or replacement.

There are limited data on surgical outcomes. The need to perform mitral valve replacement will augment mortality in this group of patients with left ventricular systolic dysfunction. Some operative failure does occur, and operative mortality can be high if left ventricular systolic dysfunction is severe. However, long-term postoperative survival can be very good.[28]

CASE 1

History

▸ 75-year-old woman evaluated for abdominal pains and electrolyte disturbances
▸ No history of chest pains or shortness of breath
▸ Past medical history is significant for volvulus, bowel obstruction, hypertension, type 2 diabetes, and hypothyroidism.

Physical Examination

▸ BP 160/70 mm Hg, HR 85 bpm, RR normal
▸ Grade 2 murmur of mitral regurgitation, no diastolic murmur
▸ S_1, S_2 normal; no gallops or rub
▸ Diffusely enlarged apex
▸ Normal venous pressures, no edema
▸ Clear chest

Impression, Management, and Outcome

▸ False aneurysm of the lateral wall
▸ Prior "silent" lateral wall infarction (missing first obtuse marginal branch of the left circumflex apparent on review of angiogram)
▸ Surgical (patch) repair was performed.
▸ Saphenous grafting of the first obtuse marginal branch
▸ Uneventful postoperative course; well at follow-up

Comments

▸ Occult presentation of a mechanical complication of a past silent myocardial infarction. The abnormal lateral wall contour on the chest radiograph led to echocardiography and the diagnosis.
▸ Lateral wall infarction is less apparent on many forms of testing. The ECG, to its credit, did show an abnormal Q wave in aVL.
▸ The repair of the false aneurysm was technically simple because the infarction was chronic (old) and the myocardium was well fibrosed and easy to sew together.

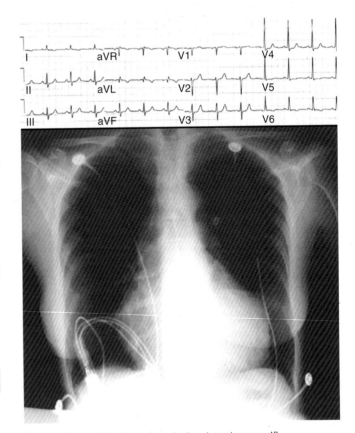

Figure 8-8. TOP, ECG shows sinus rhythm, lateral nonspecific repolarization abnormalities (V_4-V_6, I, aVL), significant Q in aVL. BOTTOM, Chest radiograph shows mildly increased cardiopericardial silhouette, no heart failure. There is a lateral bulge on the mid left heart border.

‣ The murmur at presentation, thought to be due to mitral regurgitation (which was not present on echocardiography or catheterization), was probably systolic flow into the false aneurysm. Ironically, there was postoperative mild mitral regurgitation; the repair of the lateral false aneurysm resulted in some misalignment of the infarcted anterolateral papillary muscle and mild mitral regurgitation.

‣ The diagnosis was achieved by echocardiography, by catheterization, and by surgery.
‣ The post–myocardial infarction residual systolic function was nearly normal; hence, the postoperative functional capacity was normal.

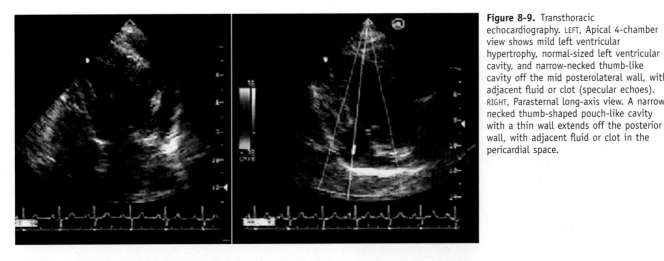

Figure 8-9. Transthoracic echocardiography. LEFT, Apical 4-chamber view shows mild left ventricular hypertrophy, normal-sized left ventricular cavity, and narrow-necked thumb-like cavity off the mid posterolateral wall, with adjacent fluid or clot (specular echoes). RIGHT, Parasternal long-axis view. A narrow-necked thumb-shaped pouch-like cavity with a thin wall extends off the posterior wall, with adjacent fluid or clot in the pericardial space.

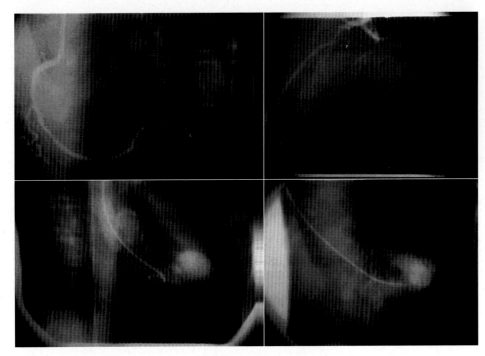

Figure 8-10. TOP LEFT, Right coronary angiography shows dominant and only minor distal disease. TOP RIGHT, Left coronary angiography shows minor disease of the left anterior descending coronary artery and minor disease of the left circumflex artery. There is uncertainty as to the paucity of marginal branches. BOTTOM LEFT, Contrast ventriculography (RAO projection) shows localized saccular outpouching from the mid left ventricular lateral wall, dyskinetic. No staining of contrast material into the pericardial space. BOTTOM RIGHT, Contrast ventriculography (LAO projection) shows localized saccular outpouching originating from the mid left ventricular lateral wall, dyskinetic.

CASE 2

History

‣ 60-year-old woman accepted in transfer with an acutely ischemic left leg
‣ 2-year history of left leg claudication
‣ The night before leg pain developed, she had several hours of nausea and vomiting.
‣ No history of chest pain or shortness of breath

‣ Past medical history is significant for hypertension and smoking (60 pack-years).

Physical Examination

‣ Shocky appearing (gray and cool); BP 60/– mm Hg
‣ Venous distention to the angle of the jaw
‣ Quiet heart sounds; no gallops, rubs, or murmurs
‣ Cold left leg
‣ pH 7.0, CK 1200

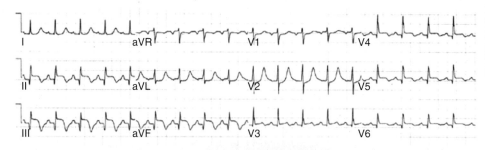

Figure 8-11. ECG shows sinus tachycardia, inferior Q waves and ST elevation, and early precordial R-wave transition: Possible posterior Q waves. ST elevation also in V_5-V_6, suggestive of acute inferior ± posterior infarction or pericarditis.

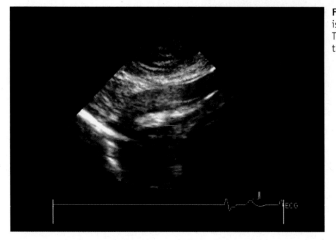

Figure 8-12. Transthoracic echocardiography, subcostal long-axis view. There is speckled soft tissue in the pericardial space consistent with blood clot. The right-sided heart cavities are very small, consistent with compression by the thrombus.

Initial Impression and Management

‣ Cause of leg ischemia was unclear, whether in situ leg arterial thrombosis secondary to shock (low flow), embolism from left ventricular mural thrombosis secondary to acute myocardial infarction (less likely with inferior myocardial infarction), embolism from undocumented atrial fibrillation, or embolism from the aorta.

‣ Shock was most likely due to acute inferior myocardial infarction complicated by right ventricular infarction (elevated neck veins) and acidosis from leg ischemia and shock.

‣ The infarct was managed medically, without fibrinolytics, because the leg required urgent operation.

‣ The leg was salvaged by femoral thromboembolectomy.

‣ Surprisingly, the hemodynamics tolerated the operation without particular problem.

‣ The blood pressure normalized within 12 hours, and shock indices normalized. It was believed that the right ventricular infarction was the dominant problem, aggravated by the acidosis.

‣ After a period of 12 stable hours, the urine output fell despite normal blood pressure; a pulmonary artery (PA) catheter was inserted to exclude treatable problems, such as hypovolemia.

‣ PA catheter insertion was difficult and prolonged and required multiple punctures. By the time the line was inserted, the blood pressure was then 70/40 mm Hg. The neck veins were again distended; there were no rubs or murmurs.

‣ PA catheter–derived hemodynamics: CVP, 34 mm Hg; PAP, 47/30 mm Hg; CI, 2.2 L/min/m² (on inotropes again); PCWP, 32 mm Hg

‣ Marked elevation and "equilibration" of diastolic pressures

‣ Scenarios considered included post–myocardial infarction rupture causing tamponade, tamponade due to other cause (such as the heparin given for the ischemic leg and possibility of thromboembolism), and reinfarction.

Subsequent Impression, Management, and Evolution

‣ Compression of the heart from blood clot; cause was unclear, whether post–myocardial infarction rupture or other cause

‣ Large thrombi complicating aortic atheroma may have been the source of the initial leg ischemia.

‣ Avoidance of IABP for blood pressure resuscitation, given the aortic thrombosis

‣ Surgical inspection of the heart and evacuation of blood clot

‣ Rather than postinfarction rupture of the heart, two punctures of the superior vena cava (SVC) from the central line were the source of bleeding and were easily sewn up.

‣ The postoperative course was uneventful.

‣ The patient refused coronary angiography.

‣ Stress testing showed only a fixed defect of the inferior wall.

‣ Seen in follow-up 2 months later, she was without angina but with NYHA class II heart failure symptoms.

Eventual Diagnosis, Management, and Outcome

‣ False aneurysm formation of the posterolateral wall

‣ The patient declined surgical repair.

‣ The blood pressure was tightly controlled, and physical exertion was curtailed to lessen risk of rupture.

‣ She survived 8 months with few symptoms, then died suddenly. No autopsy was performed.

Comments

‣ The definitive cause of leg ischemia was never established; thromboembolism from the aorta was a possibility.

‣ The right ventricular involvement by the initial inferior infarction was probably the dominant cause of shock.

‣ The low output of cardiogenic shock may have allowed simultaneous thrombosis of the heavily atherosclerotic aorta and of the femoral arteries.

‣ What was initially believed to be post–myocardial infarction rupture or tamponade was iatrogenic.

‣ Later, she developed a false aneurysm and may have eventually experienced rupture as the cause of sudden death.

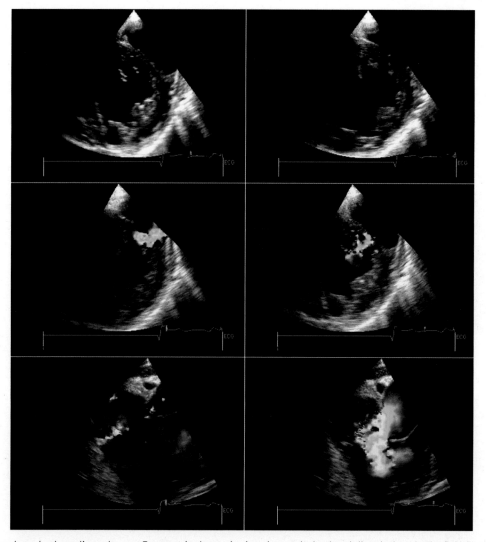

Figure 8-13. Transesophageal echocardiography. TOP, Transgastric short-axis views in systole (LEFT) and diastole (RIGHT). The fluid-filled cavity is seen between the 12-o'clock and 2-o'clock positions; it bulges prominently in systole. The neck or passageway into the cavity is seen, as is the complex breakdown of myocardium in the area. There is no pericardial fluid seen elsewhere. MIDDLE, Transgastric short-axis views with color Doppler study in diastole (LEFT) and systole (RIGHT) show systolic flow into and diastolic flow out of the false aneurysm through the narrow neck. BOTTOM, Oblique views (oriented to the lower left aspect of the heart) in systole (LEFT) and diastole (RIGHT). In systole, flow enters the saccular cavity beside the heart; in diastole, flow returns into the heart from the cavity.

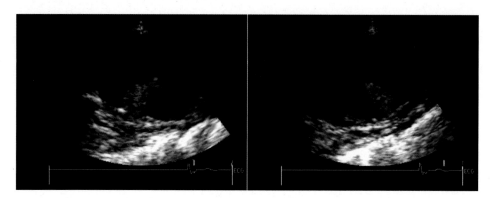

Figure 8-14. Transesophageal echocardiography. LEFT, Horizontal plane view of the distal aortic arch. There is a large and mobile protruding thrombus overlying a complex-appearing plaque. RIGHT, Vertical plane view of the distal aortic arch again shows the same large and mobile protruding thrombus overlying a complex-appearing plaque.

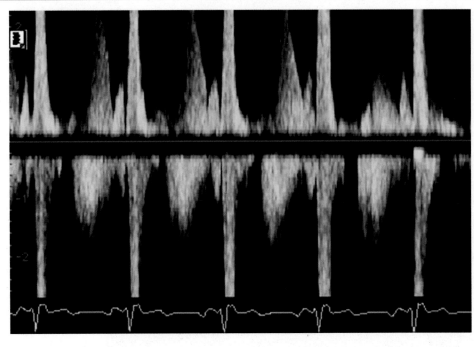

Figure 8-15. Transesophageal echocardiography spectral Doppler evaluation of flow into and out of the false aneurysm shows reciprocating or to-and-fro flow.

CASE 3

History

▸ 74-year-old man admitted with "pneumonia"
▸ Appearance of dementia and bipolar disorder
▸ No history obtainable from the patient
▸ Heavy smoker, hypertensive

Physical Examination

▸ BP 105/65 mm Hg, no pulsus paradoxus, HR 80 bpm, RR 15/min
▸ Difficult to keep calm in bed, incessantly restless (psychiatric issues)
▸ Venous distention, no edema
▸ Normal heart sounds; no gallops, rubs, or murmurs
▸ Normal troponins, CK

Impression, Management, and Outcome

▸ False aneurysm of the lateral wall, with leakage into the pericardial space; subacute rupture

▸ Prior silent lateral wall infarction in a demented patient
▸ Surgery was considered but not undertaken because of the advanced dementia. Conservative measures were undertaken.
▸ During 10 days, the false aneurysm leaked and the pericardial effusion enlarged, and tamponade developed and progressed.
▸ The patient died comfortably.

Comments

▸ The date of the infarction could never be determined, and the infarct was not represented electrocardiographically.
▸ The post–myocardial infarction false aneurysm ran the expected course (completion of rupture or evolution into tamponade).
▸ Lateral wall location (the most common), diagnosed by echocardiography
▸ There was an interval between infarction and false aneurysm, and false aneurysm leakage and death.
▸ Association of in-hospital exertion (due to psychiatric disease) and post–myocardial infarction myocardial rupture

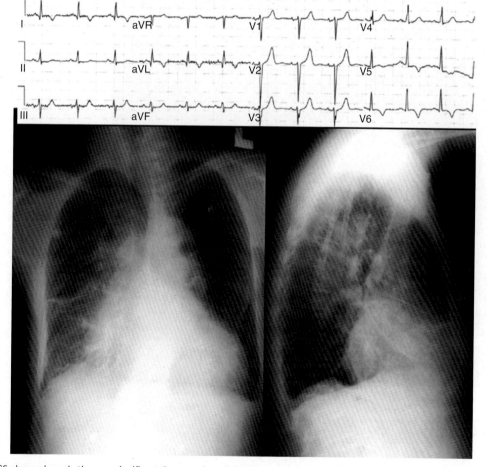

Figure 8-16. TOP, ECG shows sinus rhythm, no significant Q waves, lateral (V_5-V_6, I, aVL) T-wave inversions, and nonspecific repolarization abnormalities. BOTTOM, Chest radiograph shows mild cardiomegaly, left ventricle enlargement (rule of Rigler), and mild interstitial pulmonary edema.

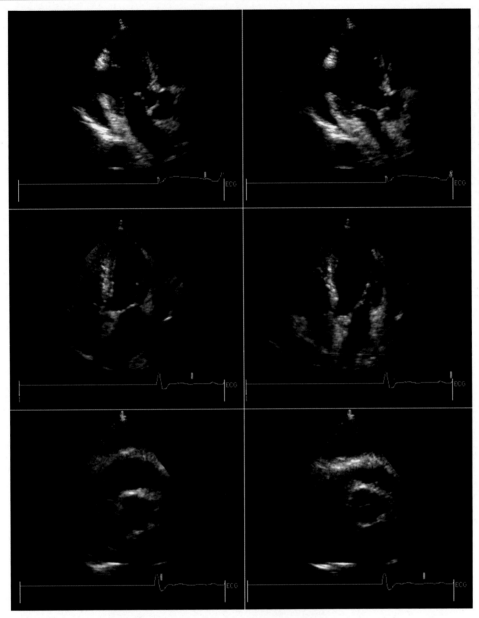

Figure 8-17. Transthoracic echocardiography. TOP, Modified apical 5-chamber views in diastole (LEFT) and systole (RIGHT) show a thumb-like extension of the left ventricular cavity into a crescent-shaped pericardial space. MIDDLE, Apical 4-chamber views in systole (LEFT) and diastole (RIGHT) show grossly normal left ventricular systolic function on this plane. There is a crescent-shaped fluid-filled cavity lateral to the mid left ventricle that appears narrowly connected to the LV cavity on the diastolic image. No right atrial inversion or right ventricle inversion on this view. BOTTOM, Parasternal short-axis views in systole (RIGHT) and diastole (LEFT) show a pericardial effusion anteriorly and to the right side of the heart. There is right atrial systolic inversion but no right ventricular or right ventricular outflow tract diastolic inversion.

CASE 4

History

▸ A 64-year-old man 6 weeks after infarction was seen for complaints of fatigue, episodes of atypical sharp epigastric pains, episodes of nausea and vomiting, and typical angina of effort (CCS class II). No heart failure symptoms.
▸ Details of previous infarction sketchy: it was apparently a non-STEMI with "5 cardiac arrests"; early post–myocardial infarction pericarditis, treated with NSAIDs; a gastroenterologist believed that the nausea was due to an ulcer from the NSAIDs.
▸ An echocardiogram unexpectedly showed myocardial rupture.

Physical Examination

▸ BP 110/80 mm Hg, no pulsus paradoxus, HR 80 bpm, RR 15/min
▸ Alert, well appearing; no venous distention, edema, or rub
▸ S_1, S_2 normal; S_4 present; apex diffusely enlarged
▸ Definite to-and-fro murmur at the apex

Impression, Management, and Outcome

▸ False aneurysm of the lateral wall
▸ Subacute rupture accounting for recurrent pericarditis; fluid or clot over the right ventricular outflow tract (away from the false aneurysm itself)
▸ Cardiac surgery for patch closure
▸ Findings at surgery: inflamed pericardium, clot over right ventricular outflow tract, large lateral false aneurysm, fibrosed (chronically infarcted) anterolateral papillary muscle
▸ Uneventful postoperative course
▸ Well at follow-up; mild M wave persists, CCS class I, NYHA class I

Comments

▸ Anatomically typical of a false aneurysm: narrow neck, wide body, location off the lateral wall
▸ Subacute rupture (clot elsewhere in the pericardial space)

8

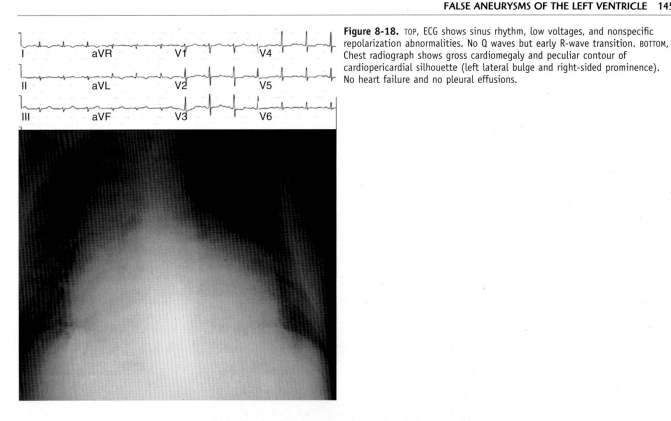

Figure 8-18. TOP, ECG shows sinus rhythm, low voltages, and nonspecific repolarization abnormalities. No Q waves but early R-wave transition. BOTTOM, Chest radiograph shows gross cardiomegaly and peculiar contour of cardiopericardial silhouette (left lateral bulge and right-sided prominence). No heart failure and no pleural effusions.

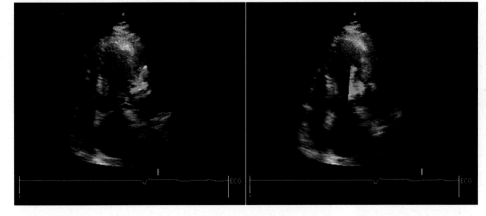

Figure 8-19. Transthoracic echocardiography in systole (LEFT) and diastole (RIGHT). There is flow in systole into and out of the cavity in diastole beside the LV, through a narrow channel. There is flow in systole into the cavity beside the LV and flow in diastole out of the cavity back into the LV. The flow that enters and exits the cavity does so through a narrow neck.

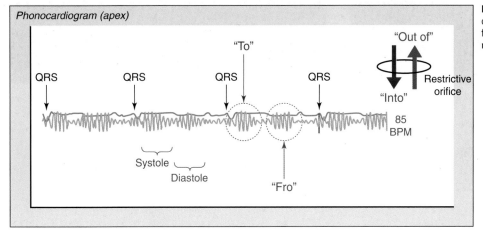

Figure 8-20. Phonocardiogram (recorded on an echo machine) shows to-and-fro flow reciprocating into and out of the restrictive orifice of the false aneurysm.

▸ History notable for recurrent pericarditis symptoms, episodes of feeling unwell, and nausea and vomiting, which may have been manifestations of subacute rupture

▸ Interestingly, no Q waves on the ECG (ECG lacks sensitivity to the lateral wall, as many tests do)

▸ The chest radiograph was so obviously abnormal that either it or the physical diagnosis findings might have led to an earlier consideration of a complication of infarction.

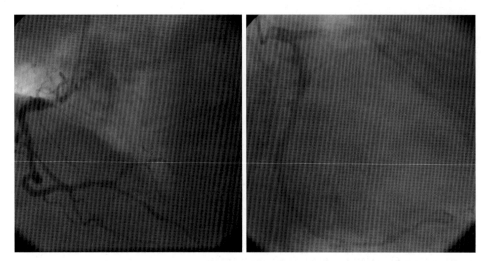

Figure 8-21. LEFT, Right coronary angiogram shows dominant right coronary artery and disease in the acute marginal branch. RIGHT, Left coronary angiogram shows mild to moderate disease of the left anterior descending coronary artery. LCx: missing first obtuse marginal.

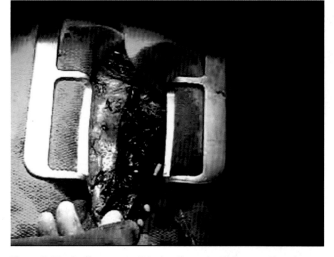

Figure 8-22. Cardiac surgery. Entering the pericardial space, there is thrombus anteriorly.

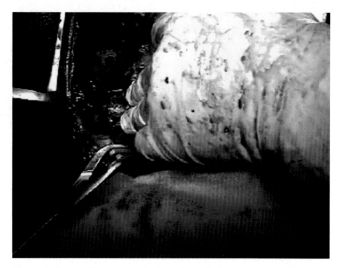

Figure 8-23. Cardiac surgery. Looking through the now opened false aneurysm, the hole (neck) of the false aneurysm is seen.

CASE 5

History

- 78-year-old man referred for angiography after infarction
- Past medical history is significant for long-standing hypertension.
- Recent anterior non-STEMI, old inferior STEMI
- Various pains since the recent myocardial infarction, some typical of angina, some atypical; occasional nausea, no vomiting

Physical Examination

- BP 155/95 mm Hg, HR 70 bpm
- No venous distention, no edema
- Normal S_1, S_2; no gallops, rubs, or murmurs
- Chest clear

Impression, Management, and Outcome

- Postinfarction false aneurysm of the posterior wall (>12 months old); subacute rupture

- Surgical (patch) repair; 3-vessel aortocoronary bypass was performed
- Surgical findings: well-scarred inferoposterior infarction, posterior false aneurysm, and a clot elsewhere in the pericardium
- Slow but uneventful postoperative course
- Well at follow-up 3 years later

Comments

- False aneurysm with subacute rupture
- Unanticipated "serendipitous" incidental diagnosis
- Very poorly seen by transthoracic echocardiography; false aneurysm and pericardial fluid both seen fairly well by transesophageal echocardiography
- False aneurysm was best seen by catheterization, which did not detect pericardial fluid
- Successful surgical repair

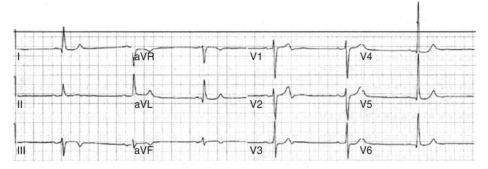

Figure 8-24. ECG shows sinus bradycardia, left ventricular hypertrophy, no Q waves, and inferior repolarization abnormalities.

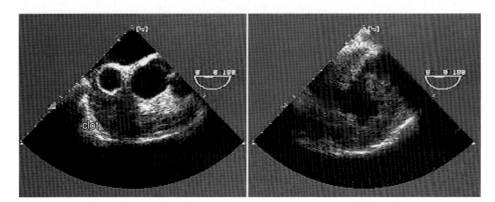

Figure 8-25. Transesophageal echocardiography. LEFT, Horizontal plane view at the level of the SVC entering the heart; there is intrapericardial clot. RIGHT, Transgastric short-axis view shows an intrapericardial clot around the SVC and aortic root (specular echoes within the pericardial space). Communication of the LV cavity with a space inferolaterally to the LV is revealed.

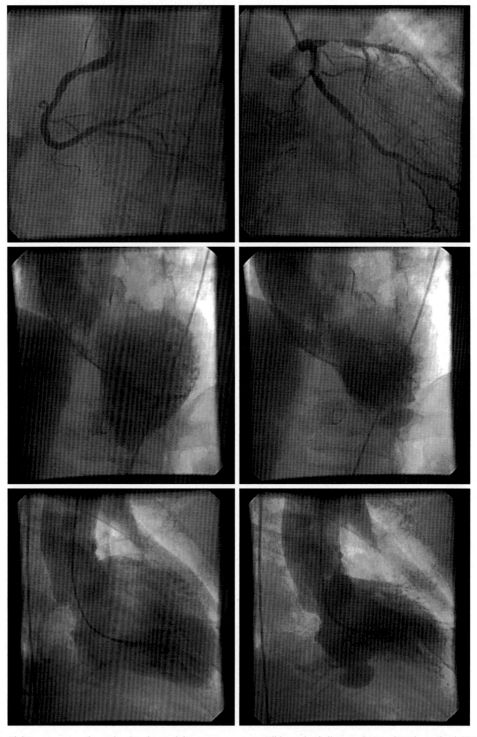

Figure 8-26. TOP LEFT, Right coronary angiography. Dominant right coronary artery. Mild proximal disease. Severe (90%) proximal PDA, moderate 50% distal RCA, severe posterolateral branch disease. TOP RIGHT, Left coronary angiography. Left anterior descending coronary artery: proximal 90%, mid 60%, severe distal disease. LCx: 50% OM1. MIDDLE IMAGES, Contrast ventriculography, left anterior oblique projection in diastole (LEFT) and systole (RIGHT). Akinetic inferior and posterior walls. A small narrow-necked cavity distends inferior to the LV in systole. BOTTOM IMAGES, Contrast ventriculography, right anterior oblique projection in diastole (LEFT) and systole (RIGHT). A small narrow-necked cavity bulges in systole.

CASE 6

History

▸ 78-year-old man was referred because of a new apical murmur; no change in usual symptoms
▸ Suffered anterior infarction 4 years before (late-presentation STEMI, post-infarction ventricular septal defect that was repaired)
▸ Usually NYHA class II congestive heart failure, CCS class I angina
▸ Past medical history is significant for hypertension and permanent pacemaker.

Physical Examination

▸ BP 100/60 mm Hg, HR 90 bpm
▸ No venous distention, no edema
▸ Diffusely enlarged and sustained apex, mesoapical impulse
▸ Apical 3/6 holosystolic murmur, no thrill; apical decrescendo diastolic murmur?
▸ Normal S_1, S_2; no gallops or rubs
▸ Clear chest

Impression, Management, and Outcome

▸ Late development of a false aneurysm at the left ventricular apex. It was unclear whether the partition of the false aneurysm from the true cavity of the left ventricle represented myocardium or patch material or both.
▸ The previous surgery surely had some influence on the findings, given that the cavity margins probably were retained by pericardial adhesions from the prior surgery.
▸ No signs of subacute rupture (clot or fluid elsewhere in the pericardium)
▸ Surgical (patch) repair was considered, but given the age and general weakness of the patient, conservative nonsurgical management was undertaken.
▸ The patient lived 2 more years.

Comments

▸ Asymptomatic development of a false aneurysm
▸ Complex anatomy, given the prior ventricular septal defect and surgical patching
▸ In his lifetime after infarction, the patient had experienced two forms of rupture (ventricular septal defect and false aneurysm) and two forms of aneurysms (well-formed true aneurysm of the left ventricle and false aneurysm).
▸ Visualization of the morphologic features was suboptimal with the imaging available at the time, and the angiography and echocardiography were more complementary than similar.
▸ Survival for years without surgery

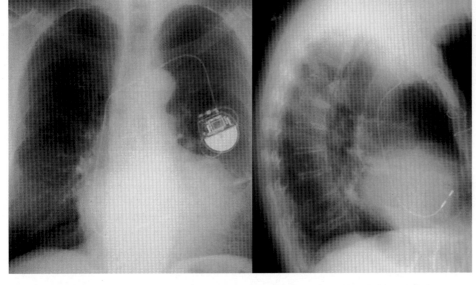

Figure 8-27. Chest radiographs show cardiomegaly, mild heart failure (vascular redistribution and interstitial edema), pacer wire, and abnormal left lateral heart bulge and contour.

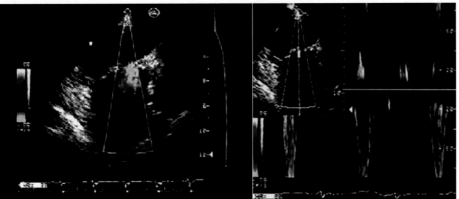

Figure 8-28. Transthoracic echocardiography. Shortened apical 4-chamber views with color Doppler study show restricted flow into and out of the apical cavity, more consistent with a false aneurysm than a true aneurysm.

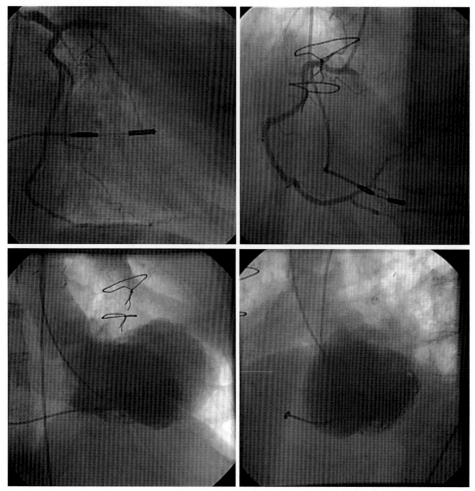

Figure 8-29. TOP LEFT, Right coronary angiography shows codominant right coronary artery and no significant disease. TOP RIGHT, Left coronary angiography. LMCA: 30%. Left anterior descending coronary artery: occluded after first septal. LCx: codominant; no significant disease. BOTTOM LEFT, Contrast ventriculography. RAO projection shows aneurysm of the anterior wall and septum. BOTTOM RIGHT, LAO ventriculogram shows aneurysm of the septum.

CASE 7

History

▸ 82-year-old woman admitted with 7 hours of pressure-like central chest pain
▸ No heart failure symptoms
▸ Past medical history is significant for hypertension.

Physical Examination

▸ BP 145/85 mm Hg, HR 70 bpm
▸ Venous distention 6 cm above the sternal angle, no edema
▸ Normal apex
▸ Normal S_1, S_2; no gallops, rubs, or murmurs
▸ Clear chest

Impression, Management, and Outcome

▸ Inferoposterior infarction complicated by small posterior left ventricular false aneurysm and probable right ventricular infarction (elevated neck veins)

▸ Surgical (patch) repair was offered, but the patient refused all testing interventions and surgery.
▸ The following week in the hospital was characterized by episodes of intermittent nonischemic chest pains of pleuritic nature, enlargement of the false aneurysm, and development of and progressive enlargement of a pericardial effusion.
▸ Tamponade developed and resulted in low-output failure. She died peacefully in her sleep.

Comments

▸ Posterior false aneurysm, detected by echocardiography
▸ Progressive enlargement and subacute rupture culminating in tamponade and death, illustrating one of the natural histories of false aneurysms (the other being sudden rupture and death)
▸ The episodes of chest pain presumably resulted from abrupt expansion of the false aneurysm, episodes of leakage into the pericardial space and pericarditis, or traction on pericardial surfaces from expansion.

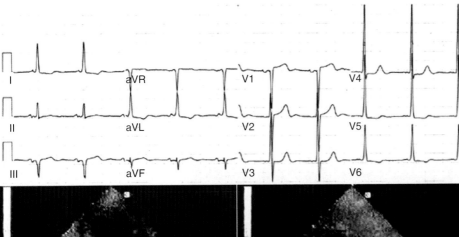

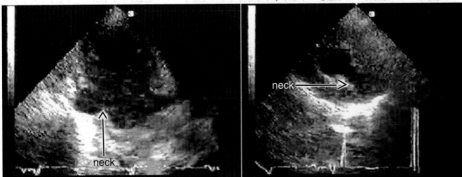

Figure 8-30. TOP, ECG shows sinus rhythm, left ventricular hypertrophy voltages, inferior Q waves (II, aVF) and ST elevation (III), and widespread nonspecific repolarization abnormalities, suggesting possible inferior infarction. BOTTOM, Transthoracic echocardiography. On the apical 2-chamber view, one sees a normally contracting anterior wall, mid posterior wall akinesis, and basal posterior dyskinesis. There is a 2-cm localized, dyskinetic cavity with a long narrow neck arising from the posterior wall.

CASE 8

History

▸ A frail 62-year-old man presented with atypical chest pains, but troponins were positive.
▸ Past medical history is significant for renal failure, hypertension, permanent pacemaker, aortocoronary bypass 14 years before, and prior infarction.
▸ Many medical complications of renal failure

Physical Examination

▸ BP 155/75 mm Hg, HR 60 bpm
▸ No venous distention, no edema
▸ Enlarged apex
▸ Split S_1, S_2; no gallops, murmurs, or rubs
▸ Chest: bibasilar crepitations

Impression, Management, and Outcome

▸ Posterolateral false aneurysm
▸ The date of the responsible infarction was unclear.
▸ Surgical (patch) repair was considered, but given the age of the patient and many comorbidities, conservative nonsurgical management was undertaken.
▸ The patient lived 7 more weeks before dying suddenly.

Comments

▸ Posterolateral false aneurysm in the most common location
▸ Silent infarction underlies the false aneurysm
▸ Background of hypertension
▸ Some of the chest pains may have been ischemic (elevated troponins), but most were probably pericardial in origin and due to traction on the pericardium by the enlarging false aneurysm.

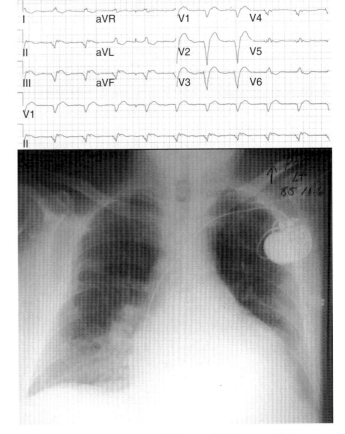

Figure 8-31. TOP, ECG shows ventricular-paced rhythm, essentially impossible to interpret with respect to infarction. BOTTOM, Chest radiograph shows cardiomegaly, interstitial pulmonary edema, and a pacemaker.

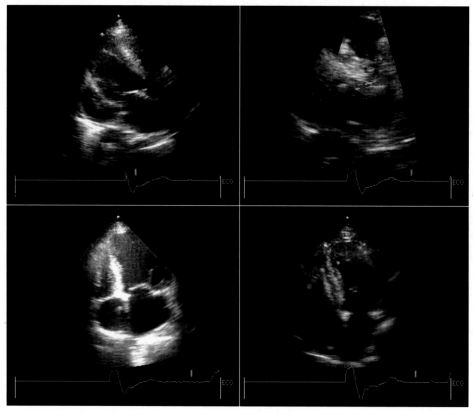

Figure 8-32. Transthoracic echocardiography. There is a fluid-filled cavity within the pericardial space adjacent to the basal posterolateral walls. The posterior wall between the fluid-filled collection and the LV cavity is dyskinetic and seen to be disarticulated on 2-dimensional imaging. There was flow apparent by color Doppler mapping (RIGHT UPPER IMAGE), through a small serpiginous channel into the cavity in systole and out of it in diastole. There is no pericardial effusion elsewhere.

CASE 9

History

▸ 78-year-old woman presented with a transient neurologic event (visual disturbance)
▸ Twelve weeks before, she had experienced a prolonged episode of chest pain.
▸ She had undergone aortocoronary bypass surgery 6 years before (no available details).

Physical Examination

▸ BP 105/70 mm Hg, HR 90 bpm, regular, venous pressure elevated with a visible V wave
▸ No edema
▸ Low pulse volumes, normal upstroke
▸ Visible and readily palpable mid-precordial systolic impulse
▸ 3/6 pansystolic murmur at the apex with axillary radiation, S_3

Impression and Outcome

▸ Probable postinfarction false aneurysm
▸ Patient refused further investigation and surgical repair

Comments

▸ In this location, it is difficult to distinguish a false aneurysm from a true aneurysm on the basis of morphologic features (neck width alone). The appearance of posterior myocardial wall disruption on the echo images added to the case that this was a false aneurysm.
▸ Pericardial adhesions from the prior bypass operation had presumably contained the false aneurysm.
▸ Heart failure state from the LV dysfunction from the recent infarction and large noncontractile (dyskinetic) false aneurysm and mitral insufficiency
▸ Mitral valve dysfunction due to severe regional distortion from the presumed false aneurysm
▸ Surgical repair may have had to entail replacement of the mitral valve.

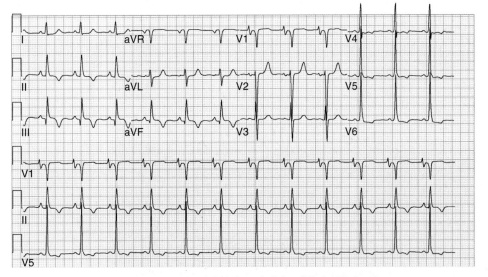

Figure 8-33. ECG shows sinus rhythm, atrial hypertrophy, Q waves inferiorly, and slighter inferior ST elevation.

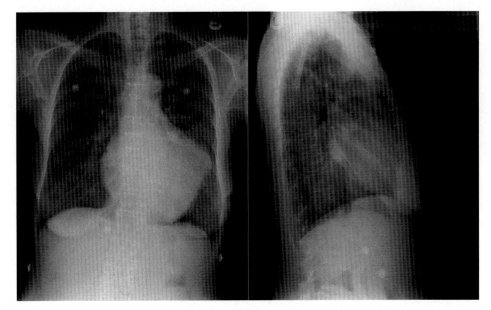

Figure 8-34. Chest radiographs. There is a conspicuous bulge along the left heart border.

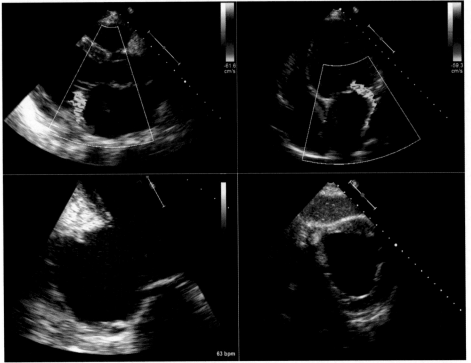

Figure 8-35. Transthoracic echocardiography. TOP LEFT, Parasternal long-axis view. The left-sided heart cavities are enlarged. There is posteriorly directed mitral insufficiency. The posterior wall was akinetic and the overall ventricular function moderately to severely depressed. TOP RIGHT, The mitral insufficiency is also laterally directed, and there is tricuspid insufficiency. Again, the left-sided chambers are dilated. BOTTOM LEFT, Zoom view of the basal posterior wall between the papillary muscle and the mitral annulus. There is a large saccular outpouching of the left ventricular cavity with mural thrombus. The myocardium of the posterior wall appears discontinuous. BOTTOM RIGHT, Subcostal cross-sectional view across the suspected false aneurysm. The mural thrombus is concentric. The diameter is approximately 9 cm.

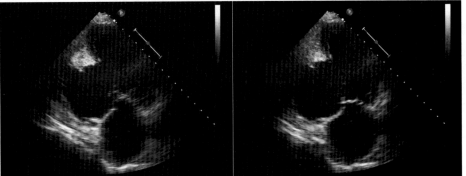

Figure 8-36. Transthoracic echocardiography. Apical 2-chamber view. There is systolic bulging of the suspected false aneurysm and what appear to be tissue strands extending off the myocardial neck.

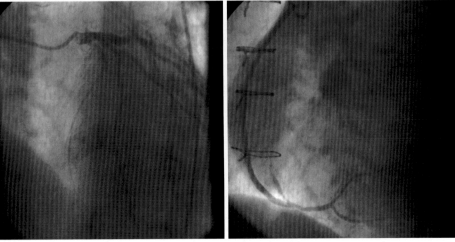

Figure 8-37. Selective coronary angiography. LEFT, LCA injection. No stenoses in the LAD or its branches. RIGHT, RCA injection reveals distal disease and distal vessels of small caliber. There is retrograde filling of a vein graft to the right coronary artery.

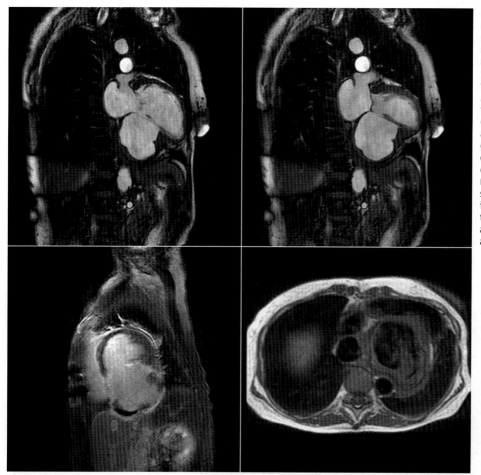

Figure 8-38. Cardiac MR. TOP IMAGES, SSFP sequences in diastole (LEFT) and systole (RIGHT). There is systolic bulging of the suspected false aneurysm, a narrow neck and wide body, and mural thrombus; the posteromedial papillary muscle appears tensely stretched over the false aneurysm. Although the myocardium is well seen and the pericardium is somewhat seen, it is not clear whether the myocardium is disrupted at the neck. BOTTOM LEFT, Inversion recovery gadolinium enhancement showing delayed enhancement through the wall of the cavity consistent with prior infarction. BOTTOM RIGHT, T1-weighted black blood sequences. The wall of the false aneurysm is better seen, as is its distinction from the mural thrombus. There is low-flow artifact within the cavity of the false aneurysm.

CASE 10

History

▸ 77-year-old man presented feeling "unwell"
▸ Past medical history is significant for hypertension and type 2 diabetes mellitus.

Physical Examination

▸ BP 100/60 mm Hg, HR 70 bpm
▸ Clear chest
▸ Normal venous pressures
▸ 3/6 apical pansystolic murmur with radiation to the axilla
▸ No gallops or pericardial rub

Management and Outcome

▸ Suspected false aneurysm
▸ Referred for surgical repair and bypass

▸ Surgery revealed a mid-basal posterolateral false aneurysm with a large volume of thrombus in it.
▸ In-hospital recovery was slow because of heart failure but eventually successful.

Comments

▸ The only murmur was of mitral insufficiency. The flow into the false aneurysm was inaudible in proximity to the mitral insufficiency. The flow out of the false aneurysm was inaudible, presumably owing to the velocity.
▸ The extent of LV dysfunction was relevant to the postoperative and postdischarge course.
▸ The responsible vessel for the lateral wall infarction was probably the large diseased obtuse marginal branch.

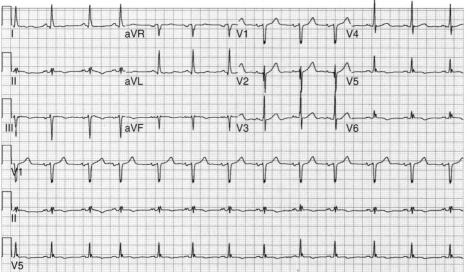

Figure 8-39. ECG shows sinus rhythm. Diffusely abnormal repolarization, including nonsignificant ST elevation in V_5 and V_6.

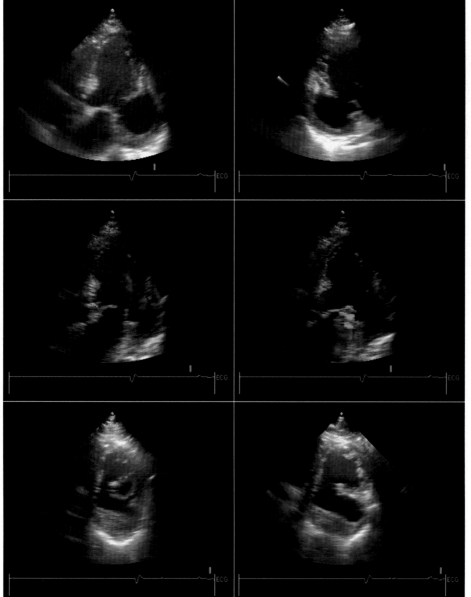

Figure 8-40. Transthoracic echocardiography. TOP LEFT, Apical 4-chamber view. There is a narrow-necked cavity arising off the basal LV wall that contains mural thrombus. TOP RIGHT, Off-plane apical 3-chamber view. The very narrow neck to the cavity is again seen. The tissue over the cavity is not papillary muscle, which is nearly off the plane of imaging. MIDDLE LEFT, There is low-velocity flow swirling out of the cavity in diastole back into the LV (note the AI). MIDDLE RIGHT, Mitral insufficiency is present. The flow into the cavity is low velocity. BOTTOM LEFT, Basal parasternal short-axis image. There is aneurysmal–false aneurysmal extension of the LV cavity posteriorly, containing a large amount of mural thrombus. BOTTOM RIGHT, Mid parasternal short-axis image. The same aneurysmal–false aneurysmal extension of the LV cavity posteriorly is seen, with a disrupted shelf of the posterior wall contributing to the narrow neck.

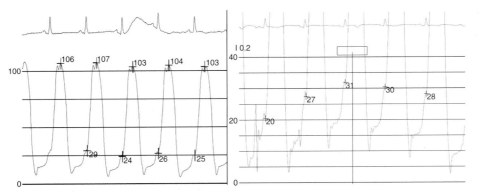

Figure 8-41. The LV systolic pressure is low, and the post–A wave end-diastolic pressure is increased, consistent with reduced LV compliance.

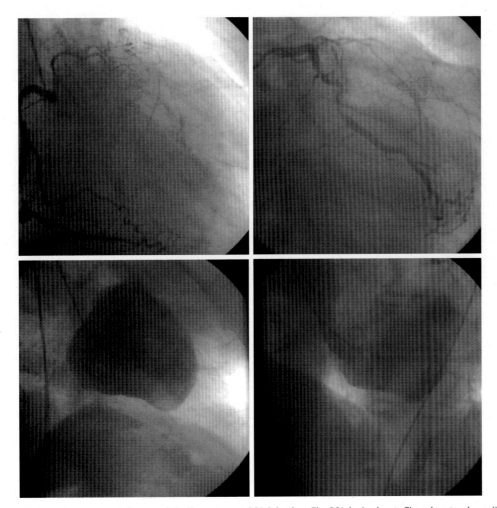

Figure 8-42. Coronary angiography. TOP IMAGES, Coronary injection. TOP LEFT, RCA injection. The RCA is dominant. There is extensive collateralization to the LAD. TOP RIGHT, LCA injection. The LAD is occluded. There is a large and significantly stenosed obtuse marginal branch. BOTTOM IMAGES, RAO (LEFT) and LAO (RIGHT) contrast ventriculography. There is severe left ventricular systolic dysfunction. On the LAO view, it is apparent that there is a bulge on the basal lateral aspect of the heart. The neck is not well seen.

References

1. Vlodaver Z, Coe JI, Edwards JE: True and false left ventricular aneurysms. Propensity for the altter to rupture. Circulation 1975;51:567-572.

2. Jiang C, Zhao R, Yang X: Six-year follow-up of a left ventricular pseudoaneurysm without surgical repair. Can J Cardiol 2007;23:739-741.

3. Butany J, Dias B, Grapa J, et al: Left ventricular pseudoaneurysm. Can J Cardiol 2002;18:1122-1123.

4. Goudevenos J, Parry G, Morritt GN: Subacute rupture of a pseudoaneurysm formed by late rupture of a true left ventricular aneurysm. Br Heart J 1989;62:225-227.

5. Coupe M, Dancy M, Pepper J: Coincidence of true and false left ventricular aneurysms after myocardial infarction. Br Heart J 1986;56:567-568.

6. Frances C, Romero A, Grady D: Left ventricular pseudoaneurysm. J Am Coll Cardiol 1998;32:557-561.

7. Gueron M, Wanderman KL, Hirsch M, Borman J: Pseudoaneurysm of the left ventricle after myocardial infarction: a curable form of myocardial rupture. J Thorac Cardiovasc Surg 1975;69:736-742.

8. Paul JF, Mace L, Caussin C, et al: Multirow detector computed tomography assessment of intraseptal dissection and ventricular pseudoaneurysm in postinfarction ventricular septal defect. Circulation 2001;104:497-498.

9. Hamilton K, Ellenbogen K, Lowe JE, Kisslo J: Ultrasound diagnosis of pseudoaneurysm and contiguous ventricular septal defect complicating inferior myocardial infarction. J Am Coll Cardiol 1985;6:1160-1163.

10. Stoddard MF, Dawkins PR, Longaker RA, et al: Transesophageal echocardiography in the detection of left ventricular pseudoaneurysm. Am Heart J 1993;125(pt 1):534-539.

11. Saner HE, Asinger RW, Daniel JA, Olson J: Two-dimensional echocardiographic identification of left ventricular pseudoaneurysm. Am Heart J 1986;112:977-985.

12. Burns CA, Paulsen W, Arrowood JA, et al: Improved identification of posterior left ventricular pseudoaneurysms by transesophageal echocardiography. Am Heart J 1992;124:796-799.

13. Esakof DD, Vannan MA, Pandian NG, et al: Visualization of left ventricular pseudoaneurysm with panoramic transesophageal echocardiography. J Am Soc Echocardiogr 1994;7:174-178.

14. Roelandt JR, Sutherland GR, Yoshida K, Yoshikawa J: Improved diagnosis and characterization of left ventricular pseudoaneurysm by Doppler color flow imaging. J Am Coll Cardiol 1988;12:807-811.

15. Spindola-Franco H, Kronacher N: Pseudoaneurysm of the left ventricle. Radiographic and angiocardiographic diagnosis. Radiology 1978;127:29-34.

16. Duvernoy O, Wikstrom G, Mannting F, et al: Pre- and postoperative CT and MR in pseudoaneurysms of the heart. J Comput Assist Tomogr 1992;16:401-409.

17. Hsu YH, Chiu IS, Chien CT: Left ventricular pseudoaneurysm diagnosed by magnetic resonance imaging in a nine-year-old boy. Pediatr Cardiol 1993;14:187-190.

18. Harrity P, Patel A, Bianco J, Subramanian R: Improved diagnosis and characterization of postinfarction left ventricular pseudoaneurysm by cardiac magnetic resonance imaging. Clin Cardiol 1991;14:603-606.

19. March KL, Sawada SG, Tarver RD, et al: Current concepts of left ventricular pseudoaneurysm: pathophysiology, therapy, and diagnostic imaging methods. Clin Cardiol 1989;12:531-540.

20. Rogers JH, De Oliveira NC, Damiano RJ Jr, Rogers JG: Images in cardiovascular medicine. Left ventricular apical pseudoaneurysm: echocardiographic and intraoperative findings. Circulation 2002;105:e51-e52.

21. Catherwood E, Mintz GS, Kotler MN, et al: Two-dimensional echocardiographic recognition of left ventricular pseudoaneurysm. Circulation 1980;62:294-303.

22. Lascault G, Reeves F, Drobinski G: Evidence of the inaccuracy of standard echocardiographic and angiographic criteria used for the recognition of true and "false" left ventricular inferior aneurysms. Br Heart J 1988;60:125-127.

23. DePace NL, Dowinsky S, Untereker W, et al: Giant inferior wall left ventricular aneurysm. Am Heart J 1990;119(pt 1):400-402.

24. Crenshaw BS, Granger CB, Birnbaum Y, et al: Risk factors, angiographic patterns, and outcomes in patients with ventricular septal defect complicating acute myocardial infarction. GUSTO-I (Global Utilization of Streptokinase and TPA for Occluded Coronary Arteries) Trial Investigators. Circulation 2000;101:27-32.

25. Kishon Y, Iqbal A, Oh JK, et al: Evolution of echocardiographic modalities in detection of postmyocardial infarction ventricular septal defect and papillary muscle rupture: study of 62 patients. Am Heart J 1993;126(pt 1):667-675.

26. Figueras J, Cortadellas J, Calvo F, Soler-Soler J: Relevance of delayed hospital admission on development of cardiac rupture during acute myocardial infarction: study in 225 patients with free wall, septal or papillary muscle rupture. J Am Coll Cardiol 1998;32:135-139.

27. Edwards BS, Edwards WD, Edwards JE: Ventricular septal rupture complicating acute myocardial infarction: identification of simple and complex types in 53 autopsied hearts. Am J Cardiol 1984;54:1201-1205.

28. Brown SL, Gropler RJ, Harris KM: Distinguishing left ventricular aneurysm from pseudoaneurysm. A review of the literature. Chest 1997;111:1403-1409.

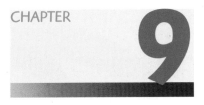

Incomplete Rupture: Intramyocardial Hematoma, Myocardial Dissection, and Subepicardial Hematoma

Postinfarction intramural hematoma is a form of incomplete myocardial rupture into but not through the necrotic myocardial wall. As the pocket communicates with the left ventricular lumen, it is pressurized and distended, and it is prone to further dissection (myocardial dissection).[1,2] Blood within it may re-enter the left ventricle through the communication in diastole; or it may flow out of it into the pericardial space, causing an effusion or tamponade; or it may flow out of it into the right ventricle, conferring septal rupture physiology.[3,4] The pocket, being within the myocardium, is not visible from the outside. It may bulge prominently into the left ventricular cavity when it is pressurized in diastole (Fig. 9-1).[5]

The incidence of postinfarction intramyocardial hematoma is unknown. The natural history is believed to be progression to rupture through the free wall or into the right ventricle. Either ventricle may develop intramyocardial hematoma.[2]

Clinical presentations that have been described include atypical postinfarction chest pains, abnormal imaging findings, cardiac rupture or tamponade, and drainage into the right ventricle with septal rupture–like physiology. Reported causes of intramyocardial hematoma other than transmural infarction include trauma, pericardiocentesis (trauma), and balloon angioplasty (trauma).

Extension of the intramyocardial hematoma up to the epicardium but not extending into the pericardial space results in a similar lesion—the subepicardial hematoma or subepicardial aneurysm (misnomer), in which the outer extension of the hematoma is retained only by epicardium (Fig. 9-2). Extension beyond epicardium into the pericardial space to be restrained only by adherent pericardium is essentially a false aneurysm.[3] Complica-

tions resulting from subepicardial aneurysms are described in Table 9-1.[3]

DIAGNOSTIC TESTING

There are no comparative studies of different imaging modalities and no sufficient contemporary imaging studies to establish the optimal means to identify intramyocardial hematomas. The ideal imaging test would accurately delineate the cavity of the intramyocardial hematoma and also depict the myocardial and pericardial layers. Echocardiography and contrast ventriculography, the tests most commonly performed to assess the acutely infarcted ventricle, may reveal an intramyocardial hematoma, but neither test is ideal. Transesophageal echocardiography is likely to be superior to transthoracic echocardiography. For contrast ventriculography to depict an intramyocardial or subepicardial hematoma, the view would have to project the hematoma free of the left ventricle. Potentially, gated cardiac computed tomography and magnetic resonance (SSFP sequences) may be useful because they delineate blood pool and myocardium well.

Other conditions with luminal extension into the myocardium (left ventricular noncompaction or isolated left ventricular abnormal trabeculation) and hypertrabeculation (blood in the deeper recesses between abnormally tall trabeculations) can mimic abnormal luminal extension if the area has a wall motion abnormality (Fig. 9-3).[6]

There are generally no hemodynamic disturbances attributable directly to the intramural hematoma. The typical coronary anatomy associations are unknown.

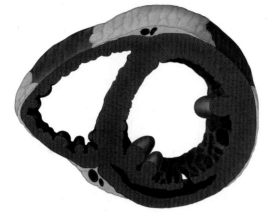

Figure 9-1. This image depicts an intramyocardial hematoma complicating a transmural inferior wall infarction. The cavity of the intramyocardial hematoma may passively bulge in systole.

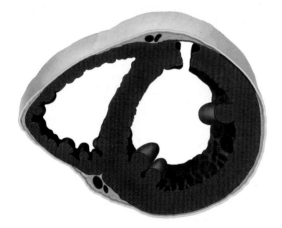

Figure 9-2. This image depicts a subepicardial hematoma complicating an anterior transmural infarction. The left ventricular blood pool has extended into the wall through an endocardial rent, up to the epicardium. The cavity has not extended into the pericardial space. This lesion may be referred to as a false aneurysm, but it is more precisely referred to as a subepicardial hematoma.

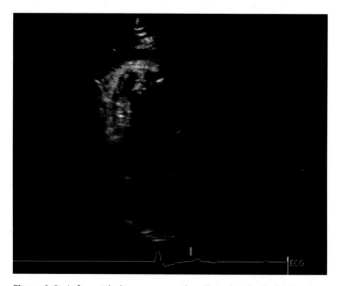

Figure 9-3. Left ventricular noncompaction. There is a luminal extension into a sinus or cavity in the apical myocardium, in an area of acute infarction-related akinesis. This finding was known from before the infarction and presumed to be isolated ventricular noncompaction.

Table 9-1. Complications of Subepicardial Aneurysms[3]

Complication	Number
Moderate to severe congestive heart failure without MR or VSD	25
Ventricular septal defect	6
True aneurysm	5
Mitral regurgitation	5
Systemic emboli	2
Ventricular arrhythmias	3
Supraventricular arrhythmias	3
Dysphagia	1
Salmonella mycotic aneurysm	1
Cardiac arrest with resuscitation and no evidence of MI	1

MI, myocardial infarction; MR, mitral regurgitation; VSD, ventricular septal defect.
From Epstein JI, Hutchins GM: Subepicardial aneurysms: a rare complication of myocardial infarction. Am J Med 1983;75:639-644.

MANAGEMENT

Surgical repair should be obtained and coronary angiography performed before surgery to plan for concurrent aortocoronary bypass grafting. Too few cases have been described for the outcomes to be known, but case reports describe operative success.

CASE 1

History

▸ 61-year-old man suffered prolonged ischemic-type chest pains 2 days before
▸ Presented with recurrent pains and shortness of breath
▸ Past medical history is significant for hypertension.

Physical Examination

▸ BP 100/50 mm Hg, HR 105 bpm, RR 18/min
▸ Alert, ashen, extremities warm
▸ Venous distention
▸ S_1, S_2 soft
▸ 5/6 pansystolic murmur at the LLSB radiating to RLSB
▸ CK 900, urine output 50 mL/hr

Clinical Impression

▸ Inferior left ventricular and right ventricular STEMI or transmural myocardial infarction
▸ Septal rupture
▸ False aneurysm or intramural hematoma of the inferior right ventricular wall
▸ Killip IV

Management

▸ IABP already inserted
▸ Inotropes
▸ Refer for surgery for exploration and repair.
▸ Perform coronary angiography on the way to surgery.
▸ Perform contrast ventriculography to try to elucidate the suspected false aneurysm or intramural hematoma.

Surgical Repair

▸ Patient was referred for septal patch closure through infarctectomy.
▸ Surgery revealed inferior and right ventricular infarction and basal inferior septal rupture. The suspected false aneurysm was not clearly seen at surgery. The right ventricular infarction was extensive and unrecognizably breaking apart at surgery.
▸ Aortocoronary bypass (saphenous vein to PDA) was performed.
▸ Perioperative course was marked by low but viable output.

Evolution and Outcome

▸ Septal rupture was repaired, and there was no evidence of shunting by color Doppler study or oximetry.
▸ There was either a persistence or redevelopment of the fifth cavity, which either recurred or was not seen at surgery as it resided within the wall. It was apparent only on echocardiographic and ventriculographic imaging because it was pressurized while being imaged.

▸ The patient remained stable and was convalescing from the first operation, with a second one planned to address the intramural hematoma and false lumen, when an abdominal viscus perforated and sepsis developed, and he died.

Comments

▸ Large (6 cm) and complex intramural hematoma originating at the inferior left ventricular wall and extending along and within the infarcted inferior wall of the left ventricle into and along the infarcted inferior wall of the right ventricle
▸ Intramural hematoma is more difficult to appreciate at surgery than a false aneurysm because it cannot be seen by surface inspection.
▸ The marked right ventricular infarction complicated the surgery and caused the breakdown of the right ventricular wall and consequently the intramural hematoma.
▸ This is a case of an extremely complicated inferior myocardial infarction: + right ventricular infarction + septal rupture + intramural hematoma.

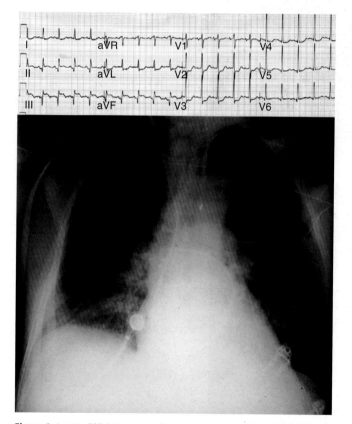

Table 9-2. Hemodynamic Profile

	Physical Examination	Echocardiography	Catheterization
RVSP	Elevated (P_2)	55 mm Hg	63 mm Hg
O_2 step-up	NA	Visualized VSD	Yes
Qp:Qs	NA	2.4:1	2.6:1
CVP	8 cm	10 mm Hg	14 mm Hg
CI, systemic	Shocky	1.4 L/min/m^2	1.6 L/min/m^2

CI, cardiac index; CVP, central venous pressure; RVSP, right ventricular systolic pressure; VSD, ventricular septal defect.

Figure 9-4. TOP, ECG (at presentation) shows sinus tachycardia, inferior Q waves and ST elevation, early R-wave transition (V_2,V_3) with resting ST depression, inferior ± posterior acute infarction. BOTTOM, Chest radiograph shows normally sized heart and interstitial pulmonary edema. PA catheter is in main right pulmonary artery, and IABP tip is in correct position.

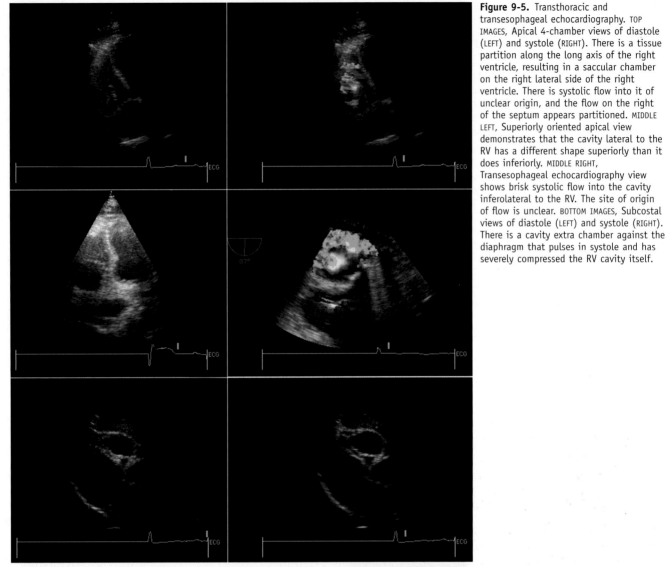

Figure 9-5. Transthoracic and transesophageal echocardiography. TOP IMAGES, Apical 4-chamber views of diastole (LEFT) and systole (RIGHT). There is a tissue partition along the long axis of the right ventricle, resulting in a saccular chamber on the right lateral side of the right ventricle. There is systolic flow into it of unclear origin, and the flow on the right of the septum appears partitioned. MIDDLE LEFT, Superiorly oriented apical view demonstrates that the cavity lateral to the RV has a different shape superiorly than it does inferiorly. MIDDLE RIGHT, Transesophageal echocardiography view shows brisk systolic flow into the cavity inferolateral to the RV. The site of origin of flow is unclear. BOTTOM IMAGES, Subcostal views of diastole (LEFT) and systole (RIGHT). There is a cavity extra chamber against the diaphragm that pulses in systole and has severely compressed the RV cavity itself.

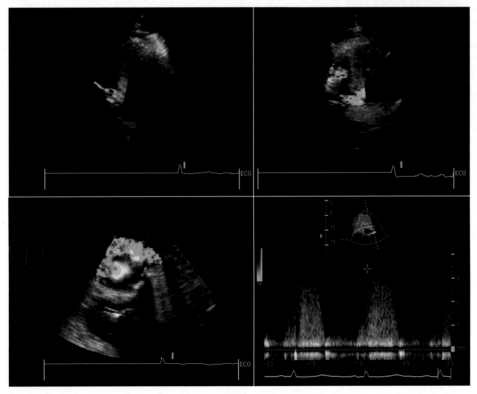

Figure 9-6. Transthoracic and transesophageal echocardiography. TOP LEFT, Apical 2-chamber view demonstrating flow in systole into the inferior wall of the left ventricle and along it. TOP RIGHT, Modified apical color Doppler study demonstrating systolic flow across the basal interventricular septum: septal rupture or flow directly into the lower aspect of the cavity inferolateral to the right ventricle. There is also a second systolic jet appearing in the more apical right ventricle. BOTTOM LEFT, Transesophageal echocardiography view showing brisk systolic jet into the cavity posterolateral to the right ventricle and inward buckling of the right ventricle wall by the pressurized cavity. BOTTOM RIGHT, Spectral display of the systolic flow into that cavity.

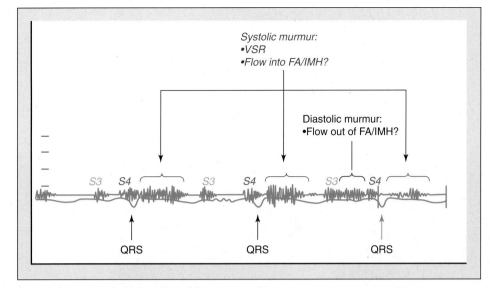

Figure 9-7. Phonocardiogram (recorded on an echo machine) shows systolic murmur consistent with septal rupture and flow into saccular cavity. Diastolic murmur may suggest flow out of saccular cavity ± S_3, S_4.

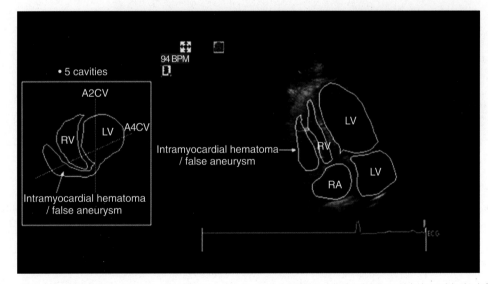

Figure 9-8. Transthoracic echocardiography, apical view. The fifth chamber is contiguous not with the right ventricle but with the left ventricle through an inferior entry and inferior diaphragmatic neck.

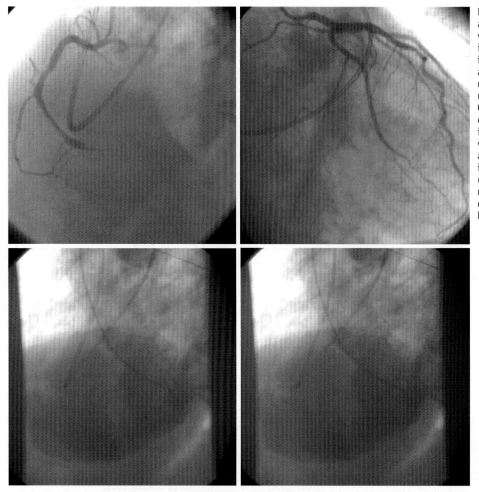

Figure 9-9. TOP IMAGES, Coronary angiography shows dominant and occluded vessel, explaining the inferior myocardial infarction and right ventricular myocardial infarction. Coronary angiography of the left anterior descending coronary artery shows mild disease. Left circumflex artery shows no significant disease. BOTTOM IMAGES, Contrast ventriculography, left anterior oblique projection. Contrast injection into the left ventricle opacifies the left ventricle and demonstrates inferior aneurysm and dyskinesis. Left ventricle injection also opacifies the right ventricle (establishing the presence of a septal rupture). There may also be opacification of a third cavity on the right side of the heart.

CASE 2

History

- 74-year-old man presented 5 days after inferior STEMI (late presentation,14 hours; no fibrinolytics)
- No heart failure symptoms
- Past medical history is significant for hypertension and type 2 diabetes.
- During 30 minutes, he became restless and had mild dyspnea but no chest pain.

Physical Examination

- BP fell from 145/80 to 85/40 mm Hg, HR rose from 60 to 110 bpm
- Venous distention
- New 4/6 pansystolic murmur at the LLSB radiating to RLSB; no thrill
- No rub
- No ECG changes; developed oliguria

Clinical Impression

- Inferior infarction with right ventricular infarction and "ventricular septal defect" extending several centimeters through the infarcted inferior right ventricular wall, indicative of an intramural hematoma

Management and Outcome

- Patient was referred for septal patch closure through right ventricular infarctectomy.

- Surgery revealed inferior and right ventricular infarction, hemorrhagic in appearance.
- Basal inferior septal rupture with tunneling of the septal rupture course through the infarcted inferior and lateral right ventricular wall and entry of the ventricular septal defect channel into the right ventricle at the lateral right ventricle
- The patient came off bypass, but the patches were seen to tear extensively, and he was put back on pump for a revision, which was successful but only for an hour. The circulation again collapsed, and by echocardiography it was seen that the patches had torn again.
- Definitive repair of the massively infarcted right ventricle was believed to be impossible.
- The patient died several hours later of low output.

Comments

- No overt herald symptoms before rupture
- Late-presentation inferior STEMI complicated by right ventricular myocardial infarction and intramural hematoma that progressed to become a "round-and-about" septal rupture; the length of the intramural hematoma tunnel from the basal posterior left ventricle into the right ventricle free wall was 9 cm.
- Painless hemodynamic deterioration consistent with intracardiac rupture
- Many adverse prognosticators: shock, markedly elevated CVP, the "100 thing" (heart rate > 100 bpm, blood pressure systolic < 100 mm Hg)

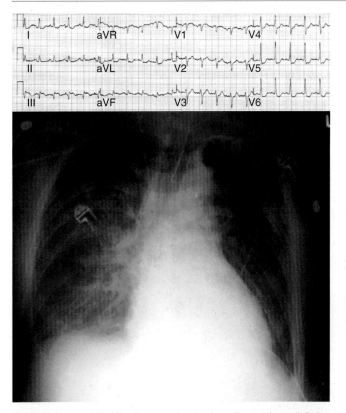

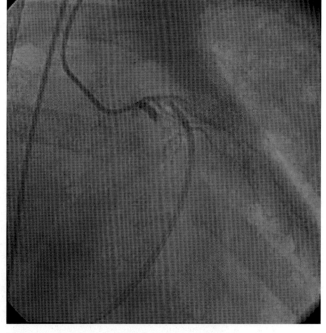

Figure 9-11. Angiogram of the left anterior descending coronary artery shows no significant disease. LCx: proximal occlusion (dominant).

Figure 9-10. TOP, ECG (day 4) shows sinus tachycardia; persistent inferior (II, III, aVF) ST elevation, suggesting acute inferior infarction and a possible aneurysm; and nonspecific anterolateral repolarization abnormalities. BOTTOM, Chest radiograph shows normally sized heart and mild pulmonary edema. IABP and ET tube are in correct position.

Figure 9-12. Elevated LVEDP (32 mm Hg), tachycardia, and hypotension (75 mm Hg). An important clue to remember is the "100 thing" (HR > 100 bpm, BP < 100 mm Hg).

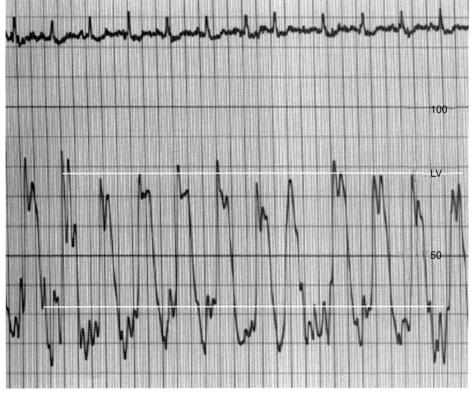

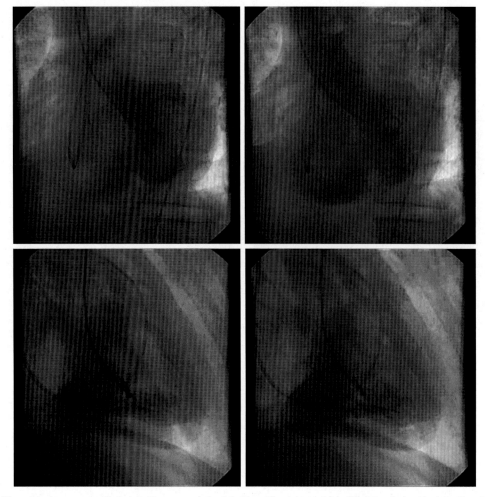

Figure 9-13. TOP, LAO ventriculogram. LEFT, Early injection. RIGHT, Later injection. The right ventricle fills later during the injection. Earlier to fill is a space inferior to the right ventricular cavity. This area achieves the densest opacification on the right side of the heart. BOTTOM, RAO ventriculogram. LEFT, Early injection. RIGHT, Later injection. The outline of the right ventricular inferior wall and of the RVOT becomes clear in the later injection. There is a denser collection of dye of uncertain etiology at the basal inferior aspect of the heart. Also visible are inferior akinesis and inferior aneurysm. Opacification of the RV, RVOT, and PA is indicative of left-to-right shunting.

Table 9-3. Hemodynamic Profile

	Physical Examination	Echocardiography	Catheterization
RVSP	Not elevated	42 mm Hg	50 mm Hg
O₂ step-up	NA	Visualized VSD	Yes
Qp:Qs	NA	NA	2.5:1
CVP	Elevated JVP	10 mm Hg	20 mm Hg
CI, systemic	Shocky	1.4 L/min/m²	1.2 L/min/m²

CI, cardiac index; CVP, central venous pressure; JVP, jugular venous pressure; RVSP, right ventricular systolic pressure; VSD, ventricular septal defect.

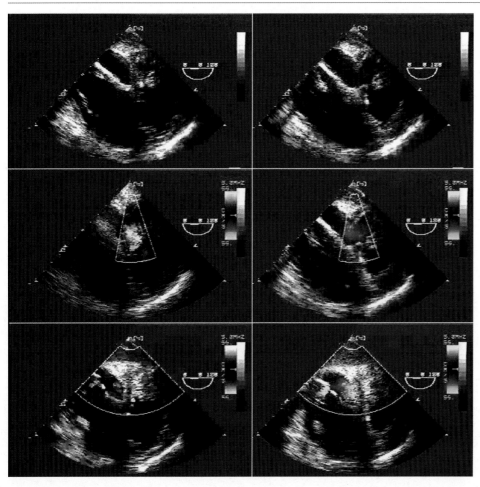

Figure 9-14. Transesophageal echocardiography, transgastric short-axis images. TOP ROW, There is a bicornuate cavity that extends into the posterior right ventricular wall and also into the left ventricular wall; it has a narrow neck arising at the basal inferior aspect of the septum. MIDDLE ROW, Systole (LEFT) flow into the neck. Diastole (RIGHT) flow out of the left aspect of the cavity. BOTTOM ROW, View more to the right side. LEFT, The continuation of the cavity extends along the posterolateral right ventricular wall. RIGHT, Flow out of the cavity into the right ventricular cavity proper.

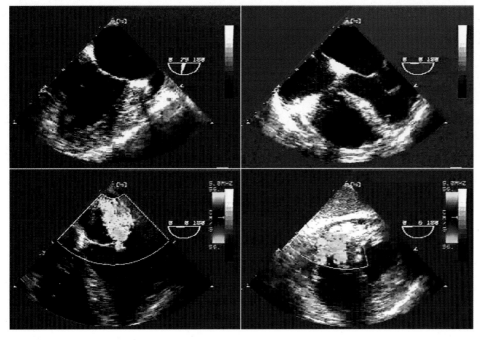

Figure 9-15. TOP LEFT, A deep extension of the left ventricular cavity has occurred inferiorly. It appears to be an aneurysm. TOP RIGHT, There is marked right ventricular dilation and rounding consistent with extensive right ventricular infarction. BOTTOM LEFT, 3+ mitral insufficiency. BOTTOM RIGHT, Brisk systolic flow in the cavity posterior to the right ventricle and dispersing into the right ventricular cavity.

References

1. Harpaz D, Kriwisky M, Cohen AJ, et al: Unusual form of cardiac rupture: sealed subacute left ventricular free wall rupture, evolving to intramyocardial dissecting hematoma and to pseudoaneurysm formation—a case report and review of the literature. J Am Soc Echocardiogr 2001;14:219-227.

2. Scanu P, Lamy E, Commeau P, et al: Myocardial dissection in right ventricular infarction: two-dimensional echocardiographic recognition and pathologic study. Am Heart J 1986;111:422-425.

3. Epstein JI, Hutchins GM: Subepicardial aneurysms: a rare complication of myocardial infarction. Am J Med 1983;75:639-644.

4. Di Bella I, Minzioni G, Maselli D, et al: Septal dissection and rupture evolved as an inferobasal pseudoaneurysm. Ann Thorac Surg 2001;71:1358-1360.

5. Vargas-Barron J, Roldan FJ, Romero-Cardenas A, et al: Two- and three-dimensional transesophageal echocardiographic diagnosis of intramyocardial dissecting hematoma after myocardial infarction. J Am Soc Echocardiogr 2001;14:637-640.

6. Stollberger C, Finsterer J, Waldenberger FR, et al: Intramyocardial hematoma mimicking abnormal left ventricular trabeculation. J Am Soc Echocardiogr 2001;14:1030-1032.

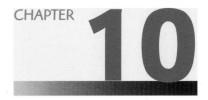

Postinfarction Pericardial Tamponade

Pericardial effusions occurring within the first 48 hours after infarction are quite common (30%). They are more commonly seen in anterior infarction and in patients with heart failure. It does not appear that the presence of pericardial effusion is associated with early pericarditis, peak creatine kinase concentration, anticoagulation, or mortality. Most effusions in this setting are small, and few effusions evolve into tamponade. Approximately 8% of them are still present at 6 months.[1]

Before the era of widespread percutaneous intervention in acute infarction cases, postinfarction pericardial tamponade was uncommon. Rapid accumulation of only a small to moderate amount of pericardial fluid may exceed the pericardial compliance reserve and result in tamponade. The pericardial compliance reserve may already be reduced by left- or right-sided heart chamber dilation from acute infarction. The presence of an abnormal heart under the effusion, and in many cases also of pulmonary or systemic venous congestion, renders atypical the physical diagnosis signs and hemodynamic findings of tamponade of acute infarction cases. For example, pulsus paradoxus is present in less than half of subacute rupture cases with tamponade.[2]

Postinfarction pericardial tamponade may result from several causes (Fig. 10-1):

- Hemorrhagic pericarditis (+ anticoagulants, antiplatelet agents, fibrinolytics)
- Iatrogenic due to instrumentation (pacemaker lead; stenting, coronary perforations)
- Free wall rupture
- Early exudative effusion
- Type A aortic dissection (causing coronary occlusion and pericardial tamponade)

The single greatest challenge in managing postinfarction tamponade cases is establishing which cases are plausibly at risk of subacute ruptures, leaking false aneurysms, and intramural hematomas and require surgical inspection and repair. The determination of which cases require surgical inspection and treatment remains a demanding clinical judgment.

Although temporal association of instrumentation with the development and recognition of tamponade suggests that the instrumentation is responsible for the occurrence of tamponade, this is not always the case, particularly in the era of primary and rescue percutaneous coronary intervention (PCI), when many cases "go directly" to the interventional catheterization laboratory and have the full scope of their problems (e.g., mechanical complications) first established there during interventional procedures. Type A aortic dissection results in myocardial ischemia by the intimal flap's partially or completely occluding a coronary ostium and may be first recognized while undergoing early angiography.[3]

No single test is able to discriminate all cases of rupture from other causes of postinfarction tamponade. Composite assessment—clinical, imaging, and in some cases hemodynamic assessment—is needed.

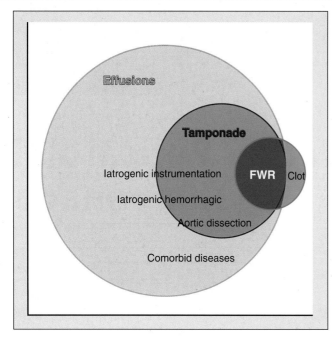

Figure 10-1. Causes of myocardial infarction–related tamponade. There are far more effusions than cases of tamponade, and many causes. Free wall rupture (FWR) may result in fluid compression of the heart or clot compression of the heart.

CASE 1

History

▸ 77 year old man, admitted with atypical chest pains, with some pleuritic features, and presyncope
▸ Past medical history is significant for four prior infarctions (the most recent an inferior STEMI 7 weeks before), ICD for sustained symptomatic VT, congestive heart failure (NYHA class III dyspnea, ejection fraction 22%), and hypertension.

Physical Examination

▸ BP 100/70 mm Hg, pulsus paradoxus 23 mm Hg, HR 80 bpm (beta-blocked), RR 18/min
▸ Appeared well
▸ Venous distention to the angle of the jaw, diminished *y* descent
▸ S_1, S_2 soft
▸ No murmurs
▸ Triphasic pericardial friction rubs
▸ First troponin mildly elevated, second and subsequent ones were not

Clinical Impression

▸ Post–inferior Q-wave myocardial infarction (completed STEMI)
▸ Clinically with pericarditis
▸ Other than an inferior aneurysm, no complications of infarction

Management

▸ Pericardiocentesis (yielded straw-colored fluid)
▸ Drained 900 mL fluid ×48 hours
▸ NSAIDs
▸ Avoidance of anticoagulant therapy

Outcome

▸ Pericarditic chest pains alleviated within 24 hours
▸ No reaccumulation of fluid
▸ Discharged 3 days later with usual symptoms

Comments

▸ Postinfarction pericarditis, pericardial effusion, and tamponade
▸ Presyncope was likely due to the tamponade.
▸ Echocardiography identified the effusion but not the clot, corroborated the tamponade, and excluded a post-MI false aneurysm.
▸ Pericardiocentesis was therapeutic and conclusively established that the fluid was not sanguineous and that rupture was not responsible.

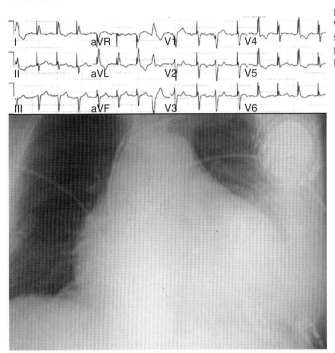

Figure 10-2. TOP, ECG shows ventricular demand pacing with PVCs and PACs. Voltages are not low. BOTTOM, Chest radiograph shows large cardiopericardial silhouette. This shape can be produced by cardiomyopathy and also by pericardial effusion. There is a fluid stripe up to the aortic arch suggestive of pericardial fluid. Also visible is ICD hardware.

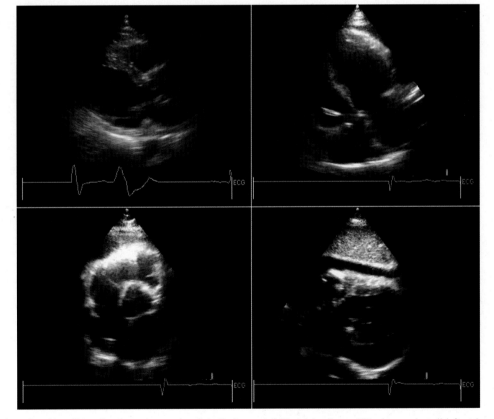

Figure 10-3. Transthoracic echocardiography views show pericardial effusion and right atrial collapse, ICD wires, and small left atrium consistent with underfilling.

CASE 2

History

▸ 66-year-old man presented with non-STEMI, without heart failure or arrhythmias
▸ Developed recurrent pains
▸ Treated with beta-blocker, ACE inhibitor, ASA, heparin, clopidogrel, IIb/IIIa inhibitors
▸ Past medical history is significant for two prior infarctions, hypertension, dyslipidemia, and type 2 diabetes.
▸ Underwent PCI to responsible lesion. Difficulty was experienced in crossing the lesion, but despite this, the procedure was angiograpically successful.
▸ Atypical chest pains developed during the next 3 days.

Physical Examination

▸ BP 90/60 mm Hg, pulsus paradoxus 35 mm Hg only, HR 105 bpm
▸ Alert, but weak appearing
▸ Low-volume pulses
▸ Venous distention to the angle of the jaw
▸ S_1, S_2 distant
▸ No murmurs
▸ Urine output low (20 mL/hr)

Clinical Impression

▸ Pericarditis, effusion, and tamponade in an ACS patient after PCI
▸ The patient was stable and recovering from the first operation, with a second one planned to address the intramural hematoma–false lumen, when an abdominal viscus perforated and sepsis developed.

Management

▸ Pericardiocentesis and drainage (therapeutic) led to prompt normalization of JVP and BP.
▸ 600 mL of bloody fluid drained. There was no ongoing drainage during the next 24 hours, so the drain was removed at that point, and the patient was discharged the following day.
▸ Low-dose NSAIDs

Outcome

▸ Discharged symptom free

Comments

▸ Pericarditis, pericardial effusion, and tamponade from combined antiplatelet and anticoagulant therapy and PCI
▸ The infarction was non-STEMI; therefore, pericarditis from the infarction was unlikely, and rupture with a small (CK 300) MI was unlikely.
▸ Bloody return of pericardial fluid does confront the operator with the possibilities of (1) intracardiac insertion of the drain and (2) myocardial rupture. Injection of saline established the intrapericardial location of the drain. The likelihood of rupture was considered low: no false aneurysm or dyskinetic segment was seen on echocardiography, the symptom and blood pressure response to drainage was large, and the fluid did not continue to drain—all factors held against rupture as an underlying cause.

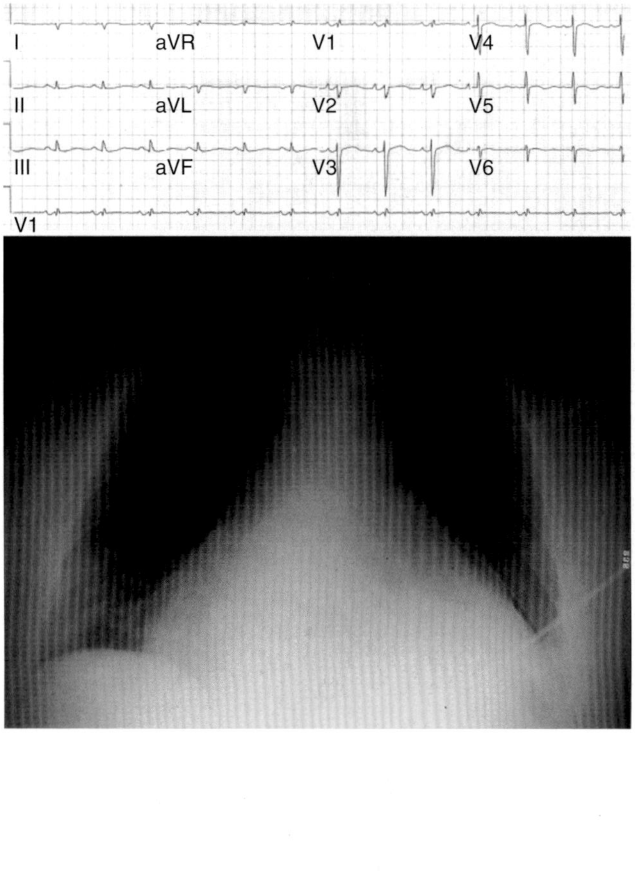

Figure 10-4. TOP, ECG on day 1 after PCI shows low voltages, right axis deviation, no electrical alternans on rhythm strip, and nonspecific repolarization abnormalities. Heart rate may be influenced by the beta-blocker use. BOTTOM, Chest radiograph shows enlarged cardiopericardial silhouette. Flask shape is consistent with pericardial fluid; globular shape is also seen with cardiomyopathy.

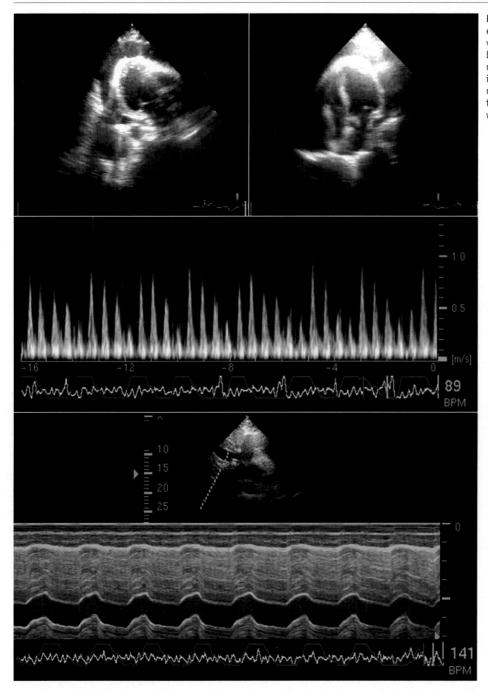

Figure 10-5. Transthoracic echocardiography views showing left ventricle inflow. With inspiration (denoted by the upward deflection of the respirometer tracing), the early diastolic inflow velocities fall 50%. Subcostal M-mode study of the IVC shows dilation of the IVC (3 cm) with failure to collapse with inspiration.

References

1. Galve E, Garcia-Del-Castillo H, Evangelista A, et al: Pericardial effusion in the course of myocardial infarction: incidence, natural history, and clinical relevance. Circulation 1986;73:294-299.
2. López-Sendón J, González A, López de Sá E, et al: Diagnosis of subacute ventricular wall rupture after acute myocardial infarction: sensitivity and specificity of clinical, hemodynamic and echocardiographic criteria. J Am Coll Cardiol 1992;19:1145-1153.
3. Hansen MS, Nogareda GJ, Hutchison SJ: Frequency of and inappropriate treatment of misdiagnosis of acute aortic dissection. Am J Cardiol 2007;99:852-856.

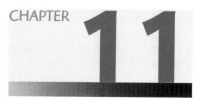
Ventricular Septal Rupture

- The incidence of VSR is 0.2% to 2%; it accounts for 4% of postinfarction cardiogenic shock cases.

- LAD occlusion and anteroapical VSR are twice as common as PDA occlusion and inferobasal VSR.

- Inferobasal VSRs are usually anatomically complex, more commonly associated with other mechanical complications, and commonly associated with right ventricular infarction.

- Typical background includes first infarction, hypertension, and little previous recognized CAD.

- Because of the shunt lesion, the right ventricle receives an excess volume load (250% of normal), and therefore right ventricular function, rather than left ventricular (systolic and diastolic) function, has the dominant influence on outcome.

- Right ventricular infarction is common in VSR cases—generally small in anteroapical VSR and often moderately sized or large in inferobasal cases.

- Diagnosis is made by clinical suspicion, appearance of a new systolic murmur, and echocardiography in conjunction with oximetric or contrast ventriculographic evidence of left-to-right flow at the ventricular level.

- Management strategy:

  - Normotensive, well-perfused cases: selective arterial vasodilators or IABP

  - Hypotensive, poorly perfused cases: IABP

  - Inotropes for patients with pulmonary congestion

  - Angiography if stability of the patient permits

  - Arrange for surgical repair early (for Killip classes I and II) or urgently (for Killip classes III and IV and cardiogenic shock cases).

Postinfarction ventricular septal rupture (VSR) is a severe but potentially salvageable mechanical complication of infarction. The term *ventricular septal defect* is more suitable to the congenital lesion, in which the hole is the entire lesion. *Postinfarction ventricular septal rupture* is a more suitable term for postinfarction lesions that comprise the hole and, importantly, a moderate or large area of necrotic myocardium as well, contributing to poor preoperative hemodynamics, poor surgery tissue, and poor postoperative hemodynamics.

Postinfarction VSR is commonly associated with other complications of infarction, such as false aneurysms, intramural or intramyocardial hematoma, right ventricular infarction, higher Killip and Forrester classes, and cardiogenic shock.

The first pathologic description of VSR was made by Latham in 1847. In 1923, Brunn first described its clinical features, and the first successful surgical repair was reported by Cooley in 1957.

Postinfarction VSR occurs in 0.2% to 2% of infarction cases and is responsible for 1% to 5% of deaths due to infarction.[1] In the era before fibrinolysis, among early and late ST elevation infarctions and ST depression infarctions, the reported incidence of septal rupture was 2%. By the time of the fibrinolytic era, more selective trials reported a 0.2% incidence of septal rupture (early, <6 hours, presentation). VSR is responsible for approximately 4% of cardiogenic shock cases and is the second most common and the second most salvageable form of myocardial rupture (Fig. 11-1).[2]

Among septal rupture cases, typical patient factors include preexistent hypertension (57%),[3] first infarction, and first presentation of coronary artery disease (CAD). The absence of chronic CAD lessens the likelihood of collateral formation and thereby increases the transmurality of infarction—the requisite substrate to achieve septal or free wall rupture. Arterial hypertension increases the physical forces generated by the left ventricle and thereby increases the likelihood of disruption and rupture of the infarct segment.

The influence of fibrinolytic and reperfusion therapy on septal rupture is bidirectional, and overall no clear effect emerges. There are data to suggest that early fibrinolysis is not associated with excess VSR; but late fibrinolysis is, possibly through hemorrhagic conversion of the infarct area. Observational data derived from 36,303 patients enrolled in fibrinolytic trials and 1295 patients in the Primary Angioplasty in Myocardial Infarction trials (PAMI-1 and PAM-2) suggest that primary angioplasty is

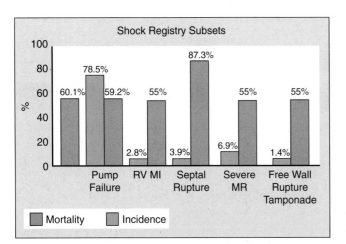

Figure 11-1. The large majority (78.5%) of SHOCK registry cases were left ventricular pump failure. Right ventricular infarction and "mechanical complications" accounted for the remainder. MI, myocardial infarction; MR, mitral regurgitation; RV, right ventricle. (From Hochman JS, Buller CE, Sleeper LA, et al: Cardiogenic shock complicating acute myocardial infarction—etiologies, management and outcome: a report from the SHOCK Trial Registry. SHould we emergently revascularize Occluded Coronaries for cardiogenic shocK? J Am Coll Cardiol 2000;36[Suppl A]:1063-1070, with permission from Elsevier.)

associated with a significantly lower incidence of VSR than is fibrinolytic use (0% versus 0.47%).[4] The apparent lower incidence of rupture with percutaneous coronary intervention (PCI) versus fibrinolytic use may be explained either by superior reperfusion rates by PCI, lessening rupture, or conversely by hemorrhagic conversion due to fibrinolytic use, especially in later infarcts, increasing rupture rates.

The natural history of nonrepaired VSR entails 75% mortality by 8 weeks: 25% die within 24 hours, 25% more die within 1 week, and another 25% die by 8 weeks. A few patients survive longer (months), and undeniably, a scant number survive for years.

Surgical repair reduces mortality. Surgical risk is heavily influenced by the preoperative hemodynamic status of the patient. In GUSTO I, 34 patients underwent surgical repair at a mean of 3.5 days after infarction. Ten percent of patients underwent later operation between 30 days and 1 year. The 30-day and 1-year mortalities were 47% and 53% for patients who underwent operation and 94% and 97% (both $P < .001$) for patients who did not undergo surgery. The GUSTO I trial observed a 27% operative and in-hospital mortality for patients with Killip class I or class II heart failure and a 100% mortality for the more advanced Killip class III and class IV heart failure.[3] Postoperative 10-year survival was 30% to 70%.

VSRs are caused by either left anterior descending (LAD) or posterior descending (interventricular) artery (PDA) occlusion (Figs. 11-2 to 11-5). In most patients, the LAD supplies the anterior two thirds of the septum along its length and the entire height of the septum at the apex, as the LAD usually wraps around the apex to supply apical septal branches from above and below. The typical lesion that is responsible for LAD-mediated VSR is in the midportion of the LAD, such that the distal septum and apex undergo infarction, but there remains sufficient functional myocardium to generate the physical forces that can result in disruption and rupture of the more distally necrotic septum. Lesions and occlusion of the proximal LAD are less likely to leave suffi-

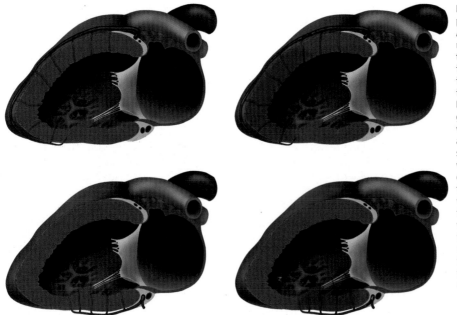

Figure 11-2. The anatomic correlates of postinfarction septal ruptures. UPPER IMAGES, Anteroapical VSR due to mid LAD occlusion and mid-distal anteroseptal, anterior, and apical transmural infarction. The LAD occlusion, being in the midportion, generates a moderate-sized infarction; but unlike a proximal LAD occlusion, it is not such a large infarction that the LV lacks sufficient functional myocardium to generate the pressures and forces to rupture its wall. Most anteroapical septal ruptures are anatomically simpler. LOWER IMAGES, Posterobasal septal ruptures are due to occlusion of whichever vessel supplies the posterior descending or interventricular artery, usually the right coronary artery, and are associated with infarction of the basal posterior septum, the basal inferior walls of the left and right ventricles, and often the right ventricular free wall as well. Typically, posterobasal septal ruptures are associated with smaller amounts of infarction of the left ventricle than of the right ventricle, and most are anatomically complex channels.

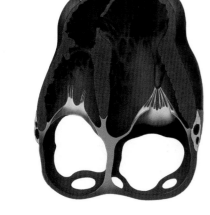

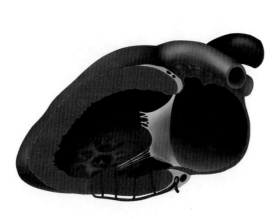

Figure 11-3. Most postinfarction septal ruptures are anteroapical, associated with distal septal and anterior and apical infarction of both the left and right ventricles, due to a mid LAD occlusion (UPPER IMAGES), or basal posterior septal, associated with infarction of the basal posterior septum and inferior walls of the left and right ventricles, due to right coronary occlusion and often with a disproportionate degree of right ventricular infarction (LOWER IMAGES).

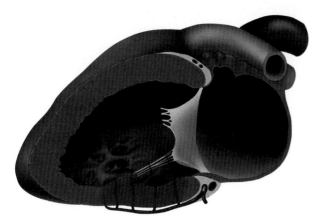

Figure 11-4. Some septal ruptures are located at neither the anteroapex nor the posterobasal portion of the septum and are in the mid septum.

cient residual functioning myocardium to generate the forces needed to disrupt and rupture the apical septum. Rupture of the anteroapical septum from LAD occlusion is 1.5 to 2.5 times more common than is rupture of the inferior septum. Occlusion of the posterior descending (interventricular) artery, or of the vessel that supplies it, results in infarction of the lower third of the septum in the basal and middle portions of the left ventricle but seldom of the apical portion of the septum that is supplied by the distal LAD as it wraps around the apex. Because right coronary artery (RCA) occlusion is generally responsible for inferior wall infarction, concurrent right ventricular infarction is common in inferior septal VSR. Thus, the large majority of VSR lesions are located in either the apical or anteroapical septum or the basal inferior portion of the septum. Among the 84 cases of septal VSR in GUSTO I, 70% were anterior, 29% were inferior, and 1% were elsewhere.[3]

The usual presentation of VSR is that of a new rough holosystolic murmur, relative hypotension, and progressive biventricular failure.[5] The murmur is almost always holosystolic and results from turbulent flow across the rupture hole. Biventricular failure results because both ventricles are compromised by the shunt and the infarction. There is less prominent pulmonary edema among VSR cases than among those with papillary muscle rupture; low output is a more prominent finding.

In VSR cases, the overall left ventricular systolic function is usually only moderately depressed. In GUSTO I, ejection fraction of VSR cases averaged 40%. That there is only moderate dysfunction can be explained because most patients had preinfarction normal ventricular function, few had prior infarction, and only a minority (11% to 36%) had underlying three-vessel CAD. Most patients have a degree of excess systolic function

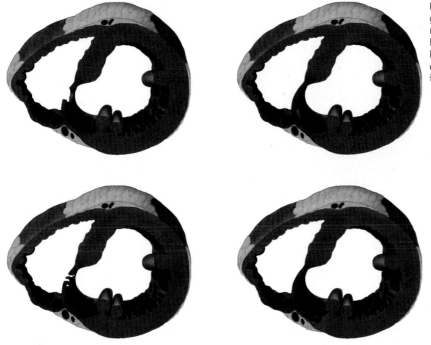

Figure 11-5. Posterobasal septal ruptures exhibit the greatest variation in anatomy and complexity. Tracts may uncommonly be single (UPPER IMAGES) and located higher or lower in the septum, or they may be sieve-like (LEFT LOWER IMAGE) or a serpiginous channel that is essentially an intramyocardial hematoma that ruptured into the right ventricle.

because of mild left ventricular hypertrophy (LVH) from prior hypertension. Severely depressed overall left ventricular systolic function is seen more commonly among cases with underlying three-vessel CAD and is a prominent aspect of early cardiogenic shock VSR cases; the inability of noninfarcted myocardium to become hypercontractile, because of ischemia, prevents compensation.

VSR lesions are described as simple or complex, terms originally used by pathologists but as of late also important for surgery and imaging:

A simple rupture of the interventricular septum is defined as a direct, through-and-through opening connecting the two ventricular chambers. Neither gross hemorrhage nor laceration are present in the tissue surrounding the septal defect. The left and right ventricular openings are at about the same horizontal level of the interventricular septum. A complex rupture of the ventricular septum is defined as an interventricular communication that ascribes an undulating or serpiginous course. The tract may enter, in part, into regions remote from the site of primary acute myocardial infarction. Branching zones with disruption of myocardial tissue and hemorrhage occur. Frequently, the openings into the two ventricles are at different planes of the ventricular septum.[6]

The location of VSR is prominently associated with the likelihood of anatomic complexity of the rupture (Fig. 11-6). Apical VSRs are complex in only 20% of cases, whereas basal VSRs are complex in all cases (100%) and usually appear to represent myocardial dissection and intramyocardial hematoma and association with false aneurysms.[7] About 20% of VSR cases are associated with another mechanical complication (papillary

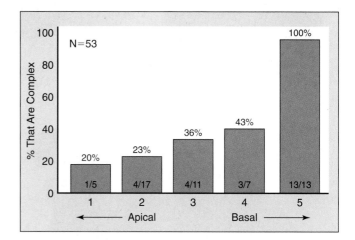

Figure 11-6. A strong relation of anatomic lesion complexity to anatomic location is present in VSR, with simpler lesions at the apex and uniformly complex lesions at the base. (From Edwards BS, Edwards WD, Edwards JE: Ventricular septal rupture complicating acute myocardial infarction: identification of simple and complex types in 53 autopsied hearts. Am J Cardiol 1984;54:1201-1205, with permission from Elsevier.)

muscle rupture, free wall rupture, false aneurysm, or aneurysm).[6]

Inferobasal septal ruptures are commonly associated with right ventricular infarction, anatomic complexity, and other ruptures. Right ventricular infarction renders the right side of the heart less capable of managing the excess volume and pressure load imparted by the shunt. Anatomic complexity also renders inferobasal septal rupture more difficult to repair surgically. The mortality of inferobasal septal rupture, repaired or nonrepaired, is greater.[3]

PATHOPHYSIOLOGY OF VENTRICULAR SEPTAL RUPTURE

Unlike papillary muscle rupture, which is the result of small infarctions, VSR is inevitably caused by a medium-sized or moderately large infarction. The average of 40% ejection fraction described in VSR series represents the net effect of akinesis and dyskinesis of the infarct zone, and generally of hyperkinesis of the noninfarcted myocardium, and it is more of an arithmetic than a pathophysiologic description of the state of the left ventricle in VSR cases. The effective forward left ventricular stroke volume is reduced by the amount of the shunt volume that crosses through the septum into the right ventricle. Typically, the shunt volume is as large as or larger than the residual left ventricular forward stroke volume. In an attempt to maintain cardiac output in the face of a severely reduced stroke volume, the heart rate elevates, and tachycardia is usual. To maintain blood pressure, peripheral vascular resistance also increases. Importantly, among VSR patients, the peripheral vascular resistance can, by virtue of past hypertension, elevate substantially, imparting a particularly poor relationship between the blood pressure and the cardiac output. As with mitral regurgitation (MR), peripheral vascular resistance has a significant effect on septal rupture hemodynamics. In the case of MR, higher impedance to left ventricular ejection increases the regurgitant volume. In the case of VSR, high impedance to ejection increases the shunt volume (Table 11-1). This has profound implications for supportive measures. If the blood pressure and peripheral perfusion are sufficient, afterload reduction by pure arterial vasodilators lessens shunt flow and improves peripheral blood flow as some proportion of the regurgitant volume becomes stroke volume. Intra-aortic balloon counterpulsation (IABP) is useful to lower systolic pressure and impedance to ejection, thereby lowering the shunt volume or fraction and augmenting diastolic pressure and thereby mean blood pressure. Therefore, in all patients with low output, IABP should be strongly considered.

Right ventricular systolic function is enormously relevant in VSR cases, as the right ventricle needs to eject a volume of blood that is two or three times normal. The right ventricle is usually mildly impaired in apical VSR and moderately or severely impaired in inferobasal VSR. Right ventricular systolic indices are far more powerful discriminators of survival than are any left-sided heart indices because right ventricular systolic dysfunction is the critical parameter responsible for maintaining cardiac output. Right ventricular infarction is the single parameter that best correlates with the development of cardiogenic shock[8]—far better than do Qp:Qs, left ventricular ejection fraction, or extent of underlying CAD.[8] Because of this, cardiogenic shock is far more common in the setting of inferior infarction with VSR than in anterior infarction with VSR (60% versus 20%; $P < .01$), and so is mortality (73% versus 30%; $P < .05$).[5]

In the case of inferobasal VSR, the right ventricle is commonly infarcted—the extent of infarction depending on the location of the RCA occlusion. In general, the posterior right ventricle is akinetic, but if the RCA occlusion is proximal before acute marginal branches, the right ventricle lateral wall may as well be akinetic, representing extensive right ventricular systolic dysfunction. To complicate matters, right atrial branches may also be affected by RCA occlusion and can result in significant right atrial infarction, depriving the right ventricle of needed preload augmentation. In cases of apical VSR, the apical right ventricle and some of the anterior right ventricle are almost always infarcted, as these areas receive blood supply from the now occluded LAD. Whereas inferobasal VSRs are prominently associated with right ventricular infarction (to their detriment), apical VSRs are less associated with right ventricular infarction (Figs. 11-7 to 11-9).[9] Right ventricular infarction is the Achilles heel of unrepaired and surgically repaired patients with postinfarction septal rupture.

Right atrial pressure is typically elevated as a result of the overfilling of the right ventricle by the shunt flow and also by any degree of right ventricular infarction. The pulmonary artery pressure reflects the total effect of increase in pulmonary artery flow, increasing pulmonary artery pressures; of elevation of the left atrial pressure, effecting backpressure through the pulmonary circuit; and of right ventricular infarction, lowering the generated right ventricular systolic pressure (RVSP). Tricuspid regurgitation due to right ventricular dysfunction (and rarely due to right ventricular papillary muscle rupture) further worsens cardiac output and increases right atrial pressure. Loss of cardiac output elicits a rise in systemic vascular resistance, which increases shunt volume.

Table 11-1. Factors Influencing Shunt Volume in Ventricular Septal Rupture

Size of hole (rupture cm²)

Right ventricular (RV) factors

   RVSP determinants (size of RV MI)

   Impedance to RV ejection (PAP, PVR)

Left ventricular (LV) factors

   LVSP determinants (usual BP, size of LV MI)

   Impedance to LV ejection (BP, aortic stenosis)

BP, blood pressure; LVSP, left ventricular systolic pressure; PAP, pulmonary artery pressure; PVR, pulmonary vascular resistance; MI, myocardial infarction; RVSP, right ventricular systolic pressure.

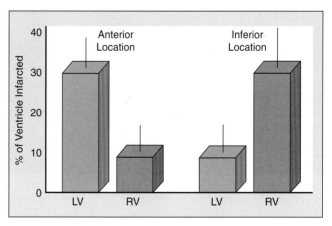

Figure 11-7. Anterior location VSR (the result of LAD occlusion) is associated with greater extent of left ventricular (LV) infarction and lesser extent of right ventricular (RV) infarction. Conversely, inferior (basal) VSR (due predominantly to RCA occlusion) is associated with lesser left ventricular infarction and far more right ventricular infarction. (From Cummings RG, Califf R, Jones RN, et al: Correlates of survival in patients with postinfarction ventricular septal defect. Ann Thorac Surg 1989;47:824-830.)

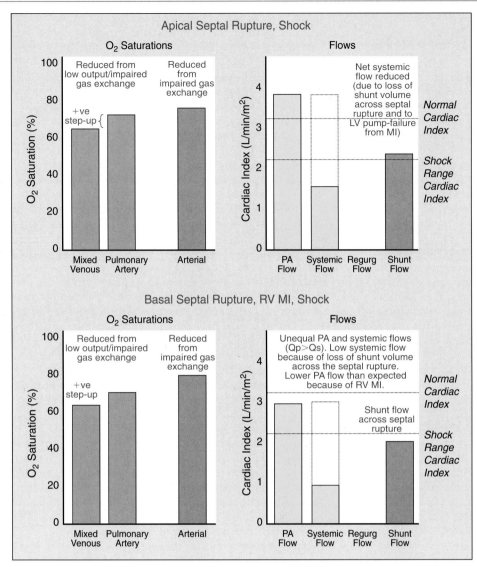

Figure 11-8. TOP, Apical septal rupture and shock hemodynamics. BOTTOM, Basal septal rupture and shock hemodynamics. Oximetry reveals low systemic saturation in VSR due to the increased tissue extraction to compensate for lessened tissue perfusion. A step-up is present at the right ventricular level due to the admixture within the RV of systemic venous return and oxygenated shunt flow through the VSR. Arterial saturations are reduced because there is increased lung water from the high intrapulmonary flow and elevated left atrial pressure. The left atrial pressure is elevated due to LV stiffness from the infarction and because of excess venous return. Pulmonary artery (PA) flow exceeds systemic arterial flow by the amount of the regurgitant volume, which typically slightly exceeds the forward stroke volume. The fact that sustaining forward flow in VSR cases is critically dependent on right ventricular function is revealed in the basal septal rupture, associated with more right ventricular infarction and lesser pulmonary or systemic output. RV MI, right ventricular myocardial infarction.

Extensive left ventricular systolic dysfunction is associated with early cardiogenic shock, as the left ventricle is without the means to compensate for the inefficiency imparted by the shunt volume and by the infarct. Such cases experience very poor survival. Extensive or global left ventricular systolic function is seen in cases with underlying multivessel CAD and in cases of truly large infarcts that complicate septal rupture.

The sum total of systemic venous return to the right side of the heart with the addition of shunt flow into the right ventricle increases the right ventricular output to be greater than that of the left side of the heart. The venerable index of pulmonary artery to systemic flow ratio (Qp:Qs) is typically 2.2 to 2.5 in VSR cases (Figs. 11-10 and 11-11). The excess venous return to the left side of the heart, coupled with the diastolic dysfunction or failure of the moderate-sized left ventricular infarction ± LVH effect, increases left ventricular diastolic pressure, leading to pulmonary venous congestion but not usually frank pulmonary edema. The substantially augmented venous return in systole leads to a significant V wave in many patients as the capacitance of the left atrium is exceeded by the excess venous return.

CLINICAL PRESENTATION OF VENTRICULAR SEPTAL RUPTURE

Most VSRs present within the 3- to 7-day window after infarction, although some occur earlier on the first day or as late as 2 weeks after infarction. Fibrinolysis and reperfusion may result in earlier rupture. A few VSR cases occur as late as 2 weeks after infarction, once the patient has been discharged. Some VSRs are detected at admission and presumably reflect infarction within the week before presentation. The usual case experiences a generalized deterioration, often with chest pain (Table 11-2). Because of the sudden development of shunt flow, the blood pressure falls, and systemic and pulmonary venous pressures increase.

A new pansystolic murmur is generally at the left lower sternal border and often radiates, as the flow across the VSR is left to right, toward the right of the lower sternum. The typical VSR pansystolic murmur is harsh and raspy. In cases in which the rupture through the septum is enormous or there is pre-terminal shock, a murmur may be absent. An associated thrill is present in

11

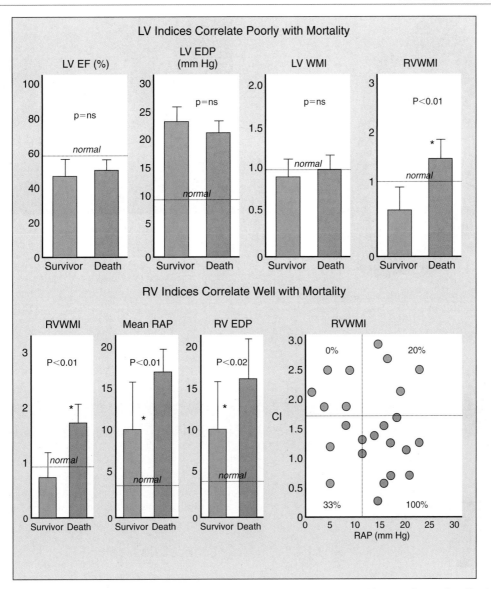

Figure 11-9. Left and right ventricular indices and correlates of survival. Left ventricular (LV) indices, neither systolic nor diastolic, do not discriminate survivors from those who die of VSR. Right ventricular (RV) indices, both systolic and diastolic, do correlate with outcome. The combination of severe elevation of right ventricular diastolic pressure and low cardiac index predicts exceedingly poor outcome. EDP, end-diastolic pressure; EF, ejection fraction; RAP, right atrial pressure; WMI, wall motion index. (Data from Moore CA, Nygaard TW, Kaiser DL, et al: Postinfarction ventricular septal rupture: the importance of location of infarction and right ventricular function in determining survival. Circulation 1986;74:45-55.)

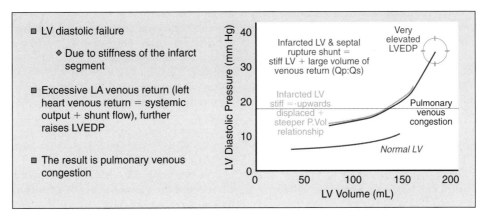

Figure 11-10. The left ventricular diastolic pressure is elevated in VSR cases because of both the up-shifting of the LV passive pressure:volume relation curve, due to loss of compliance from acute infarction, and the significant rightward displacement, due to excess venous return. LVEDP, left ventricular end-diastolic pressure.

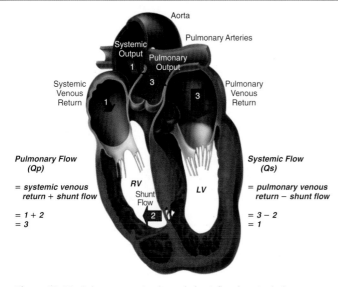

Figure 11-11. Pulmonary, systemic, and shunt flow in a typical anteroapical septal rupture.

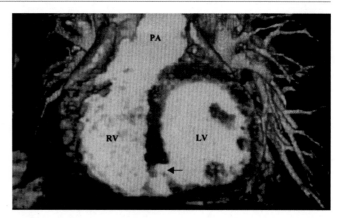

Figure 11-12. Coronal view in the plane of the pulmonary artery with 3D rendering technique showing a VSD (*arrow*) that was responsible for the right-to-left shunt found on Doppler ultrasonography. (From Paul JF, Macé L, Caussin C, et al: Multirow detector CT assessment of intraseptal dissection and ventricular pseudoaneurysm in postinfarction ventricular septal defect. Circulation 2001;104:497-498, with permission.)

Table 11-2. Clinical Presentations of Ventricular Septal Rupture

Murmur

Thrill

Jugular venous pressure elevation

Hemodynamically stable

Biventricular heart failure

Cardiogenic shock

Pulseless electrical activity

Other

many patients, particularly if the blood pressure is sustained and the VSR defect is restrictive in physiology. Third heart sounds are common and reflect high left and right atrial pressures. Signs of pulmonary congestion are generally present but usually are not prominent. Right-sided heart failure signs abound because of the combined effects of right ventricular volume overloading and right ventricular infarction. A systolic murmur is present in 98% and a thrill in 48%, and jugular venous pressure is elevated more than 7 cm in 69%.[8]

Blood pressure and heart rate are insightful parameters, and the number 100 is a useful benchmark (the "100 thing")—patients with systolic blood pressure below 100 mm Hg and heart rates above 100 bpm face substantially greater mortality. The presence of hypotension despite tachycardia occurs from failure of available compensatory mechanisms and represents circulatory failure. Mean systolic blood pressure and heart rates among VSR survivors are 110 ± 20 mm Hg and 87 ± 18 bpm; among non-survivors, they are 93 ± 19 mm Hg ($P < .01$) and 104 ± 25 bpm ($P < .05$).[10]

Data from GUSTO I documented that most (>90%) patients who were to develop VSR had only Killip class I or II hemodynamics at the time of presentation.[3]

DIAGNOSTIC TESTING FOR VENTRICULAR SEPTAL RUPTURE

Postinfarction VSR is suggested by the physical examination findings, but objective testing is required to establish the diagnosis and in particular to distinguish it from postinfarction MR and from papillary muscle rupture.

Echocardiography

Echocardiography is the test of choice because it is accurate, portable (it can be performed at the bedside or in the catheterization laboratory), and contrast free. About half of septal ruptures are obvious, large, and easily visualized holes; however, some are less easily directly visualized because they are tracts through tissue, some are multichanneled, and some are sieve-like. Therefore, septal rupture is detected more easily by color Doppler flow imaging that reveals the abnormal turbulent blood flow converging into the septum, traversing the septum, and dispersing into the right ventricle.[11] One series described a sensitivity of 58% by 2-dimensional imaging alone and 100% by color Doppler flow mapping.[12] Because the VSR generally occurs through an aneurysm that displaces into the right ventricle, views need to be angulated toward the right side. Useful echocardiographic views to image VSR are basal short-axis view, apical 4-chamber view, and subcostal long-axis view (for inferobasal VSR), and low parasternal long-axis view, apical 4-chamber view, and subcostal long-axis view (for anteroapical VSR).

Other goals for echocardiography in VSR cases are (1) to characterize the site and extent of left ventricular infarction and the site and extent of right ventricular infarction; (2) to establish or to refute the presence or absence of other complications, such as ruptures (papillary muscle rupture, false aneurysm, intramural hematoma, free wall rupture), MR, effusions, and clots; and (3) to calculate hemodynamic parameters, such as forward systemic cardiac index and RVSP.

Cardiac Computed Tomography

Advances in gated, multidetector cardiac computed tomography (CT) have enabled more robust delineation of the tract or channel responsible for the VSR shunt flow and associated false aneurysms or other complex postinfarction complications.[13] These details may be useful in planning surgery. However, CT does entail a large load of contrast material and lacks the ability to detect flow, unlike contrast ventriculography, Doppler echo, and CMR SSFP sequences.

Angiography and Catheterization Hemodynamics

Recurrent ischemia (26%), reinfarction (6%), and perioperative ischemia occur in VSR cases.[3] Angiography is indicated to identify multivessel CAD that may adversely influence the perioperative course and long-term course should the patient survive to discharge. Obtaining angiography is predicated on sufficient stability of the patient to justify the delay in obtaining surgical repair.

Catheterization is indicated to diagnose septal rupture if this happens to be the most expedient means, as it may be when the diagnosis is first suspected when the patient is in the catheterization laboratory or in the setting after repair, in which recurrent ventricular septal defect (patch leak) is often easily detected if there is a pulmonary artery catheter line in place. Otherwise, in the current era, heart catheterization is usually unnecessary to diagnose VSR. Formerly, catheterization for pressures and waveforms, oximetry, and ventriculography were central in the diagnosis of septal rupture and its distinction from MR; however, they no longer are.

Performance of catheterization, oximetry, or ventriculography may increase time delay in obtaining surgery, and contrast ventriculography may accentuate the tendency to renal insufficiency, which is extremely common in septal rupture cases. Furthermore, catheterization is not diagnostic of septal rupture, oximetry has false-positives and false-negatives, the calculation of Qp:Qs is not necessary for the management of VSR, and contrast ventriculography is less accurate in depicting associated complex post–myocardial infarction complications such as false aneurysms. Renal insufficiency is a marker of mortality.

The majority of septal rupture cases have underlying single- or two-vessel CAD (see Table 7-2), but angiographic three-vessel CAD is present in about one quarter of cases.[14]

As would be expected, VSR cases have an approximately 2:1 ratio of LAD disease to RCA disease (64% versus 26%) and very little responsible left circumflex disease (2%).[3] VSR cases are non-reperfusion cases; the GUSTO I trial tabulated that infarct-related arteries had 61% only TIMI 0 or I flow, stenoses in 100%, and occlusion in 57%.[3]

Right-sided heart balloon flotation catheterization is often useful to optimize hemodynamics and can be used to diagnose VSR by an O_2 step-up. The following are usual right-sided heart hemodynamic findings:

- Elevated right atrial pressure from right ventricular diastolic failure, ± tricuspid regurgitation
- Elevated pulmonary artery (PA) pressure from elevation of pulmonary capillary wedge pressure (PCWP; backpressure), V or VA waves, and high flow
- Elevated PCWP from left ventricular diastolic failure and high pulmonary venous return
- Increased (right-sided) cardiac output (note that in VSR, pulmonary and systemic flows are not interchangeable; therefore, PA catheter–derived flows are not to be interpreted as systemic flow)

Significant V waves are common in VSR, in the absence of concurrent mitral insufficiency, and reflect venous return exceeding atrial compliance. In a series of six patients with postinfarction septal rupture, all six had an O_2 step-up consistent with a ventricular septal defect, five of six had large V waves on PA catheterization, and none had mitral insufficiency by either contrast ventriculography or echocardiography. Therefore, V waves are not specific for mitral insufficiency in the postinfarction setting.[15,16]

Oximetry, by establishing a step-up from the right atrium to the right ventricular levels, indicates left-to-right shunting at the ventricular level (Figs. 11-12 and 11-13). A threshold of more than 5% is used when fluoroscopic guidance of sampling is employed or more than 10% if fluoroscopic guidance is not employed. Oximetric sampling may be performed by one or more techniques: (1) fluoroscopic guidance of sampling; (2) pressure and waveform guidance of sampling; and (3) use of the right atrial and distal PA catheter ports. The bedside PA catheter technique of proximal and distal port sampling is the easiest, and it is probably accurate to establish the presence of a shunt if a delta of more than 10% is used; but it is the least accurate means to localize the level of shunting because it may be anywhere between the two sample sites, and it is not without false-positives with respect to septal rupture. Other causes of step-ups may occur at the atrial level if there is an atrial septal defect, at the ventricular level if there is a congenital ventricular septal defect or other shunt into the right ventricle, or into the pulmonary artery if there is a patent ductus arteriosus or massive mitral insufficiency.

Inflation of a 7-French balloon catheter in the main pulmonary artery has been performed to successfully resuscitate the blood pressure of postinfarction septal rupture patients.[17]

MANAGEMENT OF VENTRICULAR SEPTAL RUPTURE

VSR is a class I ACC/AHA indication for each of the following[18]:

- Balloon flotation right-sided heart catheter monitoring
- IABP
- Early coronary angiography
- Emergency or urgent cardiac surgical repair
- Emergency or urgent coronary artery bypass graft surgery

Management of VSR patients with *adequate* tissue perfusion:

- Airway and breathing, mechanical ventilation if needed
- Vasodilators (nitroprusside, hydralazine, nitroglycerin) ± inotropes

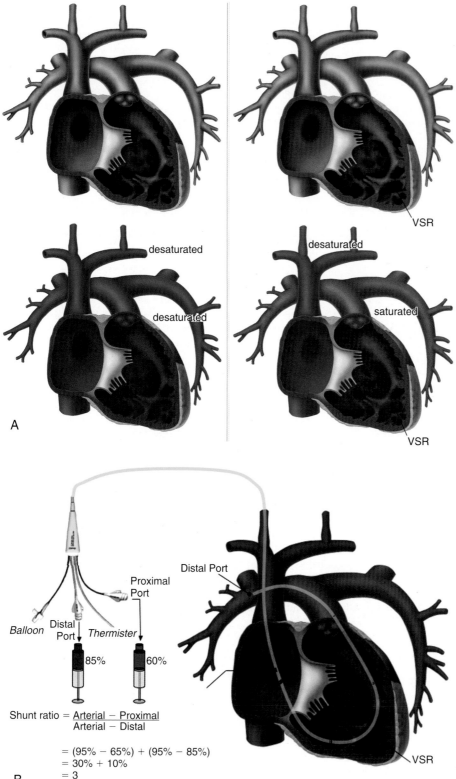

Figure 11-13. A, Right-sided views of an intact heart (LEFT IMAGES) and of a heart with an apical ventricular septal level defect or rupture. Lower images depict expected blood oxyhemoglobin saturation in the respective chambers and vessels. In an intact heart, the oxyhemoglobin saturation is essentially identical throughout. In a heart with a septal defect, introduction of saturated left-sided heart blood through the defect or rupture at the septal level increases the oxyhemoglobin saturation within the right ventricle and pulmonary arteries. **B,** Bedside calculation of the shunt ratio by sampling of blood from the two ports of a pulmonary artery flotation catheter.

desaturated

desaturated

VSR

desaturated

saturated

VSR

A

Distal Port

Proximal Port

Balloon   Distal Port   *Thermister*

85%   60%

Shunt ratio = $\dfrac{\text{Arterial} - \text{Proximal}}{\text{Arterial} - \text{Distal}}$

= (95% − 65%) + (95% − 85%)
= 30% + 10%
= 3

B

VSR

- Coronary angiography
- Early surgery (within 1 or 2 days)
- Consideration, if clinically stable and well, of delayed repair

Management of VSR patients with *inadequate* tissue perfusion:

- Airway and breathing, mechanical ventilation as needed
- IABP
- Inotropes are preferable because vasodilators are seldom tolerated
- ± Coronary angiography if stability allows
- Emergent surgery

Efforts to stabilize VSR cases are directed at maintenance of organ function, by optimizing hemodynamics, until surgical repair is obtained and are not to delay surgery. Afterload reduction, by selective arterial vasodilators in patients with adequate blood pressure and IABP in those without, recovers into forward stroke volume a proportion of shunt volume, thereby increasing systemic blood flow and reducing pulmonary congestion (blood flow, blood volume, and lung water) and optimizing gas exchange. When needed, inotropic agents can be used to optimize contractile function of stunned and hibernating myocardium.

IABP is the most effective means to improve systemic cardiac output and to alleviate pulmonary edema by reducing shunt flow and increasing systemic flow (Fig. 11-14). Selective arterial vasodilators (hydralazine[19] or nitroprusside) may be used to reduce the shunt flow, depending on heart rate and blood pressure. Inotropes may be useful if the patient is hypotensive or congested. Of note, many patients cannot be adequately stabilized, and prolonged episodes to do so will delay surgery.

Surgical Repair

The goals of surgical repair are to exclude the right ventricle from the left ventricle by suturing patches around the site of rupture. Concurrent aortocoronary artery bypass grafting is performed as well. Surgical repair techniques are numerous and variable, depending on the location and size of the infarct and the rupture and the presence of associated lesions, and they are best adapted to the case and to the surgeon's experience (Figs. 11-15 to 11-18). Patching of the rupture excludes the left ventricular cavity and

restores its integrity. A patch may be (but is not always) placed in the right ventricle as well. Patches are usually placed by entering the left ventricle through an infarctectomy (resection of portions of infarcted tissue). Buttressing of the repair to reduce the tension within it is commonly performed. Placement of patches solely on the right ventricular side is prone to early patch leak.[1]

Surgical repair entails high mortality (27% of non–cardiogenic shock and more than 50% of cardiogenic shock—100% in GUSTO I,[3] 81% operative mortality in the SHOCK trial), but undeniably there is a salvage rate. Surgical mortality is influenced by the severity of preoperative congestive heart failure (CHF) and hemodynamics (Table 11-3; Figs. 11-19 to 11-22).[20] Five-year survival of patients who initially survive surgery is above 50%.[21]

The optimal timing of surgery has been debated for decades. Overall, early (urgent or emergent) repair is preferable because most patients steadily deteriorate, and the strategy of waiting weeks for fibrosis of the myocardium to facilitate surgery leaves few patients to operate on. Killip class III and IV cases should undergo emergency surgery because organ failure will ensue and dominate the postoperative course.

Percutaneous device closure as a potential alternative to surgery for repair of VSR has been proposed by some (Figs. 11-23 and 11-24), borrowing from the success of congenital ventricular septal defect closures,[22] but the experience is limited and the technique unproven. Case reports and small series have established that device closure can be successful.[23,24] Closure of congenital ventricular septal defects is a different proposition because

Table 11-3. Predictors of Mortality in Ventricular Septal Rupture

Location (73% inferior versus 30% anterior, $P < .05$)

Right ventricular failure (RA pressure > 12 mm Hg, presence of severe RV systolic and septal dysfunction on echocardiography)

Shock (cardiogenic shock of any description, systemic CI < 1.75 L/min/m²)

Early onset (<7 days)

CI, cardiac index; RA, right atrial; RV, right ventricular.
From Moore CA, Nygaard TW, Kaiser DL, et al: Postinfarction ventricular septal rupture: the importance of location of infarction and right ventricular function in determining survival. Circulation 1986;74:45-55.

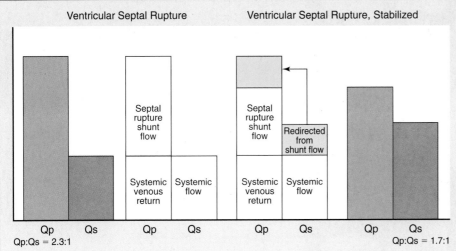

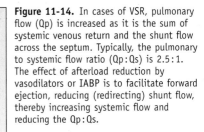

Figure 11-14. In cases of VSR, pulmonary flow (Qp) is increased as it is the sum of systemic venous return and the shunt flow across the septum. Typically, the pulmonary to systemic flow ratio (Qp:Qs) is 2.5:1. The effect of afterload reduction by vasodilators or IABP is to facilitate forward ejection, reducing (redirecting) shunt flow, thereby increasing systemic flow and reducing the Qp:Qs.

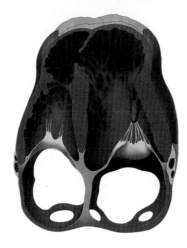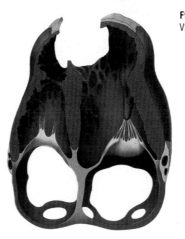

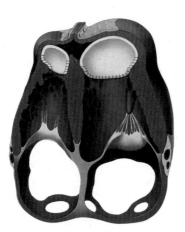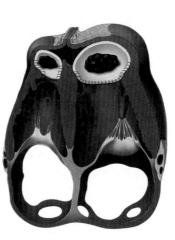

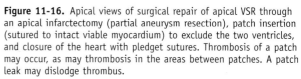

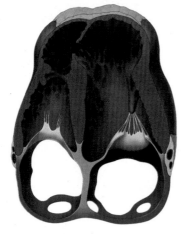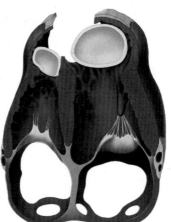

Figure 11-16. Apical views of surgical repair of apical VSR through an apical infarctectomy (partial aneurysm resection), patch insertion (sutured to intact viable myocardium) to exclude the two ventricles, and closure of the heart with pledget sutures. Thrombosis of a patch may occur, as may thrombosis in the areas between patches. A patch leak may dislodge thrombus.

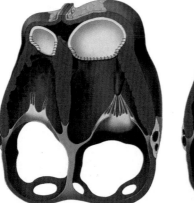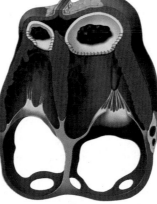

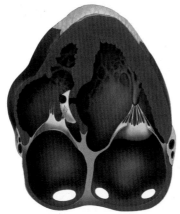

Figure 11-17. Schematic representation of surgical repair of basal VSR.

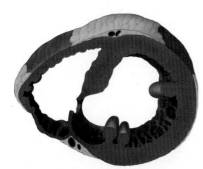
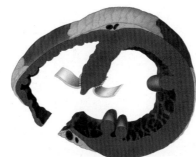
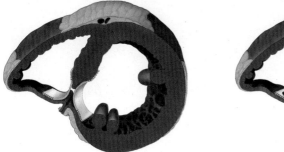
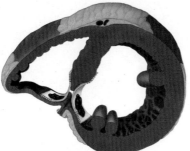

Figure 11-18. Short-axis views of surgical repair of a posterobasal VSR through a basal infarctotomy, small infarctectomy (partial aneurysm resection), patch insertion (sutured to intact viable myocardium) to exclude the two ventricles, and closure of the heart with pledget sutures. Thrombosis of a patch may occur, as may thrombosis in the areas between patches. A patch leak may dislodge thrombus.

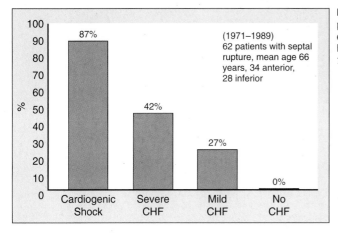

Figure 11-19. Preoperative congestive heart failure (CHF) severity clearly predicts operative mortality. (Data from Deville C, Fontan F, Chevalier JM, et al: Surgery of post-infarction ventricular septal defect: risk factors for hospital death and long-term results. Eur J Cardiothorac Surg 1991;5:167-174.)

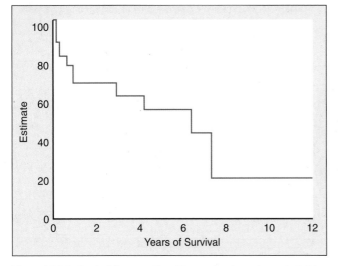

Figure 11-20. Survival for more than 10 years has been demonstrated in VSR cases that underwent repair. (From Cummings RG, Califf R, Jones RN, et al: Correlates of survival in patients with postinfarction ventricular septal defect. Ann Thorac Surg 1989;47:824-830.)

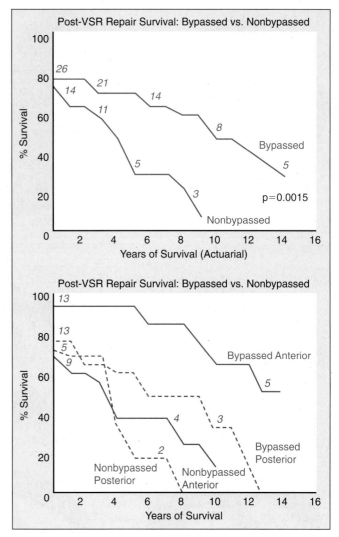

Figure 11-22. Observational data suggest that aortocoronary bypass grafting is associated with better outcomes, whether for anterior or inferior VSR. (From Muehrcke DD, Daggett WM Jr, Buckley MJ, et al: Postinfarct ventricular septal defect repair: effect of coronary artery bypass grafting. Ann Thorac Surg 1992;54:876-882. Copyright Elsevier, 1992.)

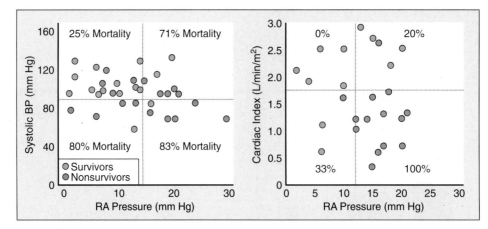

Figure 11-21. Surgical mortality can be predicted by several clinical and hemodynamic parameters. Severe low output in the setting of markedly elevated right atrial (RA) pressure as a sign of a large rupture with severe right-sided heart failure is the best predictor. Hypotension in the setting of markedly elevated right atrial pressure is a less accurate predictor, given the variable correlation of blood pressure to cardiac index. (LEFT PANEL from Held AC, Cole PL, Lipton B, et al: Rupture of the interventricular septum complicating acute myocardial infarction: a multicenter analysis of clinical findings and outcome. Am Heart J 1988;116[pt 1]:1330-1336, with permission from Elsevier. RIGHT PANEL from Moore CA, Nygaard TW, Kaiser DL, et al: Postinfarction ventricular septal rupture: the importance of location of infarction and right ventricular function in determining survival. Circulation 1986;74:45-55.)

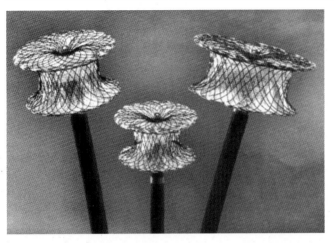

Figure 11-23. Nitinol wire ventricular septal closure devices. Note the thick stem, suitable for deployment across a normal muscular septum. (Image courtesy of AGA Medical Corporation.)

there is no associated myocardial necrosis, and seating of a device is more straightforward. Furthermore, a device is highly unlikely to rupture infarcted myocardium, whereas it may in postinfarction VSR cases. Complex rupture anatomy (multiple channels, long channels, and associated lesions such as false aneurysms and intramural hematomas) is a disadvantage for the device closure technique.

11

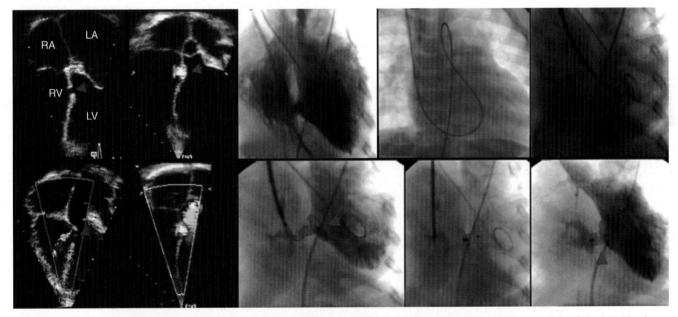

Figure 11-24. Echocardiographic (LEFT) and fluoroscopic (RIGHT) images of a congenital ventricular septal defect closure. (Courtesy of Ziyad M. Hiyazi, MD, Chicago, Illinois.)

CASE 1

History

▸ 65-year-old man with "CHF"
▸ Admitted to a community hospital with CHF (class II-III), an "MR" murmur, and a displaced apex
▸ No history of chest pains; complained of indigestion 2 weeks ago
▸ Past medical history is significant for type 2 diabetes, hypertension, remote smoker

Physical Examination

▸ BP 100/60 mm Hg, HR 102 bpm, RR 16/min
▸ Well appearing when at rest, fatigues and becomes ashen walking in the room; extremities warm
▸ JVD 8 cm (V waves)

▸ Apex enlarged and displaced
▸ S_1 normal, S_2 increased split, S_3
▸ Pansystolic murmur 3/6 maximal halfway between the apex and LLSB, radiating to the RLSB; no diastolic murmur; no thrill
▸ Urine output 60 mL/hr

Clinical Impression and Management Plan

▸ Silent inferoposterior and inferior septal infarction in an adult diabetic
▸ Postinfarction septal rupture; no MR
▸ Systolic BP of 100 mm Hg in a "hypertensive" individual indicative of the reduction in cardiac function brought on by the infarction and shunt
▸ Early surgical repair
▸ Adequate hemodynamics to obtain angiography before surgery

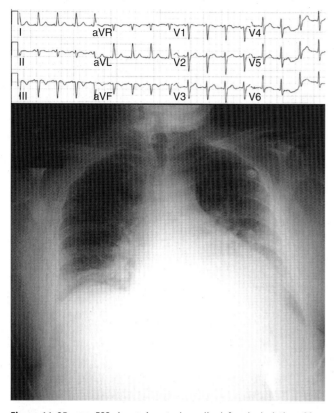

Figure 11-25. TOP, ECG shows sinus tachycardia, left axis deviation, QS waves in leads III, aVF also with T-wave inversion. Inferior infarction of indeterminate age. No ECG evidence of LVH. BOTTOM, Chest radiograph shows cardiomegaly, interstitial edema, and prominent hilar edema.

Cardiac Surgery

▸ Surgery revealed infarction of the inferoposterior wall and inferior septum, mid inferior septal rupture.
▸ The right ventricle did not appear infarcted.
▸ Closure of VSR (infarctectomy, patches) was performed as well as an aortocoronary bypass × 3 (SV to LAD, OM, PDA).

Outcome

▸ Uneventful intraoperative course and early postoperative period
▸ 24 hours later, the pansystolic murmur recurred and hemiparesis occurred.
▸ The patient survived, with neurologic disability.
▸ CCS class I, NYHA class II at follow-up
▸ The patch leak and its murmur persist. The size of the leak is not a hemodynamic problem.

Comments

▸ Silent transmural infarction (NIDDM) underlies the unrecognized VSR.
▸ Common difficulty in distinguishing VSR and MR by physical examination
▸ Difficulty in identifying pulmonary congestion without chest radiography
▸ Coronary angiography identified three-vessel disease in this patient without habitual angina.
▸ The patient was sicker initially than thought—a common retrospective conclusion in VSR cases.
▸ Postoperative patch leak (common)
▸ Survival, but with comorbidity

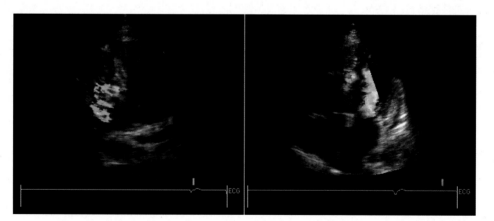

Figure 11-26. Transthoracic echocardiography with color Doppler flow mapping. LEFT, Apical 4-chamber view with inferior angulation. There is a jet within the body of the RV, although the origin of the jet is not seen on this view. RIGHT, Apical 4-chamber view. Flow convergence into and across the septum is visualized on another plane of imaging, indicating the septal rupture.

11

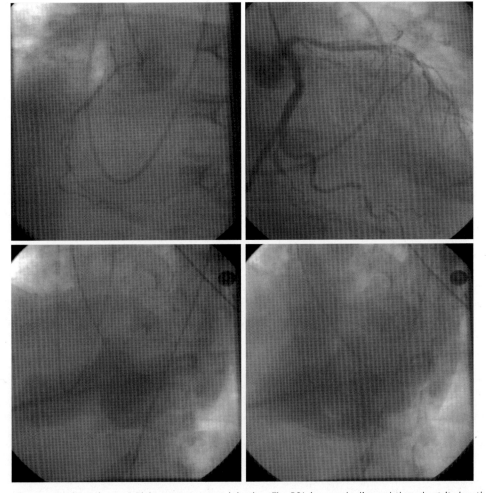

Figure 11-27. TOP ROW, Coronary angiography. LEFT, Right coronary artery injection. The RCA is severely diseased throughout its length. RIGHT, Left coronary artery injection. There are significant stenoses in the mid LAD and of a large obtuse marginal branch of the left circumflex artery. BOTTOM ROW, Contrast ventriculography, LAO projection. LEFT, Earlier frame. RIGHT, Later frame during the injection. The RV clearly opacifies early and later after injection. The inferior wall is dilated and was akinetic, as was the inferior wall of the right ventricle. The right ventricle is also dilated because of its infarction.

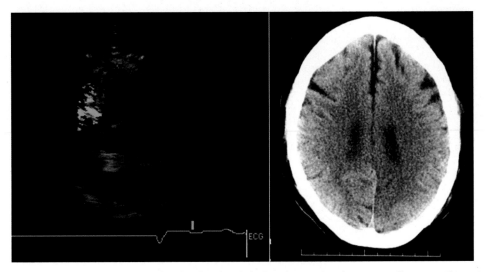

Figure 11-28. LEFT, Transthoracic echocardiography, apical 4-chamber view. Color Doppler mapping demonstrates flow across the septum, indicating a patch leak. RIGHT, Contrast-enhanced CT scan of the head. There is an enhancing region in the right occiput, consistent with infarction, presumed thromboembolism from the patch.

CASE 2

History

- 67-year-old man admitted with late-presentation anterolateral STEMI (no fibrinolytics)
  - Pains during the last 2 days but none in the last 6 hours
  - Short of breath
  - CK 2700
- Past medical history is significant for hypertension, chronic renal failure, previous renal transplantation, and abdominal aortic aneurysm (3 cm).
- Hypotensive at admission, progressive heart failure and shock during 12 hours—IABP inserted

Physical Examination

- BP 88/60 mm Hg, HR 108 bpm, RR 18/min
- Ashen appearance, extremities cool
- Central venous distention, no edema
- S_1, S_2 reduced; S_3 present; no rubs
- 3/6 pansystolic murmur radiating to RLSB, no diastolic murmurs
- Apex enlarged and sustained; crepitations at both bases
- Urine output 20 mL/hr

Clinical Impression and Management Plan

- Anteroseptal myocardial infarction, late presentation
- Postinfarction septal rupture of the anterior apex
- No other mechanical complications of infarction
- Cardiogenic shock
- Emergent surgical repair
- Obtain angiography before surgery

Cardiac Surgery and Postoperative Course

- The patient lost blood pressure by the time he arrived in the operating room and had to be resuscitated as he was being put on the pump.

- Surgical findings: an anterior apical septal rupture (almost 1.5 cm); infarction of the distal anterior wall and septum and apex; and an apical aneurysm
- Closure of VSR (infarctectomy, patches) and an aortocoronary bypass × 2 (SV to LAD coronary artery, PDA) were performed.
- After a tenuous and prolonged postoperative course, the patient was discharged home 2 months later.
- During the next 3 months, progressive congestive symptoms (NYHA class III) and a new apical pansystolic murmur with axillary radiation developed.

Second Cardiac Surgery and Eventual Outcome

- The heart failure was due to severe MR from adverse cavitary remodeling and the left ventricle dysfunction. Because it was severe despite medical therapy, the patient was referred for mitral valve replacement surgery.
- Surgery found an apical aneurysm but normal mitral apparatus (no papillary muscle rupture).
- Mechanical mitral replacement and apical aneurysmectomy were performed.
- Slow but progressive postoperative course
- Discharged home with improved heart failure symptoms, but still with shortness of breath (NYHA class II)

Comments

- Typical background of hypertension, no known prior CAD, first infarction
- Late-presentation STEMI (completed)
- Early septal rupture and early cardiogenic shock. Cardiogenic shock was due to the left ventricular dysfunction from the infarction and the large septal rupture defect.
- In this case, IABP afforded only transient stabilization. The time to obtain angiography first was clinically relevant, as the patient was arresting by the time that he was in the operating room.
- Adverse remodeling of the infarct segment resulted in severe mitral insufficiency.

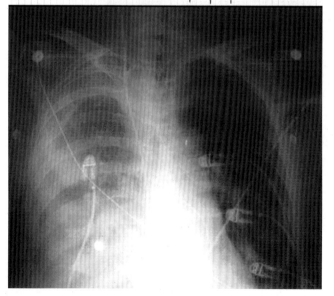

Figure 11-29. TOP, ECG shows sinus rhythm, low voltages (<5 mm in all standard limb leads); Q waves I, aVL; minimal precordial R waves; ST elevation V_2-V_6, I, ? II, III, aVF. Anterolateral infarction, possible aneurysm. BOTTOM, Chest radiograph shows pulmonary edema, endotracheal tube in correct position, PA catheter tip in main pulmonary artery, IABP tip in correct position.

11

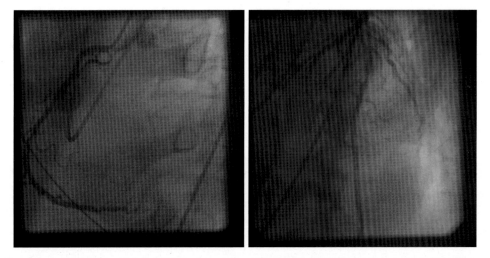

Figure 11-30. Selective coronary angiography. LEFT, The right coronary artery is dominant with moderate disease. RIGHT, The left coronary artery injection reveals proximal severe LAD disease. The left circumflex artery was without angiographically significant disease.

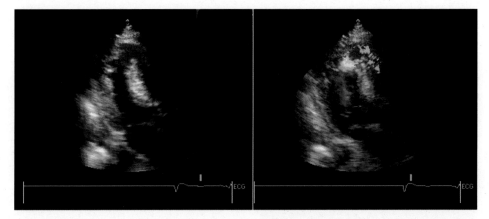

Figure 11-31. Transthoracic echocardiography. Both images show steep parasternal long-axis views. There is obvious disruption (>1 cm) of the distal septum. There was dyskinesis of the distal left ventricular walls and hypercontractile function of the proximal segments. Color Doppler flow mapping reveals the expected flow across the septum and into the right ventricle.

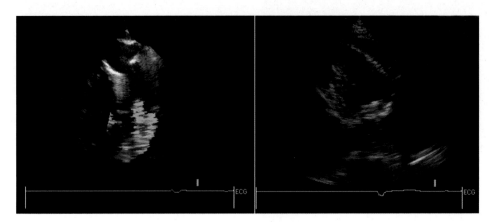

Figure 11-32. Transthoracic echocardiography. LEFT, Apical 4-chamber view with color Doppler mapping. There has been adverse remodeling of the left ventricle. The distal half of the left ventricle is an aneurysm. There is no residual (or recurrent) ventricular septal defect. There is now severe MR from "tenting" of the mitral leaflets. RIGHT, After mitral valve replacement and aneurysmectomy. The left ventricular cavity is much smaller because of the aneurysmectomy and loss of volume loading from the mitral insufficiency. The left ventricular systolic function had reduced.

CASE 3

History

▸ 72-year-old homeless man with two syncopal episodes
▸ No chest pains, no shortness of breath
▸ Past medical history is significant for smoking
▸ Inferior STEMI, given fibrinolytic in the emergency department

Physical Examination

▸ BP 80/50 mm Hg, HR 95 bpm
▸ Weak appearing, distressed
▸ No crepitations
▸ 1/6 systolic murmur at apex
▸ Apex not displaced or enlarged
▸ Venous pressure 9 cm above the sternal angle, no edema
▸ CK 310, MB positive; troponins elevated
▸ Urine output 15 mL/hr

Clinical Impression

▸ Inferior and right ventricular infarction; mid inferior septal rupture
▸ Cardiogenic shock from large septal rupture and extensive right ventricular infarction

Evolution and Outcome

▸ Within a half hour, a PEA arrest occurred from which the patient could not be resuscitated.

Comments

▸ Unknown past medical history, unknown onset of infarction, probably late presentation
▸ Cardiogenic shock from VSR and large right ventricular infarction
▸ The 1/6 systolic murmur was probably due to the VSR, although not initially thought to be so. The severe shock, low flow, and large defect did not generate the usual conspicuous murmur.
▸ Classic myocardial rupture at a hinge point
▸ The occurrence of PEA may have been further tearing of the septal rupture, right or left ventricular rupture, or another mechanical complication.

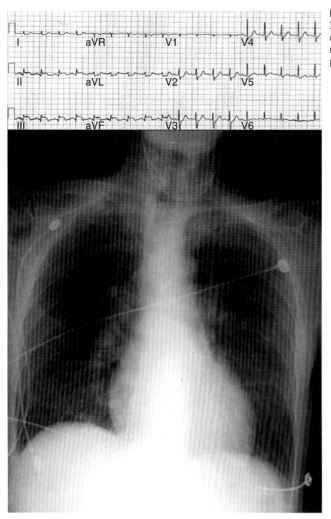

Figure 11-33. TOP, ECG shows sinus tachycardia, inferior ST elevation (II, III, aVF), ST depression V_2-V_3 and early R-wave dominance, and lateral ST depression (I, aVL). Inferior ± posterior acute infarction. BOTTOM, Chest radiograph shows normal cardiopericardial silhouette, mild interstitial pulmonary edema, and hyperinflated lungs (possible COPD).

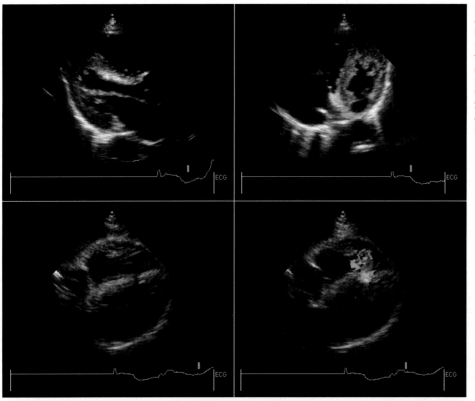

Figure 11-34. Transthoracic echocardiography. TOP LEFT, Parasternal long-axis view. The right ventricle is prominently dilated. The posterior wall of the LV is akinetic. TOP RIGHT, Apical 4-chamber view angulated to the right. The right ventricle is severely dilated. The inferior septum is dyskinetic. BOTTOM ROW, Subcostal long-axis view. There is flow across a defect in the septum in diastole (LEFT) and in systole (RIGHT).

11

CASE 4

History

▸ 75-year-old woman
▸ Late-presentation inferior myocardial infarction (14 hours after pain onset); no finbrinolytics, no clinically detected right ventricular infarction
▸ Initially heart failure free
▸ Previous hypertension; no prior known CAD
▸ Day 4 after myocardial infarction, deteriorated (without chest pain)

Physical Examination

▸ BP 90/60 mm Hg, HR 105 bpm, RR 24/min
▸ Weak, warm extremities
▸ Venous distention to angle of the jaw
▸ Normal S_1, S_2; S_3 present
▸ 4/6 pansystolic murmur (new) at the LLSB with radiation to right side of the chest
▸ Crepitations over the lower half of the lung fields
▸ Urine output 45 mL/hr

Clinical Impression and Management Plan

▸ Inferior wall and inferior septal infarction and aneurysm; postinfarction septal rupture of the inferior septum, apex; posterior right ventricular infarction; and cardiogenic shock

▸ Plan was for an emergent surgical repair and angiography before surgery.

Cardiac Surgery

▸ Surgery found a basal inferior infarction and aneurysm, basal inferior septal rupture, and basal right ventricular infarction.
▸ Closure of VSR (infarctectomy, patches) and an aortocoronary bypass × 1 (SV to PDA) were performed uneventfully.

Postoperative Course and Outcome

▸ Postoperatively, there was no murmur, and the hemodynamics were good.
▸ On postoperative day 6, late postoperative sepsis and shock developed.
▸ On postoperative day 9, she died of acidosis and renal failure.

Comments

▸ Late-presentation myocardial infarction, previously hypertensive patient
▸ Usual association of basal inferior septal rupture and right ventricular myocardial infarction
▸ Lesser right ventricular myocardial infarction explained by mid, not proximal, RCA occlusion
▸ Despite the age of 75 years, the initial postoperative course was smooth.
▸ Sepsis determined the outcome.

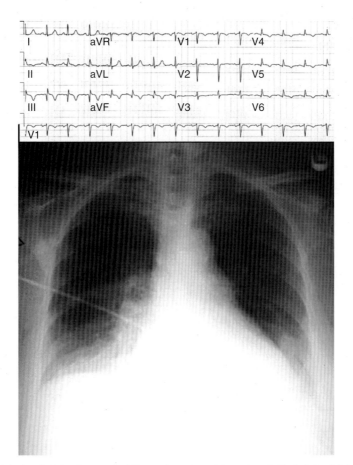

Figure 11-35. TOP, ECG shows sinus rhythm, inferior Q waves, and T-wave inversions; T inversions V_4-V_6. Inferior infarction. BOTTOM, Chest radiograph shows cardiomegaly and mild interstitial pulmonary edema.

11

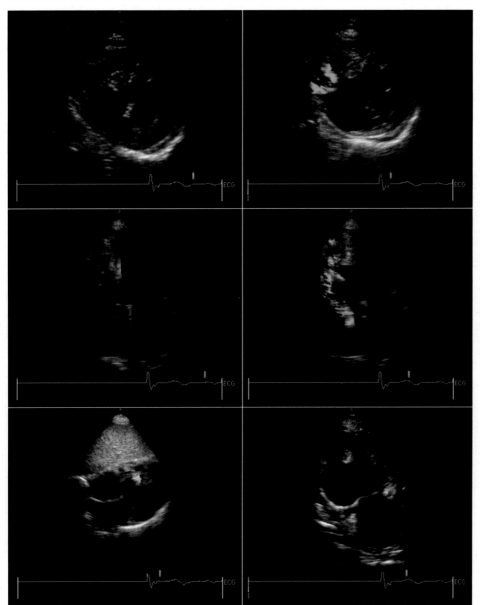

Figure 11-36. Transthoracic echocardiography. TOP LEFT, Parasternal short-axis view. Aneurysm, thinning and marked dyskinesis of the inferior wall and inferior septum. Akinesis of the inferior wall of the right ventricle. No tissue defect of the septum appreciated on 2-dimensional imaging. TOP RIGHT, Color Doppler flow mapping reveals two sites of flow through the aneurysmal segment of the inferior septum, indicating complex septal rupture. MIDDLE ROW, Apical 4-chamber view and color Doppler views in diastole (LEFT) and systole (RIGHT). Aneurysmal deformation of the basal inferior septum is apparent. Flow across it into the right ventricle is seen in systole. The right ventricle was also dilated and akinetic in its inferior and lateral walls. BOTTOM LEFT, Subcostal long-axis view with color Doppler mapping demonstrates shunt flow through the aneurysmal segment of the inferior septum at several sites, indicating complex septal rupture through the aneurysm. BOTTOM RIGHT, Apical 2-chamber view shows an aneurysm (wide-necked area of dilation in both systole and diastole) of the basal and mid inferior wall of the left ventricle.

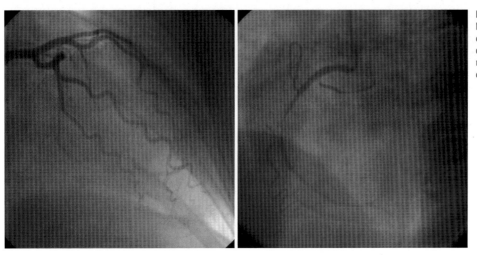

Figure 11-37. Coronary angiography. No significant stenoses within the left coronary artery. The right coronary artery is dominant and with a 95% stenosis in its midportion, with slow flow and distal competitive flow.

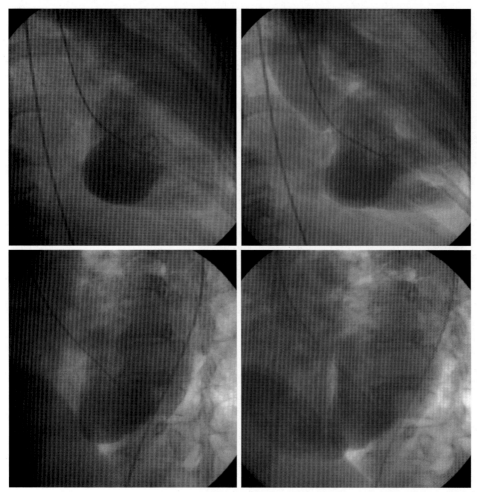

Figure 11-38. Contrast ventriculography. TOP ROW, RAO projection. BOTTOM ROW, LAO projection. LEFT IMAGES, Early injection. RIGHT IMAGES, Later injection. This test shows basal inferior aneurysm, mid inferior akinesis, and distal inferior and apical hypokinesis. Contrast appears in the right ventricle, establishing a ventricular septal defect. The right ventricle is dilated and akinetic at least in the inferior portions. There is also mitral or tricuspid regurgitation, and at least one atrium opacifies.

CASE 5

History

▸ 82-year-old woman transferred for management 5 days after inferior wall myocardial infarction; had received thrombolytics at hour 6 for an acute anterior STEMI
▸ Initially Killip class I
▸ One recurrence of angina
▸ Past medical history of hypertension

Physical Examination

▸ BP 128/75 mm Hg, HR 100 bpm, RR 32/min
▸ JVP 8 cm above the sternal angle
▸ S_1, S_2 normal; S_3
▸ 3/6 holosystolic murmur radiating to RLSB, thrill present
▸ Apex enlarged and sustained
▸ Crepitations over the lower half of the lung fields

Clinical Impression and Management Plan

▸ Anterior apical septal infarction and aneurysm
▸ Postinfarction septal rupture of the apical septum

▸ Killip III hemodynamics
▸ There was consensus that nonsurgical conservative and comfort measures would be best.
▸ Diuretics and as much hydralazine as possible were instituted, as tolerated by the blood pressure. There was surprisingly little renal insufficiency.

Outcome

▸ The patient survived 9 more weeks, with most of it at home, bedridden but comfortable and able to interact with her family.

Comments

▸ Usual background of hypertension, no known CAD, first myocardial infarction
▸ Anteroapical VSR, without significant right ventricular infarction
▸ Hemodynamically well tolerated
▸ Hemodynamics manageable with selective arterial vasodilators
▸ In terms of cardiac repair, this patient stood a good chance of successful surgery; but in terms of her ability to be weaned postoperatively, she stood little chance.
▸ The survival of 11 weeks after infarction attests to the possibility of short-term survival in about a quarter of cases.

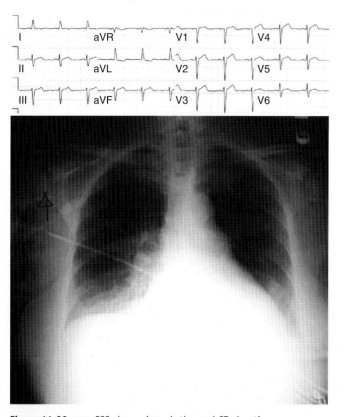

Figure 11-39. TOP, ECG shows sinus rhythm and ST elevation across precordial leads. BOTTOM, Chest radiograph shows cardiomegaly and mild interstitial pulmonary edema.

Table 11-4. Hemodynamic Profile

	Native	After Hydralazine
Blood pressure	130/773 mm Hg	105/60 mm Hg
RVSP from TR and VSR	55 mm Hg	45 mm Hg
Qp:Qs	2.2:1	1.6
Systemic CI	2.0 L/min/m^2	2.6 L/min/m^2
Symptoms (NYHA class)	IV	III

CI, cardiac index; RVSP, right ventricular systolic pressure; TR, tricuspid regurgitation; VSR, ventricular septal rupture.

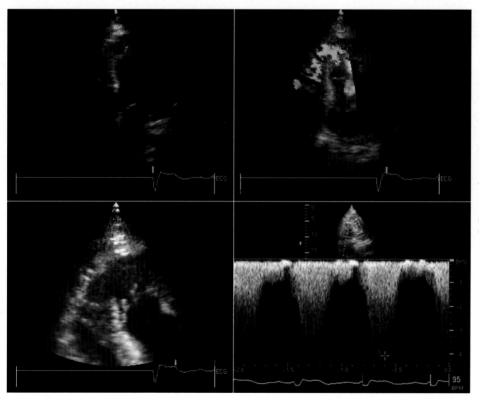

Figure 11-40. Transthoracic echocardiography. TOP LEFT, Apical 4-chamber view. Localized distal septal dyskinesis. Tissue disruption at distal septum. TOP RIGHT, Flow across the septum into the RV demonstrated by color Doppler flow mapping. BOTTOM LEFT, Zoom view of the distal septum better reveals the anatomic disruption, which has some complexity. BOTTOM RIGHT, Spectral display of holosystolic flow across the ventricular septal defect. There is a 60 mm Hg gradient from the left ventricle into the right ventricle. (RVSP = blood pressure$_{systolic}$ $- 4 \times V^2 = 58$ mm Hg. RVSP from tricuspid regurgitation jet = 58 mm Hg.) Other Doppler-derived information included a cardiac index of 2.0 L/min/m^2 and a Qp:Qs of 2.2:1.

CASE 6

History

- 75-year-old woman, young-appearing for age, very active and well
- Presented to a community hospital at hour 9 of an anterior STEMI
  - Initially hypertensive, 180/110 mm Hg, and with mild pulmonary edema
  - Received a fibrinolytic, as chest pain was ongoing (although subsiding), after control of blood pressure by IV nitroglycerin
- Past medical history is significant for hypertension.
- Mild pulmonary edema resolved spontaneously. She was heart failure free and with high-normal blood pressure for 2 days. On day 3, there was an abrupt fall in blood pressure from 155 to 105 mm Hg systolic, agitation, and a new murmur, and she was transferred for evaluation and care.
- CK: 3300

Physical Examination

- BP 105/80 mm Hg, HR 105 bpm, RR 24/min
- Venous distention: 10 cm above the sternal angle
- Normal S_1, S_2; S_3 present
- Pansystolic murmur at the LLSB (5/6) with radiation to right side of chest, thrill present
- Apex enlarged and sustained (mesoapical impulse.)

Clinical Impression and Management Plan

- Anterior apical septal infarction and aneurysm
- Postinfarction septal rupture of the apical septum
- Killip III hemodynamics
- Plan was for early surgical repair and angiography before surgery

Cardiac Surgery Findings

- Surgical findings: an anterior and apical septal aneurysm and infarct, and an apical septal rupture
- Closure of VSR (infarctectomy, patches) followed by an aortocoronary bypass × 1 (SV to LAD coronary artery), performed uneventfully

Postoperative Course and Outcome

- Postoperatively, there was no murmur, no step-up, and the CO and PCWP were normal
- Uneventful until the fourth postoperative day, when the pansystolic murmur recurred
- The systemic cardiac index fell from 2.6 L/min/m^2 to 2.1 L/min/m^2, and step-up was demonstrated. No organ dysfunction ensued, and the patient remained stable.
- She was discharged CCS class I and NYHA class II and remained stable at follow-up.

Comments

- Typical background of first infarction, no known previous CAD, chronic hypertension
- Classic abrupt painless hemodynamic deterioration due to septal rupture
- New-onset murmur and thrill
- Hypertension during the infarction may have contributed to the occurrence of rupture.
- The systolic blood pressure of 105 mm Hg was associated with severely reduced systemic CI and represented a 40% fall from the patient's usual hypertensive blood pressure.
- Postoperative patch leak (small)
- Survival

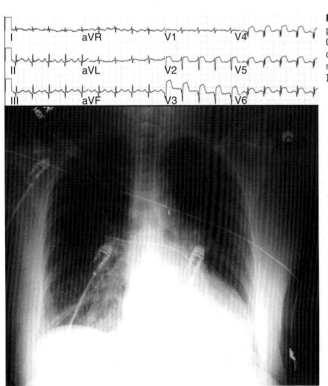

Figure 11-41. TOP, ECG shows sinus tachycardia, left atrial abnormality, precordial ST elevation (present for 4 days), Q waves V_2-V_6, and also inferior Q waves. Anteroseptal infarction recent. Inferior Q waves may be from the distal portion of the LAD coronary artery around the apex. BOTTOM, Chest radiograph shows borderline cardiomegaly and interstitial pulmonary edema. IABP is in correct position at distal arch.

11

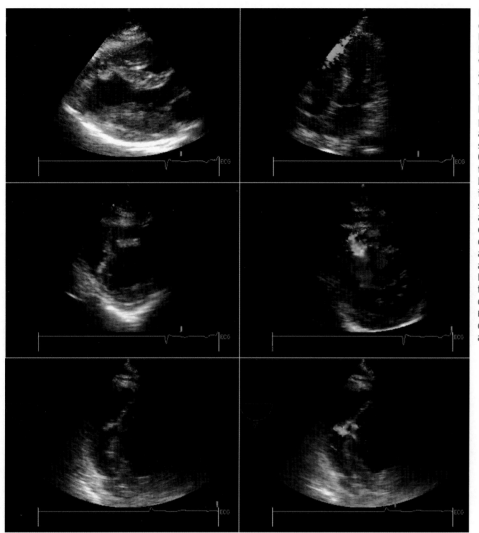

Figure 11-42. Transthoracic echocardiography. TOP LEFT, Parasternal long-axis view. Dynamic contraction of the basal septum and basal and mid posterior walls. Akinetic mid to distal septum and apex and inferior apex with aneurysm formation. Obvious flow across a septal rupture at the margin of the aneurysm. Normal mitral valve appearance. No pericardial fluid. TOP RIGHT, Dyskinetic aneurysm and disruption of the distal septum. Dyskinetic and aneurysmal apex. Color Doppler flow mapping demonstrates flow across the anterior septum. Dynamic basal lateral wall and dynamic basal inferior septum. MIDDLE LEFT, Parasternal short-axis view shows LVH, akinesis of anterior wall and mid and anterior septum, definite disruption of the mid septum, dynamic inferolateral walls, akinetic anterior right ventricle, and akinetic anterior left ventricle. MIDDLE RIGHT, Parasternal short-axis view. Color Doppler flow mapping demonstrates flow across the disruption of the mid anterior septum. BOTTOM ROW, Postoperative images demonstrate a partial patch dehiscence, allowing flow again across the septum.

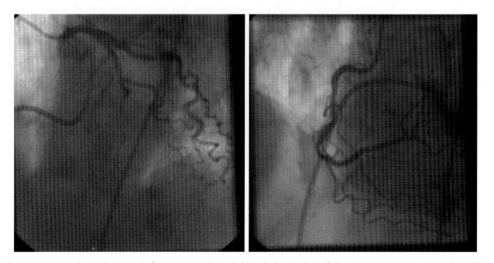

Figure 11-43. Selective coronary angiography. LEFT, Left coronary artery. Subtotal obstruction of the LAD coronary artery in the midportion. RIGHT, Right coronary artery is dominant and without angiographic disease.

CASE 7

History

▸ 74-year-old woman transferred because of postinfarction chest pain, acute pulmonary edema, and possible new murmur; had presented at hour 11 and received fibrinolytic at hour 12

Physical Examination

▸ Stoic, but weak looking
▸ BP 95/65 mm Hg, HR 110 bpm, RR 18/min (mildly labored)
▸ Low-volume pulse, normal upstroke
▸ Warm extremities
▸ Venous distention to angle of jaw, no edema
▸ S_1, S_2 normal; S_3 present
▸ Apical 4/6 pansystolic murmur with widespread radiation; no thrill
▸ Crepitations at lung bases

Clinical Impression and Management Plan

▸ Inferoposterior myocardial infarction with postinfarction septal rupture or mitral regurgitation (papillary muscle rupture?)
▸ Right ventricular myocardial infarction, low output with little likelihood of reperfusion
▸ Acute pulmonary edema due to septal rupture, papillary rupture, MR, or reinfarction
▸ Management plan included IABP at bedside, PA catheter for pressures, oximetry, and bedside echocardiography

Table 11-5. Right-Sided Heart Hemodynamics

	Native	**IABP**
Heart rate	102 bpm	88 bpm
CVP	15 mm Hg	15 mm Hg
PAP	42/20 mm Hg	38/20 mm Hg
PCWP	14 mm Hg	14 mm Hg
CI (right-sided)	2.5 L/min/m²	2.6 L/min/m²

CI, cardiac index; CVP, central venous pressure; IABP, intra-aortic balloon counterpulsation; PAP, pulmonary artery pressure; PCWP, pulmonary capillary wedge pressure.

Table 11-6. Oximetry

Positive (>10%) step-up: proximal 48%, distal 76%

Shunt ratio (Qp:Qs) = $Sat_{arterial} - Sat_{venous}$ / $Sat_{arterial} = Sat_{PA}$ = (92 − 48 / 92 − 76) = 2.7

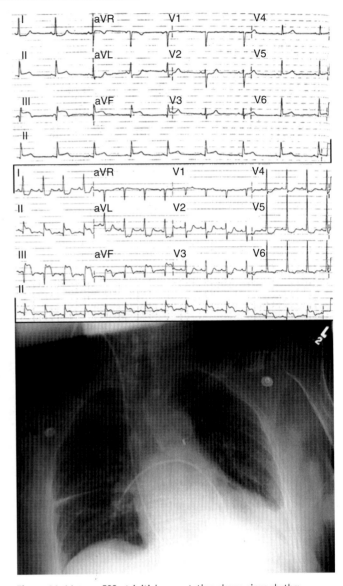

Figure 11-44. TOP, ECG at initial presentation shows sinus rhythm, inferior Q waves (III, aVF) and ST elevation, ST depression in lateral leads, minor ST depression V_2. MIDDLE, ECG at time of worsening shows sinus tachycardia, inferior Q waves and increased ST elevation, early precordial R-wave transition and ST depression (possible posterior myocardial infarction), and lateral ST depression (increased). BOTTOM, Chest radiograph shows borderline cardiomegaly, interstitial pulmonary edema, and IABP in correct position at distal arch.

Table 11-7. Hemodynamic Profile

	Physical Examination	**Echocardiography**	**Catheterization**
RVSP	Elevated (P_2)	55 mm Hg	40 mm Hg
O_2 step-up	NA	Yes (shunt seen)	Yes
Qp:Qs	NA	—	2.7:1
CVP	8 cm (JVD)	10 mm Hg	15 mm Hg
CI, systemic	Near shocky	1.6 L/min/m²	1.4 L/min/m²

CI, cardiac index; CVP, central venous pressure; JVD, jugular venous distention; RVSP, right ventricular systolic pressure.

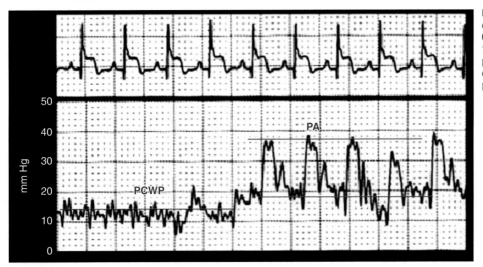

Figure 11-45. Right-sided heart catheterization shows sinus tachycardia, Q waves, and ST elevation. PCWP, 14 to 15 mm Hg; no V waves. Mildly elevated pulmonary systolic pressure but disproportionately elevated diastolic pressure.

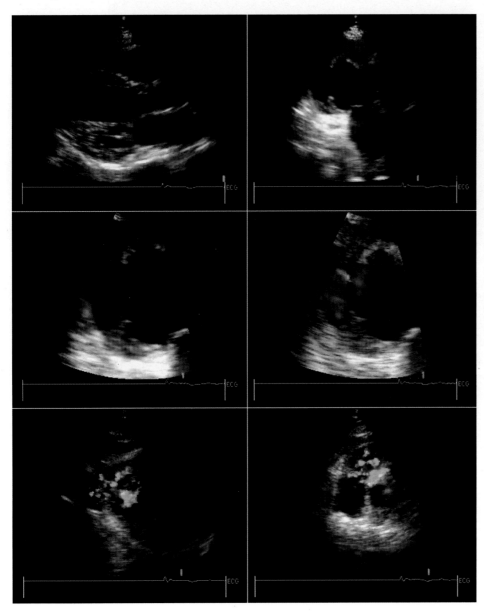

Figure 11-46. Transthoracic echocardiography. TOP LEFT, Parasternal long-axis view. There is akinesis of the basal and mid and posterior walls. The mitral leaflet appearance and motion are normal, as is the appearance of the posteromedial papillary muscle. No pericardial effusion. TOP RIGHT, Apical 2-chamber view. The inferior wall is akinetic from base to apex. There is a cavity within the inferior wall—false aneurysm and intramural hematoma. MIDDLE LEFT, Zoom apical 2-chamber view. The cavity within the inferior wall is seen. MIDDLE RIGHT, Zoom apical 2-chamber view and color Doppler mapping. The cavity within the akinetic inferior wall is seen to fill with flow. BOTTOM LEFT, Parasternal short-axis view and color Doppler mapping. There is akinesis of the inferior and posterior walls. The inferior septum has a complex appearance. Color Doppler mapping demonstrates that there is systolic flow across the complex-appearing inferior septum, demonstrating septal rupture. BOTTOM RIGHT, Off-axis apical view. Color Doppler mapping demonstrates flow across the thinned septum. There is akinesis of the adjacent right ventricle.

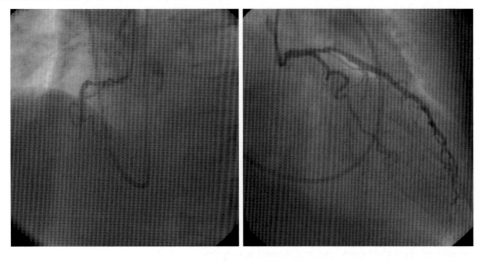

Figure 11-47. Selective coronary angiography. LEFT, The right coronary artery is occluded proximally. RIGHT, There is only an angiographically mild proximal LAD coronary artery stenosis.

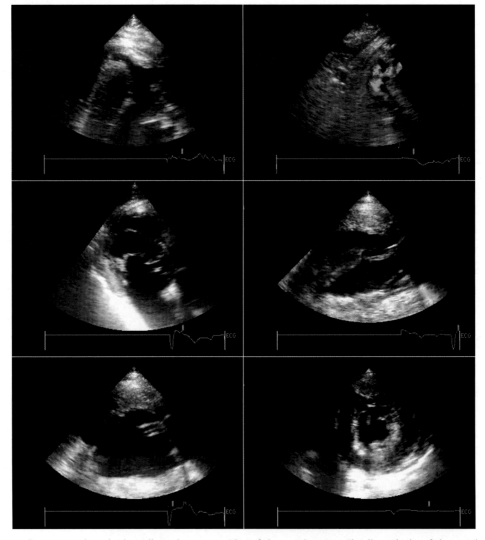

Figure 11-48. Intraoperative transesophageal echocardiography. TOP LEFT, View of the septal rupture. The discontinuity of the septal rupture is evident. TOP RIGHT, Color Doppler flow mapping depicts the flow across the septal rupture into the distal right ventricle. MIDDLE LEFT, Vertical transgastric view of the right ventricle, which is dilated and akinetic anteriorly. MIDDLE RIGHT, Transgastric long-axis view of the left ventricle. The posteromedial and anterolateral papillary muscles are intact. BOTTOM LEFT, View of the inferior wall of the left ventricle. An outpouching of the lumen into the akinetic inferior wall is seen, representing an intramural hematoma or false aneurysm. BOTTOM RIGHT, Transgastric short-axis view. Patches are seen closing the VSR and intramural hematoma.

Clinical Impression and Management Plan

‣ Posterior, inferior, inferior septal, and posterior right ventricular infarction
‣ Postinfarction rupture of the inferior basal septum
‣ False aneurysm or intramural hematoma of the inferior wall beside the septal rupture
‣ Low output
‣ Plan was to proceed to early surgical repair; angiography before surgery

Cardiac Surgery

‣ Surgery revealed left ventricular infarct, right ventricular infarct (hemorrhagic appearance); septal rupture.
‣ The basal left ventricle was too disrupted for the false aneurysm to be recognized.
‣ Infarctectomy and patch closure of septal rupture and pseudoaneurysm were performed.

Outcome

‣ Oximetry demonstrated a small residual VSR shunt.
‣ Refractory right ventricular failure dominated the postoperative course.
‣ Anuria ensued, followed by multiorgan failure and death 5 days postoperatively.

Comments

‣ Background of hypertension, no known CAD
‣ Complicated inferior myocardial infarction: low-output shock, right ventricular myocardial infarction, VSR, false aneurysm
‣ Low-output shock dominantly caused by right ventricular infarction + VSR rather than by left ventricular infarction per se. Lower than expected RVSP and PAP (given the severity of the low output) were consistent with right ventricular myocardial infarction (right ventricular systolic failure), as was the elevated CVP (right ventricular diastolic failure).
‣ Diagnosis of septal rupture and right ventricular myocardial infarction from PA catheter, confirmed and further delineated by echocardiography.
‣ Lack of substantial improvement with IABP pointed to the right ventricular infarction as dominating the hemodynamics; left ventricular infarction and VSR would likely have benefited more.
‣ Patch leak (small)
‣ The combination of severely elevated CVP + low output, as well as prominent right ventricular infarction, predicted elevated surgical risk.
‣ Right ventricular failure determined the ultimate outcome.

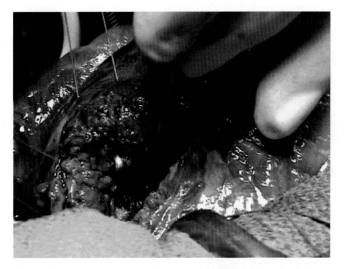

Figure 11-49. Surgical findings. Septal rupture hole.

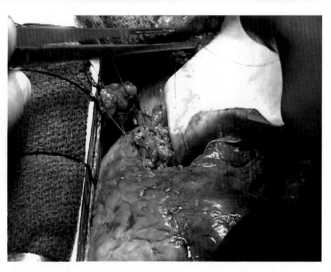

Figure 11-50. Surgical findings. Patches are being sewn into place, through an infarctectomy. Note the discoloration of infarct territory.

CASE 8

History

‣ A 51-year-old man presented with 2 hours of severe infarction-like chest pain and associated inferior ST elevation. Killip I; received tPA at 2.5 hours
‣ No resolution of chest pain; in fact, substantial worsening and ST elevation increase from 3 to 8 mm in II, III, aVF
‣ Transferred for consideration of rescue percutaneous transluminal coronary angioplasty (PTCA)

Physical Examination

‣ Distressed with pain, diaphoretic, obese
‣ BP 115/75 mm Hg, HR 90 bpm, RR 12/min
‣ JVP 8 cm above the sternal angle, no fall with inspiration
‣ No rubs or murmurs

‣ Apex neither enlarged nor displaced
‣ Chest clear
‣ No edema, periphery warm
‣ No bruits

Clinical Impression

‣ Inferior STEMI with right ventricular myocardial infarction, Killip class I
‣ Hour 4 (2 hours after tPA)—presumed failure to reperfuse RCA
‣ Plan was to attempt a rescue PTCA of the infarct-related vessel

In-Hospital Evolution

‣ No recurrences of ischemic chest pain; remained Killip I
‣ CK 9800
‣ 1 day of pleuritic pericarditic-type pains, resolved with NSAIDs
‣ Discharged home 3 days later as CCS class I, NYHA class I

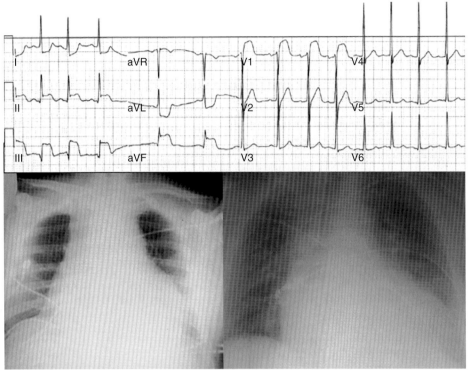

Figure 11-51. TOP, ECG shows sinus rhythm with marked sinus arrhythmia; LVH voltage; inferior (II, III, aVF) ST elevation and V_1 ST elevation and lateral ST depression, suggesting acute inferior myocardial infarction and right ventricular myocardial infarction. BOTTOM LEFT, Chest radiography shows borderline cardiomegaly, no left-sided heart failure. BOTTOM RIGHT, Chest radiograph at the time of deterioration—interstitial edema and pulmonary vascular engorgement.

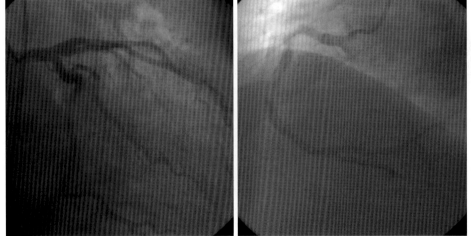

Figure 11-52. Coronary angiography. LEFT, LCA view shows no angiographic disease. RIGHT, RCA PCI. Dominant RCA. Proximal RCA lesion dilated, but there is a large bulk of thrombus in the artery, and the run-off is poor.

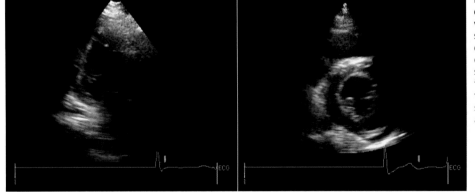

Figure 11-53. Transthoracic echocardiography. LEFT, Apical 2-chamber view. The posterior wall is akinetic and slightly dilated, but intact, as is the overlying posteromedial papillary muscle complex. RIGHT, Parasternal short-axis view shows akinesis of the inferior septum, inferior wall, and posterior wall as well as the posterior right ventricle. There is a small pericardial effusion. Myocardial walls appear intact.

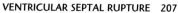

11

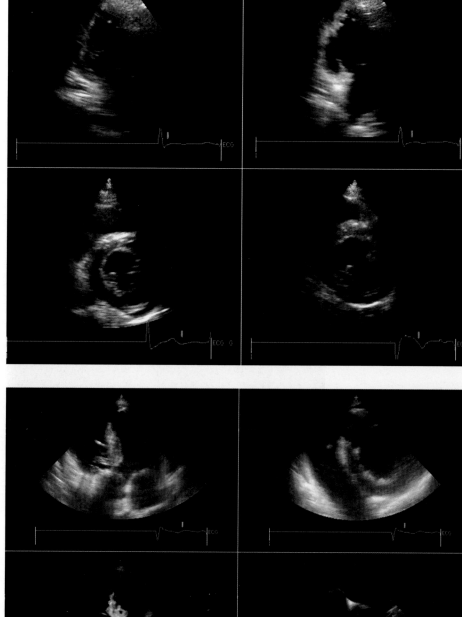

Figure 11-54. Transthoracic echocardiography, before septal rupture (LEFT IMAGES) and on return with septal rupture (RIGHT IMAGES). TOP IMAGES, Apical 2-chamber views. TOP LEFT, Akinetic, slightly dilated posterior LV wall—intact. TOP RIGHT, Further dilated posterior wall with a cavity now in the posterior wall in the basal and middle portions. BOTTOM IMAGES, Parasternal short-axis views at the mid LV level. BOTTOM LEFT, The walls all have normal thickness and no apparent disruption. BOTTOM RIGHT, On return, there is now gross distortion and disruption of the inferior wall and inferior septum with an aneurysm or false aneurysm, probable frank disruption (rupture) of the septum, and a false aneurysm or intramyocardial hematoma within the posterior wall.

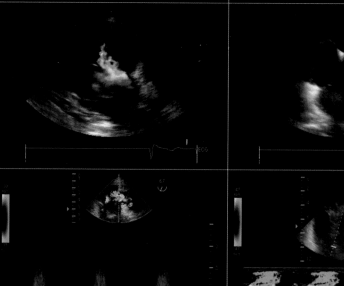

Figure 11-55. Intraoperative transesophageal echocardiography. TOP LEFT, Transgastric 4-chamber view from the apex. There is akinesis of the right ventricle. The defect in the septum is again obvious and revealed to be a straight-through rupture. TOP RIGHT, Transgastric short-axis view of the mid basal left ventricle. The defect in the inferior septum is again obvious. MIDDLE LEFT, There is flow into and across the septal rupture. MIDDLE RIGHT, The right ventricle is severely dilated and akinetic. BOTTOM LEFT, Spectral display of flow across the ventricular septal defect. There is both systolic and diastolic flow across the ventricular septal defect. BOTTOM RIGHT, Phonocardiogram and color M-mode study. Note the ECG on the bottom as a timing reference. The color M-mode study shows flow throughout systole and into diastole. The phonocardiogram also shows a murmur in systole and a shorter one in diastole.

Postdischarge Evolution

▸ 6 days after discharge, developed a single, sudden lance of chest pain and immediately felt "unwell" (weakness and mild shortness of breath)
▸ Presented to local hospital with new pansystolic murmur, venous distention, mild CHF
▸ Transferred for management

Physical Examination

▸ Ashen appearance, diaphoretic, extremities not warm
▸ BP 95/65 mm Hg, HR 95 bpm (on metoprolol), RR 18/min
▸ JVD 10 cm above the sternal angle, no edema
▸ Crepitations in lower third of the chest
▸ 5/6 mid-precordial pansystolic murmur, thrill present
▸ S_3, parasternal; vague parasternal lift

Clinical Impression

▸ Cardiogenic shock and postinfarction septal rupture
▸ Right ventricular myocardial infarction
▸ Inferior wall intramural hematoma or false aneurysm extension of the inferior septal aneurysm
▸ Plan consisted of IABP + dobutamine
▸ BP rose to 105/70 mm Hg, HR 100 bpm
▸ PCWP fall precipitated a decision to proceed with emergent surgery.

Cardiac Surgery

▸ Surgery revealed inferior and posterior infarction; right ventricular infarction.
▸ Basal septal rupture and posterior intramyocardial hematoma
▸ Infarctectomy and patch closure of septal rupture and pseudoaneurysm were performed.

Postoperative Course and Outcome

▸ Immediate postoperative course brittle due to right ventricle failure (prior infarction + preoperative right ventricle failure + bypass protection issues)
▸ On postoperative day 3, there was a recurrence of murmur and small O_2 step-up; recurrence of transseptal flow demonstrated.
▸ Persistent cardiogenic shock hemodynamics, no recovery
▸ Cardiac transplantation process initiated. The patient died of circulatory failure before arrangements could be made.

Comments

▸ Inferior myocardial infarction complicated by basal septal rupture, posterior intramural hematoma, right ventricular infarction, and late postdischarge septal rupture
▸ Although the occlusion of the RCA was opened by angioplasty, there was poor flow because of massive distal embolization of thrombus.
▸ Eventual death was determined by right ventricle failure.

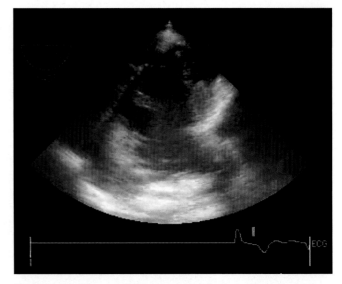

Figure 11-56. Intraoperative transesophageal echocardiography. Patch material now excludes the left ventricular cavity, and the heart will be closed.

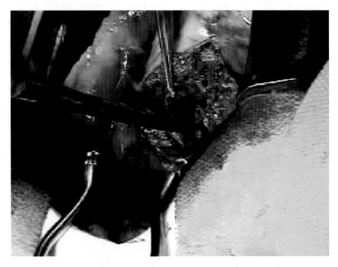

Figure 11-57. Cardiac surgery. The patch now excludes the left ventricular cavity, and the heart will be closed. The right ventricle (dark cavity) will communicate with the space behind the patches.

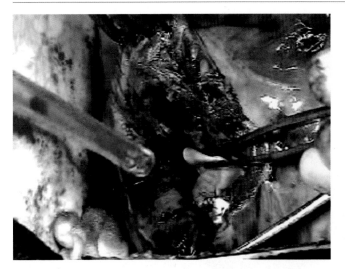

Figure 11-58. Cardiac surgery. Through the infarctotomy, the patch is sewn in along its margin to seal off the left ventricle.

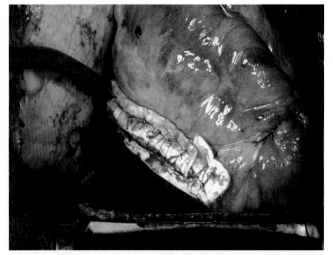

Figure 11-59. Surgical findings. The incision through the infarct is sewn together with mattress material to better hold the sutures.

CASE 9

History

▸ 75-year-old man seen in clinic; followed up previously for angina pectoris, CCS class II
▸ Recent myocardial infarction at another hospital

  ▸ No records available
  ▸ Seen in follow-up to the infarction
  ▸ Described a 15-day stay with 8 days in the ICU critically ill
  ▸ No angina or dyspnea since discharge

Physical Examination

▸ BP 145/80 mm Hg, HR 70 bpm
▸ Normal venous pressure and contour
▸ Heart sounds normal; 4/6 pansystolic murmur at the left sternal border with radiation to the right sternal border; no thrill
▸ Chest clear

Clinical Impression

▸ Cardiogenic shock at the other hospital may have been due to right ventricular infarction and clinical recovery from right ventricle infarction.

▸ Postinfarction septal rupture, probably late and out of the hospital
▸ Right ventricular myocardial infarction

Management and Outcome

▸ There was considerable debate about closure of the septal rupture because his operative risks were ideal, and the infarcted tissues would have scarred up to become easy to operate with. A closure device was considered as well. In the end, the patient refused any form of procedure.
▸ He remains without angina or left- or right-sided heart failure 2 years later.

Comments

▸ Inferior basal septal rupture and right ventricular infarction complicating RCA occlusion
▸ The rupture probably happened after discharge from the other hospital, or it may have been misdiagnosed clinically as MR.
▸ Exceptionally well tolerated septal rupture
▸ Continues to do very well without surgery

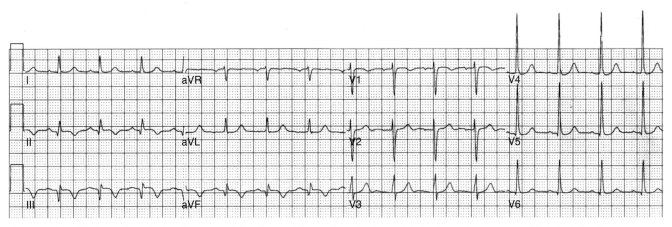

Figure 11-60. ECG shows sinus rhythm, Q waves, ST elevation, and T-wave inversion in the inferior leads, signifying recent inferior infarction.

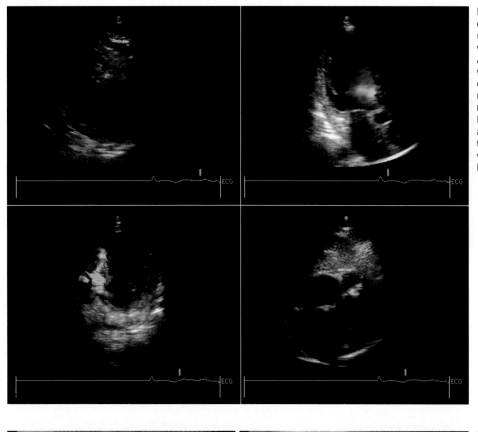

Figure 11-61. Transthoracic echocardiography. TOP LEFT, Akinesis and mild dilation of the inferior and posterior walls. TOP RIGHT, Apical 2-chamber view. Akinesis and mild dilation of the posterior wall; the posteromedial papillary muscle complex appears intact, and there is normal mitral valve coaptation and no MR. BOTTOM LEFT, Off-axis apical view. Color Doppler flow mapping depicts the flow into and across the basal inferior septum into the RV. BOTTOM RIGHT, Subcostal long-axis view with color Doppler flow mapping. Flow across the basal septum is present.

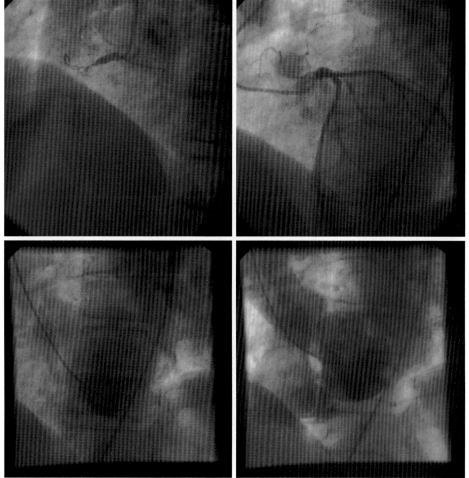

Figure 11-62. TOP ROW, Selective coronary angiography. LEFT, RCA injection reveals complete occlusion proximally. RIGHT, LCA injection demonstrates disease in the first and second diagonals. The posterior descending artery fills through the left coronary injection. BOTTOM ROW, Contrast ventriculography (LAO projection). LEFT, Early frame, RIGHT, Later frame during the injection. Contrast material can be seen first filling the left ventricle, which has an inferior cavity, then filling the right ventricle, through an inferior defect. The right ventricle is grossly dilated and was akinetic, as was the inferior wall of the left ventricle.

11

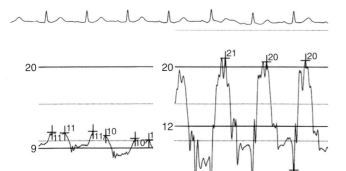

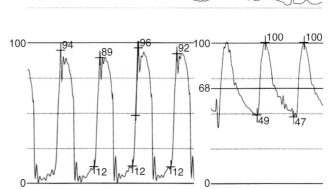

Figure 11-63. Right-sided heart catheterization: pulmonary capillary wedge pressures (LEFT), pulmonary artery pressures (RIGHT). The pulmonary capillary pressures are normal (mean of 10 mm Hg). There is no increased V wave. The pulmonary artery pressures are also normal or low.

Figure 11-64. Left-sided heart catheterization: left ventricular pressures (LEFT), aortic pressures (RIGHT). Left ventricle: 95/10 mm Hg—LV systolic hypotension, diastolic pressures normal. Aortic pressures are 100/48 mm Hg, suggesting systolic and diastolic hypotension.

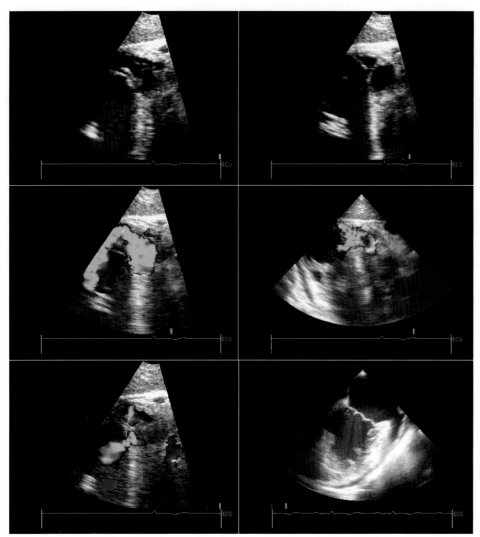

Figure 11-65. Transesophageal echocardiography. TOP IMAGES, Transgastric short-axis views of the septal rupture revealing its anatomic complexity. MIDDLE IMAGES, Color Doppler flow mapping reveals the flow across the septum. BOTTOM LEFT, Color Doppler mapping suggests that the tract is in fact not single as it had appeared on the middle images. BOTTOM RIGHT, Long-axis view from the lower esophagus. There is an aneurysm of the basal inferior wall. The left atrial appendage is distended from high left atrial pressure.

CASE 10

History

▸ 66-year-old woman, presented at hour 16 after a chest pain episode; received fibrinolytic because of residual pain and STEMI
▸ Past medical history is significant for hypertension. No angina.

Physical Examination

▸ BP 105/70 mm Hg, HR 90 bpm, slightly distressed
▸ Extremities warm, venous pressures mildly elevated
▸ 4/6 pansystolic raspy murmur at LLSB with widespread radiation; no thrill; S_3 present
▸ Rales at lung bases

Clinical Impression and Management Plan

▸ Anteroapical infarction, aneurysm, and VSR
▸ Killip II
▸ IABP inserted
▸ Decision for early surgery after angiography

Cardiac Surgery

▸ Surgery revealed anterior and septal infarction and apical septal rupture.
▸ Infarctectomy and patch closure of septal rupture and pseudoaneurysm were performed.

Outcome

▸ Survival
▸ NYHA class III

Comments

▸ Anterior infarction and anteroapical VSR
▸ Lesser right ventricular infarction with apical VSR
▸ Killip II entails lower operative mortality
▸ Postoperative CHF symptoms from persistent LV dysfunction

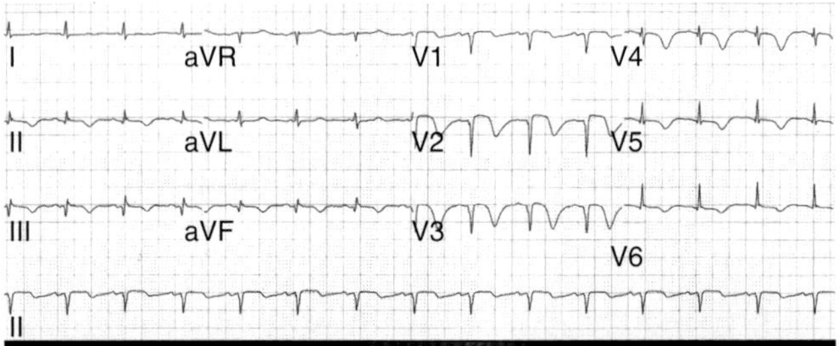

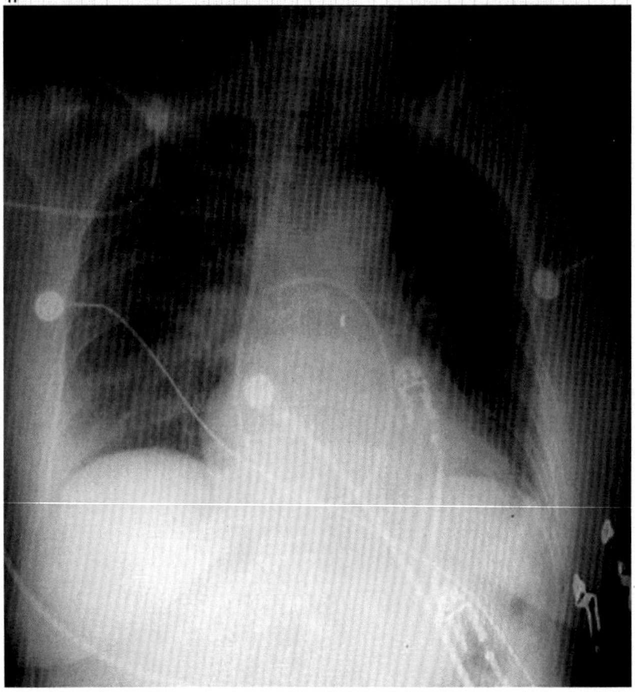

Figure 11-66. TOP, ECG shows sinus rhythm, Q waves V_2-V_4: II, III, and aVF. Resting ST elevation and T-wave inversion in the anterior leads. BOTTOM, Chest radiograph shows mild cardiomegaly, interstitial edema, PA catheter in the right main PA, and IABP tip too low.

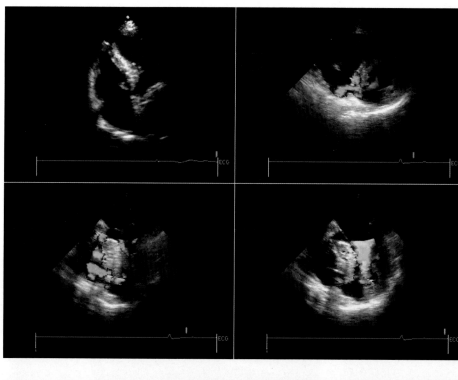

Figure 11-67. TOP LEFT, Transthoracic echocardiography, apical 4-chamber view. The right ventricle is akinetic in its lateral portions. The distal septum appears to be disarticulated. TOP RIGHT, Transesophageal echocardiography, transgastric view of the left ventricle and right ventricle. Color Doppler study demonstrates flow through the septum in two channels. BOTTOM LEFT, Transesophageal echocardiography, 4-chamber view. BOTTOM RIGHT, Color Doppler mapping. There is systolic flow across the distal anterior septum.

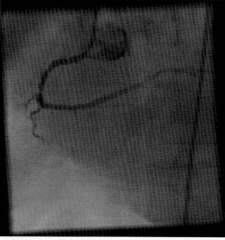
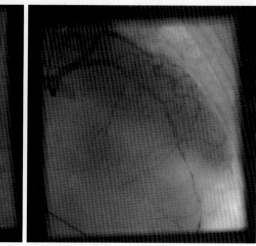

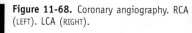

Figure 11-68. Coronary angiography. RCA (LEFT). LCA (RIGHT).

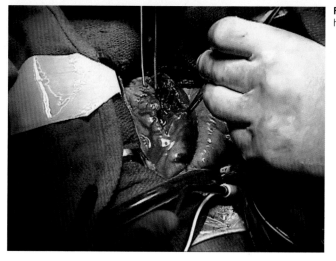

Figure 11-69. Cardiac surgery. Hemorrhagic appearance of the outside of the heart.

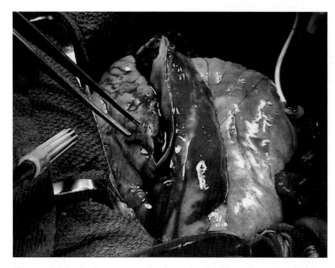

Figure 11-70. Cardiac surgery. Patch partly sewn into place to exclude the left and right ventricles.

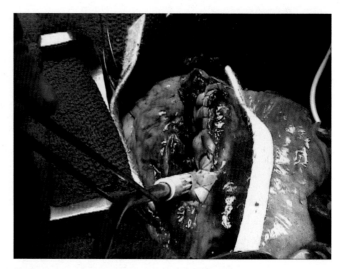

Figure 11-71. Cardiac surgery. Patch excluding the ventricles.

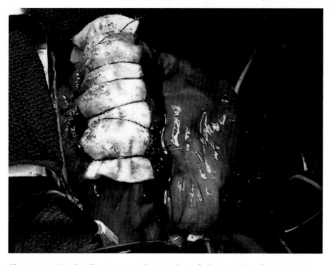

Figure 11-72. Cardiac surgery. Oversewing of the outside of the heart with mattress sutures to hold the infarcted tissue and the repair together.

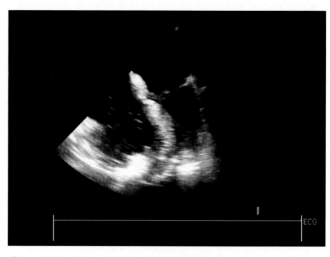

Figure 11-73. Intraoperative transesophageal echocardiography after repair, 4-chamber view. The ventricles are now smaller as the apical portions have been involved in the repair.

CASE 11

History

▸ 76-year-old woman, previously active and well, transferred with post–anterior STEMI septal rupture
▸ Presented that morning with an anterior STEMI at hour 9 and received tPA at hour 10
  ▸ Initially Killip class I; but 7 hours after the tPA, she became "uncomfortable."
  ▸ Systolic blood pressure fell from 150 to 95 mm Hg, there was a definite new murmur, and echocardiography performed at that time confirmed a septal rupture.

Physical Examination on Arrival

▸ BP 95/65 mm Hg, HR 85 bpm, RR 13/min (comfortable breathing)
▸ Low-volume pulse, normal upstroke
▸ Warm extremities, alert
▸ Venous pressure 3 cm above the sternal angle, no edema
▸ S_1, S_2 normal; S_3 present; no rubs
▸ Blowing apical pansystolic murmur 4/6 with radiation across the lower sternum into the right chest; no thrill; no diastolic murmurs
▸ No crepitations at lung bases (1/4)
▸ Initial urine output 60 mL/hr

Clinical Impression and Management Plan

▸ Anteroseptal myocardial infarction with postinfarction septal rupture with a bifurcating channel that could potentially be addressed by percutaneous closure device
▸ No pulmonary congestion; adequate peripheral perfusion (stable and normal creatinine); reasonable cardiac index noninvasively
▸ IABP for stabilization
▸ Deliberation of early versus late surgery and of closure device attempt to "buy time" until later surgery, when the necrotic myocardium would be better to sew patches to

▸ Opted for closure device attempt; proceed to cardiac surgery if device unsuccessful or complicated

Evolution

▸ The deployment of the device was unsuccessful in sealing the ventricular septal defect.
▸ Also, a pericardial effusion was developing with some tamponade features, so the decision was made to proceed directly to surgical repair.

Cardiac Surgery

▸ Surgery revealed left ventricular infarction, hemorrhagic appearance, apical right ventricular infarct, and septal rupture.
▸ Closure device was well seated but not sealing the ventricular septal defect, and there was also a bloody pericardial effusion.
▸ Patch closure of septal rupture was performed.
▸ Integrity of the patch was confirmed by intraoperative transesophageal echocardiography.

Postoperative Course and Outcome

▸ Postoperatively, there was a prominent need for inotropes.
▸ A new pansystolic murmur developed that was confirmed by echocardiography as a small patch leak.
▸ The O_2 step-up was very small.
▸ The patient died 4 days later from low output, which was not fully understood. Although the heart cavities were reduced by the patching, the systolic function was not obviously critically poor. The recurrent ventricular septal defect shunt did not appear large.

Autopsy Findings

▸ Apical left ventricular infarction, hemorrhagic appearance
▸ Apical right ventricular infarct
▸ Small patch leak around septal rupture
▸ Extensive pulmonary embolism

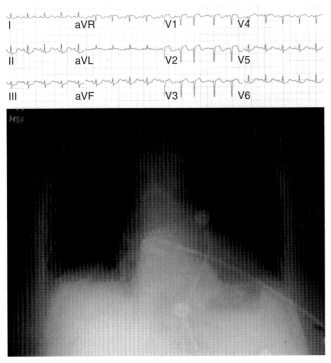

Figure 11-74. TOP, ECG shows sinus rhythm with PACs, Q waves V_1, V_2: II, III with resting ST elevation, and ST depression II, III, aVF, indicating evolved anteroseptal infarction. BOTTOM, Chest radiograph shows normal heart size and no left-sided heart failure.

▸ Thrombus at the right ventricular apex and behind the patch on the right ventricular side
▸ Deep venous thrombosis (DVT) in the vessels beside the IABP
▸ Presumed cause of death was pulmonary embolism from the DVT and patches exacerbating the postinfarction, post-pump low-output state.

Comments

▸ Anterior myocardial infarction, apical septal rupture
▸ Initial stability did not endure.

▸ The difficulty in sustaining a patient for several weeks before going to the operating room was well exemplified. Although reasonable in intention, it is very difficult to do as comorbidities develop.
▸ Initial success with surgical closure not sustained—recurrence of patch leak
▸ Pulmonary embolism from leg veins and from the right ventricular apex

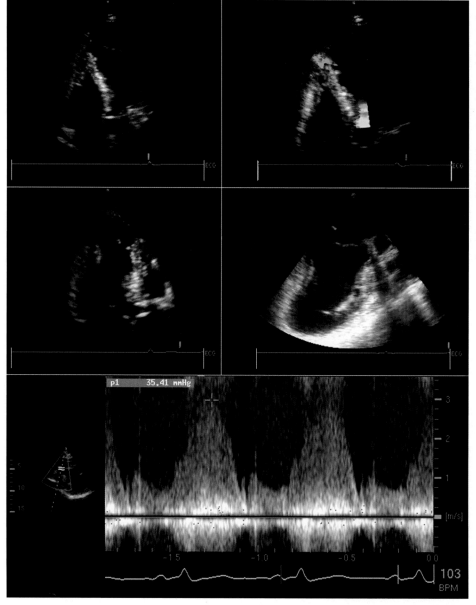

Figure 11-75. Transthoracic echocardiography. TOP LEFT, Apical 4 chamber view. In addition to dilation and aneurysm formation of the apex, there is some degree of distortion of the cavity at the apex where the septum joins it. TOP RIGHT, Color Doppler flow mapping demonstrates flow through the septum into the very most apical portion of the RV. MIDDLE LEFT, Apical 3-chamber view demonstrating the apical aneurysm. MIDDLE RIGHT, Corresponding transesophageal echocardiography 3-chamber image also showing the apical aneurysm. BOTTOM, Spectral display of the flow across the septum, which although clearly enhanced in systole is also present in diastole. The RVSP was 55 mm Hg calculated from this ($BP_{systolic}$ − gradient) and 60 mm Hg by the tricuspid regurgitation velocity. Other Doppler-derived data included a systemic cardiac index of 2.1 L/min/m^2.

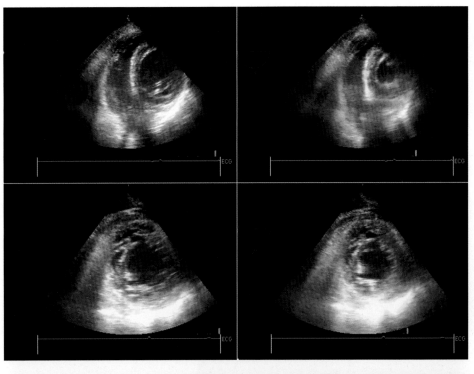

Figure 11-76. Transesophageal echocardiography transgastric views of LV function in diastole (LEFT IMAGES) and systole (RIGHT IMAGES). TOP IMAGES, Basal–mid ventricular views. BOTTOM IMAGES, Apical views. There is brisk contraction of the basal and mid ventricle and akinesis of the apical portion in the area of the aneurysm. As well, tissue disruption through the septum is present in the apical portion.

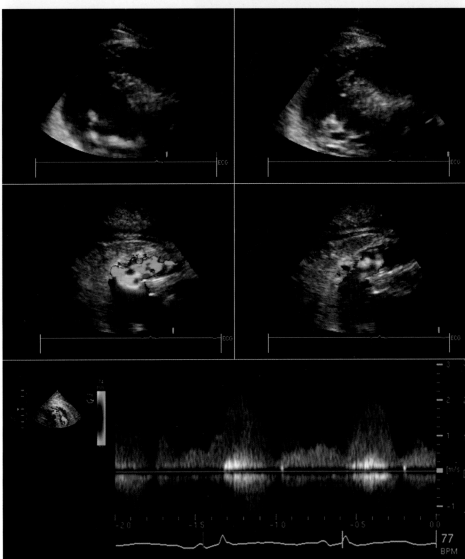

Figure 11-77. Transesophageal echocardiography. Deep transgastric near-vertical views of the apical portion of the septum in systole (LEFT) and diastole (RIGHT) reveal that the septal rupture defect is patent in both systole and diastole and has flow through it in both systole (greater) and diastole (less). BOTTOM IMAGES, Spectral display of flow across the ruptured septum.

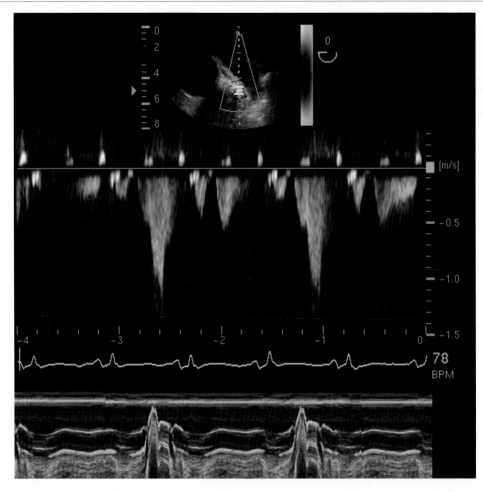

Figure 11-78. Transesophageal echocardiography: spectral flow profile of IABP-augmented (1:2) LAD coronary artery flow. The M-mode study depicts the balloon opening each second cardiac cycle. Associated with this is augmentation of the flow in the LAD coronary artery, sampled by transesophageal echocardiography pulsed wave Doppler.

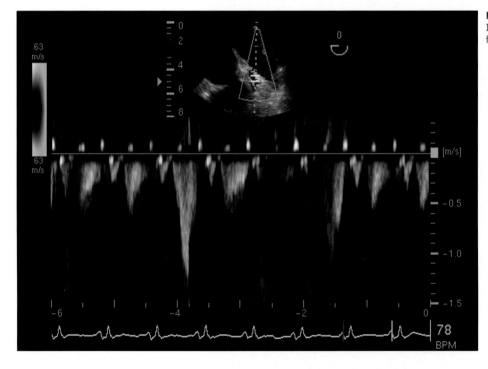

Figure 11-79. Spectral flow profile of IABP-augmented (1:3) LAD coronary artery flow.

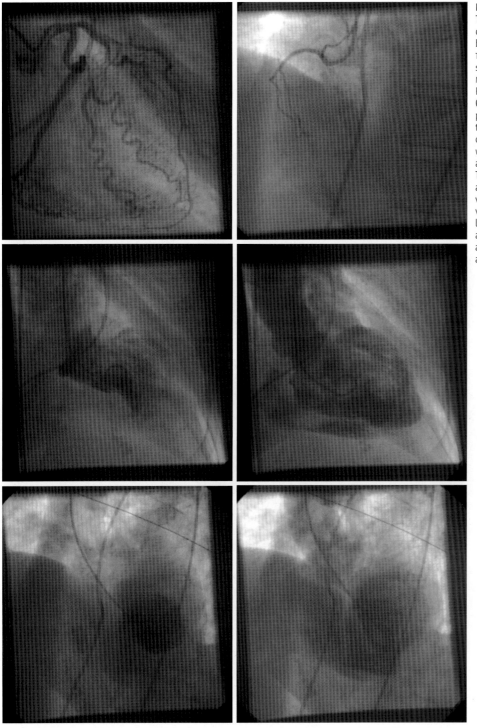

Figure 11-80. TOP LEFT, LCA injection. There is an 80% stenosis of the LAD coronary artery after the first septal branch. The circumflex artery is dominant. TOP RIGHT, RCA injection. Nondominant, supplying only right ventricular branches. MIDDLE IMAGES, Early- and late-frame views, RAO contrast ventriculography. Opacification of the right ventricle and pulmonary artery occurs after injection into the left ventricle, establishing the presence of a ventricular septal defect. The anterior wall, apex, and distal inferior wall are akinetic or dyskinetic and aneurysmal. There is no MR. BOTTOM IMAGES, Early- and late-frame views, LAO contrast ventriculography. Opacification of the right ventricle occurs after injection into the left ventricle. The basal distal septum is aneurysmal. The right ventricle is dilated and akinetic. IABP in the descending aorta.

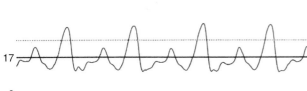

Figure 11-81. Cardiac catheterization: pulmonary capillary wedge pressure. Mean "wedge" pressure of 17 with tall V waves. The tall V waves are due to the increased venous return to the left atrium exceeding its compliance reserve.

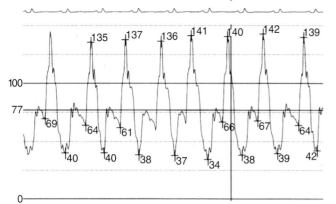

Figure 11-82. Cardiac catheterization: IABP-augmented aortic pressure. Native pressure 75/40, augmenting to 135 mm Hg.

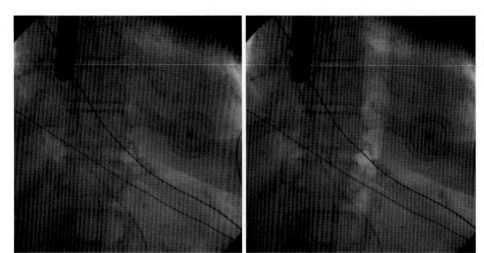

Figure 11-83. Closure device deployment attempt. The opened closure device is seen. There is a transesophageal echocardiography probe in the esophagus. The right image, acquired in diastole, reveals the inflated intra-aortic balloon.

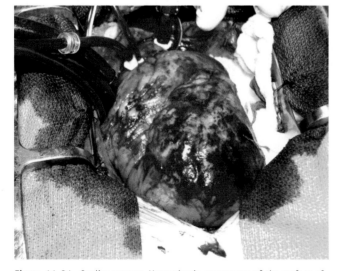

Figure 11-84. Cardiac surgery. Hemorrhagic appearance of the surface of the anterior wall and anteroapex.

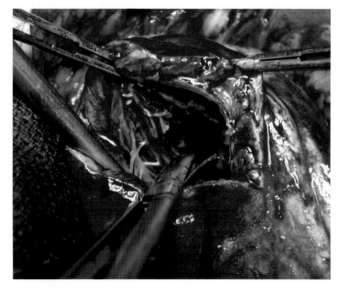

Figure 11-85. Cardiac surgery. Through the apical infarctectomy, the septal rupture is exposed. The dark space beyond the septal defect is the right ventricular cavity.

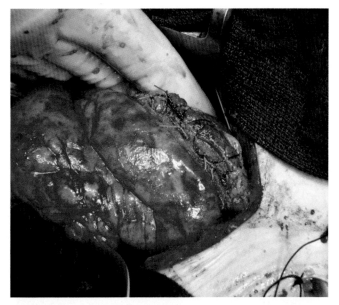

Figure 11-86. Cardiac surgery. Oversewing of the outside of the heart with mattress sutures to hold the infarcted apical tissue and the repair together.

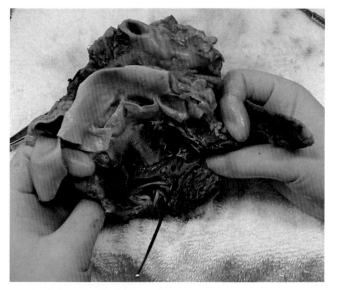

Figure 11-87. Autopsy findings. The residual ventricular septal defect leak behind and beside the patches is demonstrated by passage of a probe through the septal defect.

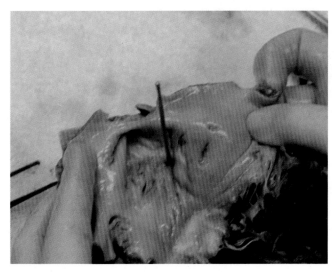

Figure 11-88. Autopsy findings. There was clinically unrecognized "probe patency" of a patent foramen ovale.

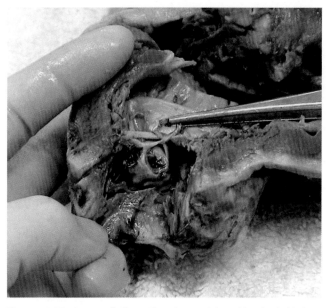

Figure 11-89. Autopsy findings. There is organizing white clot behind and around the patches on the right ventricle side of the patching. The forceps is holding a piece of thrombus.

CASE 12

History

▸ 52-year-old man transferred with post–inferior STEMI septal rupture
▸ Presented that morning with an inferior STEMI at hour 9 and received tPA at hour 10
  ▸ Initially Killip class I with jugular venous distention; 7 hours later, he became distressed.
  ▸ Systolic blood pressure fell from 145 to 70 mm Hg, and there was a definite new murmur.

Physical Examination

▸ Distressed, cool extremities, agitated
▸ BP 70/45 mm Hg, HR 105 bpm, RR 20/min (increased respiratory effort)
▸ Low-volume pulse, normal upstroke
▸ Venous pressure to the angle of the jaw, no edema
▸ S_1, S_2 normal; S_3 present
▸ Blowing holosystolic murmur 4/6 at the lower sternum into the right side of the chest; no thrill; no diastolic murmurs; no rubs
▸ Crepitations at lung bases (1/4)
▸ Urine output < 10 mL/hr

Clinical Impression and Management Plan

▸ Inferior myocardial infarction complicated with right ventricular infarction
▸ Basal septal rupture

▸ Cardiogenic shock from right ventricular dysfunction, left ventricular dysfunction, and shunt
▸ Management plan consists of IABP, urgent surgical repair, and PTCA of RCA to alleviate right ventricular dysfunction before cardioplegia

Cardiac Surgery

▸ Surgery revealed left ventricular and right ventricular infarction, hemorrhagic appearance, marked right ventricular dilation, and a basal septal rupture.
▸ Patch closure of septal rupture was performed.
▸ Integrity of the patch was confirmed by intraoperative transesophageal echocardiography.

Outcome

▸ Nonsustainable hemodynamics postoperatively
▸ The patient died within 2 hours before heart transplantation could be initiated

Comments

▸ Complicated inferior septal rupture, associated with a severe right ventricular infarction
▸ Early cardiogenic shock
▸ The associated right ventricular infarct was massive and exacerbated by the cardioplegic bypass.

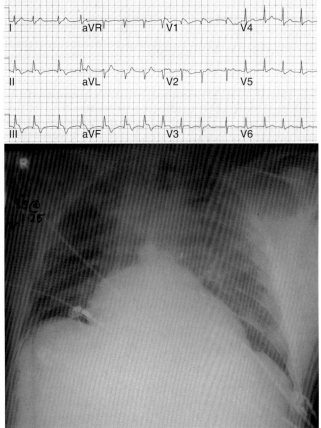

Figure 11-90. TOP, ECG shows sinus rhythm, ST elevation in leads II, aVF, aVL, V_1-V_3, indicating inferior myocardial infarction and possible right ventricular myocardial infarction. BOTTOM, Chest radiograph shows pulmonary edema, ET tube, PA catheter tip in main PA, and IABP tip positioned low.

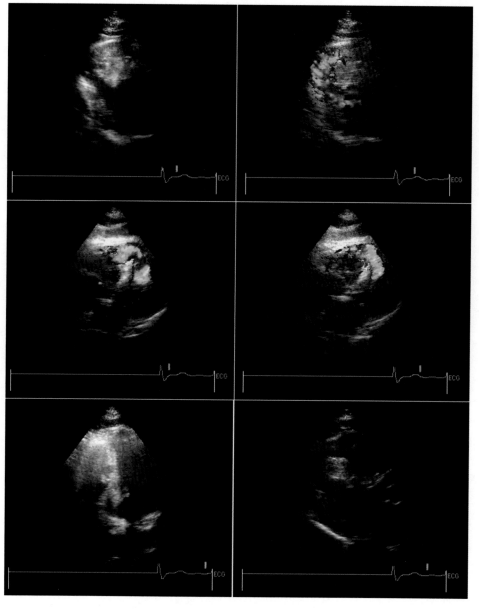

Figure 11-91. Transthoracic echocardiography. TOP ROW, Parasternal short-axis views. The 2-dimensional view (TOP LEFT) shows the defect through the septum in this case. Color Doppler mapping (TOP RIGHT) reveals the flow across is crossing through the defect from the LV into the RV. MIDDLE ROW, Subcostal long-axis views revealing prominent systolic flow across the septum. BOTTOM LEFT, Apical 4-chamber view revealing distorted septal appearance in the basal and middle portions and also RV dilation and rounding consistent with infarction. BOTTOM RIGHT, Parasternal long-axis view shows no pericardial effusion.

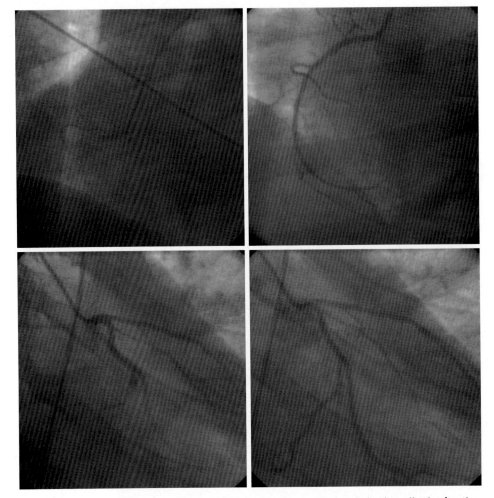

Figure 11-92. Coronary angiography. TOP LEFT, Right coronary angiogram shows complete proximal occlusion immediately after the conus branch. TOP RIGHT, After coronary stenting and restoration of flow. BOTTOM, Left coronary angiogram shows no significant disease.

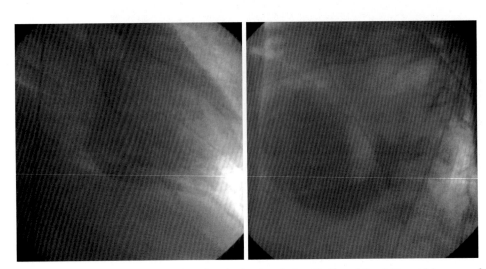

Figure 11-93. Contrast ventriculography: RAO projection (LEFT), LAO projection (RIGHT). Opacification of the right ventricle occurs after injection into the left ventricle, establishing the presence of a ventricular septal defect. The basal inferior left ventricle is akinetic. The right ventricle is akinetic. No MR. IABP in the descending aorta.

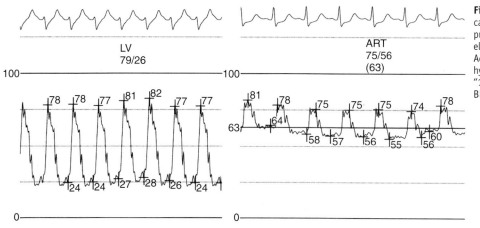

Figure 11-94. Left-sided heart catheterization. LEFT, Left ventricular pressure. Tachycardia, systolic hypotension, elevation of diastolic pressures. RIGHT, Aortic pressure. Note tachycardia, systolic hypotension, and small pulse pressure (the "100 thing": heart rate > 100 bpm, systolic BP < 100 mm Hg).

11

CASE 13

History

▸ A 64-year-old man 3 weeks after inferior STEMI, who had developed a posterior septal rupture 2 weeks before transfer. He was initially stable, but evidence of low output developed during those 2 weeks (rising creatinine).
▸ Past medical history is significant for steroid-dependent asthma.

Physical Examination on Arrival

▸ BP 100/62 mm Hg, HR 98 bpm, RR 13/min (dyspneic)
▸ Low-volume pulse, normal upstroke
▸ Warm extremities, alert
▸ Venous pressure 8 cm above the sternal angle, no edema
▸ S_1, S_2 normal; S_3 present; no rubs
▸ Blowing apical holosystolic murmur 4/6 with radiation across the lower sternum into the right side of the chest; no thrill; no diastolic murmurs
▸ No crepitations at lung bases (1/4)
▸ Urine output 35 mL/hr

Clinical Impression and Management Plan

▸ Inferior myocardial infarction complicated by extensive right ventricular infarction, septal rupture through a complex passage, and cardiogenic shock
▸ IABP for stabilization and coronary angiography
▸ Monitor for a few days to see if IABP increases cardiac output to retrieve renal function; if creatinine does not fall, proceed with surgery.
▸ Creatinine did fall by 25% with IABP. With this improvement, the patient was cleared for surgery.

Cardiac Surgery and Postoperative Course

▸ Surgery revealed a small inferior infarction, large right ventricular infarction, hemorrhagic appearance, basal inferior septal rupture, and false aneurysm or intramural hematoma extending from the rupture site.
▸ Patch closure of septal rupture was performed.
▸ Integrity of the patch was confirmed by intraoperative transesophageal echocardiography.
▸ In the postoperative period, the patient improved slowly but steadily.

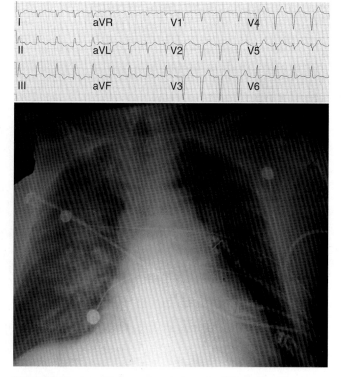

Figure 11-95. TOP, ECG shows sinus tachycardia, RAD, resting ST elevation in the inferior leads, and Q waves V_1-V_3. BOTTOM, Chest radiograph shows mild cardiomegaly and interstitial and alveolar edema.

- No recurrent murmur or patch leak
- 2 weeks in the ICU, 5 weeks on the ward
- Worsening shortness of breath occurred during 2 weeks, without apparent pneumonia or left-sided heart failure Marked venous distention. No rub, no murmur.

Clinical Impression and Management Plan

- Borderline shock from right ventricular dysfunction
- Considerable likelihood of pulmonary embolism, but a test is needed to make a positive diagnosis. No tamponade.
- Heparin anticoagulation started.
- CT scan PE protocol requested.
- Consideration of catheter-directed thrombolysis

Evolution

- Within 24 hours, there was complete alleviation of dyspnea and fatigue, concurrent with complete angiographic resolution of the pulmonary embolism.
- Anticoagulation was started.
- A small stroke occurred, confirmed to be ischemic by CT scanning.
- Another echocardiogram was performed.

Outcome

- With anticoagulation, the soft tissue mass, a presumed thrombus, resolved. There were no recurrent (recognized) emboli. Blood cultures were consistently negative, and there never accrued evidence that the mass was a vegetation.

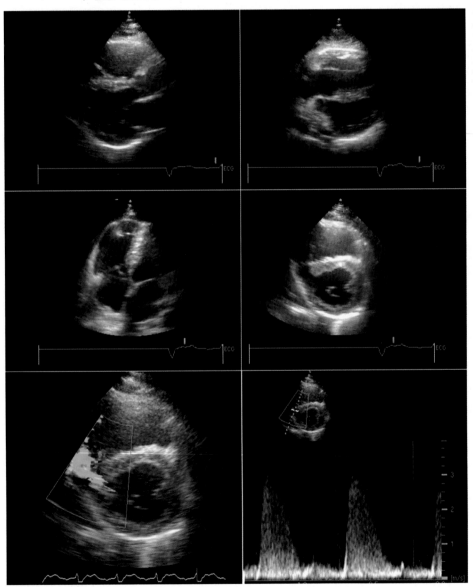

Figure 11-96. Transthoracic echocardiography. TOP LEFT, Parasternal long-axis view. The RVOT is markedly dilated and akinetic. The left ventricular cavity is small, and all wall segments on this plane are normal or hypercontractile. The posterior wall contracts but is hypokinetic. The mitral appearance is normal. There is no pericardial effusion. TOP RIGHT, Subcostal long-axis view. The right ventricle is again strikingly dilated and akinetic along the entire free wall. The left ventricle is hypercontractile. MIDDLE LEFT, Apical 4-chamber view. The right ventricle is strikingly dilated and akinetic along the entire free wall. The left ventricle is hypercontractile. MIDDLE RIGHT, Parasternal short-axis view at the base. The anterior wall, lateral wall, and posterior walls contract. The inferior wall is akinetic. There is an obvious clear-cut opening of the left ventricle into a cavity (of several centimeters in size) in the inferior septum that communicates with the right ventricle. This complex disruption may be an intramural hematoma that ruptures into the right ventricle and creates a ventricular septal defect shunt. BOTTOM LEFT, Parasternal short-axis view at the base with color Doppler mapping, which demonstrates flow across the septal rupture. BOTTOM RIGHT, Spectral profile of flow across the septal rupture. Systolic-only flow across the septal rupture.

- Several weeks later, the patient was discharged from the hospital.
- At follow-up, he is angina free and with class II dyspnea.

Comments

- Inferoposterior septal rupture, right ventricular myocardial infarction, and false aneurysm complicating inferior STEMI and proximal RCA occlusion
- Gradual (inexorable) worsening during period of attempted medical therapy is typical.

- IABP restored cardiac output and renal function and improved the preoperative condition.
- Difficult, long, but meticulous surgery achieved successful (and enduring) patch closure of both the VSR and false aneurysm.
- Leg DVT was on the side of the IABP, which was in for 2 weeks.
- Hard-fought and challenging postoperative course with multiple comorbidities: DVT, near-massive pulmonary emboli, arrhythmias, left ventricular thrombus, and stroke, but eventual survival with most quality of life intact.

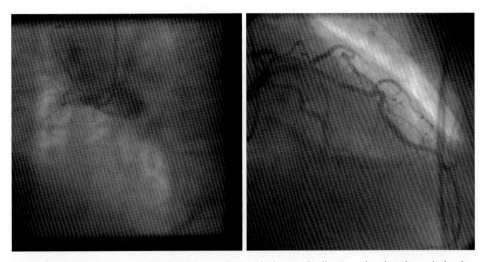

Figure 11-97. Coronary angiography. RCA injection (LEFT) reveals a complete occlusion proximally. Note also that the occlusion is proximal to right ventricle acute marginal branches, explaining the concurrent right ventricular infarction. Injection of the LCA (RIGHT) identifies only very mild proximal LAD coronary artery disease. The distal RCA fills by collaterals from the left injection.

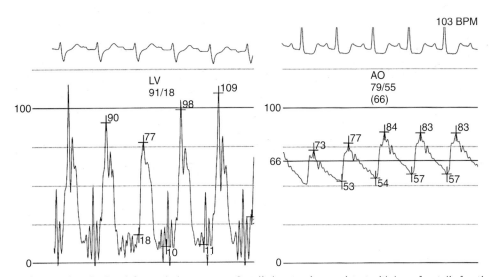

Figure 11-98. Left-sided heart catheterization: left ventricular pressures. Systolic hypotension consistent with loss of systolic function and of shunt flow to the right ventricle. Elevated diastolic pressures consistent with diastolic failure from the infarction and excess venous return from the elevated pulmonary blood flow. The aortic pressure tracing demonstrates tachycardia, systolic hypotension, and small pulse pressure consistent with small forward stroke volume (30 mL). There is respiratory variation of both the LV and aortic arterial pressure tracings.

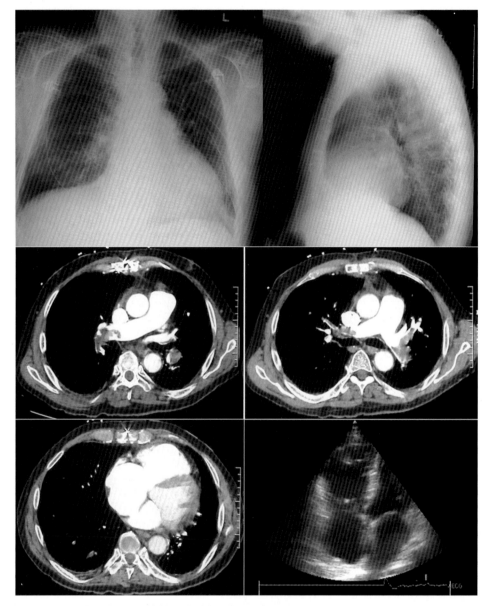

Figure 11-99. TOP, Chest radiographs show clear lung fields and mild cardiomegaly. MIDDLE, Contrast-enhanced CT scan axial images. Clot is present in the right main PA, nearly occluding it, and also as a "saddle embolus" of the left PA bifurcation and extensively filling the left lower lobe pulmonary artery. BOTTOM LEFT, CT image depicts severe dilation of the right side of the heart, which is an adverse prognosticator. The interatrial septum is deviated to the left side, consistent with right atrial pressure > left atrial pressure. BOTTOM RIGHT, Corresponding and corroborative transthoracic echocardiography depiction of RV dilation and systolic dysfunction.

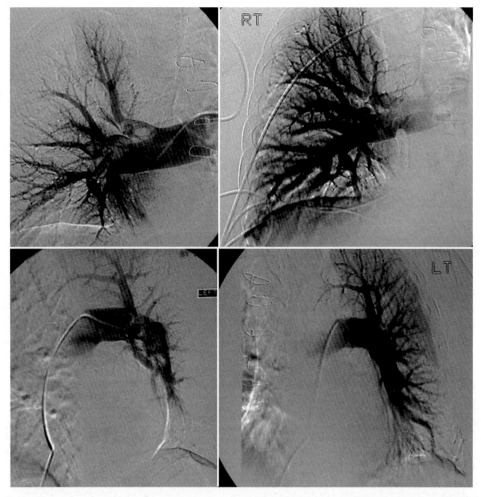

Figure 11-100. TOP, Right pulmonary angiograms. BOTTOM, Left pulmonary angiograms. Images on the left are taken before tPA infusion, and images on the right are after tPA infusion. Before infusion, there is a large burden of thrombus in the right and left pulmonary arteries. The large burden of thrombus in the left PA, virtually occluding the right lower PA, is seen to nearly entirely dissolve with 12 hours of infusion of tPA to the right side. Views of the left PA reveal residual thrombus still, which after a further 16 hours of left-sided selective catheter infusion has dissolved.

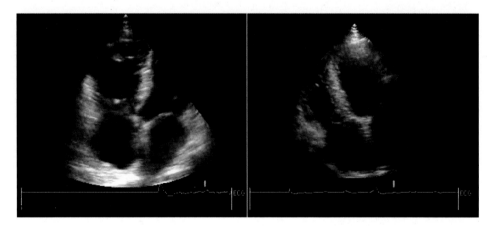

Figure 11-101. Transthoracic echocardiography before (LEFT) and after (RIGHT) tPA infusion to thrombolyse pulmonary embolism. Before tPA, the right ventricle is again strikingly dilated and akinetic, but the pattern is different from what it was due to the right ventricular infarction. Now the apex of the right ventricle is especially dilated and akinetic, whereas before it was the only part of the right ventricle contracting. This is consistent with submassive pulmonary embolism. After PA tPA infusion, the RV has nearly normalized in size and systolic function.

References

1. Heitmiller R, Jacobs ML, Daggett WM: Surgical management of postinfarction ventricular septal rupture. Ann Thorac Surg 1986;41:683-691.

2. Menon V, Webb JG, Hillis LD, et al: Outcome and profile of ventricular septal rupture with cardiogenic shock after myocardial infarction: a report from the SHOCK Trial Registry. SHould we emergently revascularize Occluded Coronaries in cardiogenic shocK? J Am Coll Cardiol 2000;36(Suppl A):1110-1116.

3. Crenshaw BS, Granger CB, Birnbaum Y, et al: Risk factors, angiographic patterns, and outcomes in patients with ventricular septal defect complicating acute myocardial infarction. GUSTO-I (Global Utilization of Streptokinase and TPA for Occluded Coronary Arteries) Trial Investigators. Circulation 2000;101:27-32.

4. Kinn JW, O'Neill WW, Benzuly KH, et al: Primary angioplasty reduces risk of myocardial rupture compared to thrombolysis for acute myocardial infarction. Cathet Cardiovasc Diagn 1997;42:151-157.

5. Moore CA, Nygaard TW, Kaiser DL, et al: Postinfarction ventricular septal rupture: the importance of location of infarction and right ventricular function in determining survival. Circulation 1986;74:45-55.

6. Edwards BS, Edwards WD, Edwards JE: Ventricular septal rupture complicating acute myocardial infarction: identification of simple and complex types in 53 autopsied hearts. Am J Cardiol 1984;54:1201-1205.

7. Di Bella, I, Minzioni G, Maselli D, et al: Septal dissection and rupture evolved as an inferobasal pseudoaneurysm. Ann Thorac Surg 2001;71:1358-1360.

8. Radford MJ, Johnson RA, Daggett WM Jr, et al: Ventricular septal rupture: a review of clinical and physiologic features and an analysis of survival. Circulation 1981;64:545-553.

9. Cummings RG, Reimer KA, Califf R, et al: Quantitative analysis of right and left ventricular infarction in the presence of postinfarction ventricular septal defect. Circulation 1988;77:33-42.

10. Held AC, Cole PL, Lipton B, et al: Rupture of the interventricular septum complicating acute myocardial infarction: a multicenter analysis of clinical findings and outcome. Am Heart J 1988;116(pt 1):1330-1336.

11. Kishon Y, Iqbal A, Oh JK, et al: Evolution of echocardiographic modalities in detection of postmyocardial infarction ventricular septal defect and papillary muscle rupture: study of 62 patients. Am Heart J 1993;126 (pt 1):667-675.

12. Fortin DF, Sheikh KH, Kisslo J: The utility of echocardiography in the diagnostic strategy of postinfarction ventricular septal rupture: a comparison of two-dimensional echocardiography versus Doppler color flow imaging. Am Heart J 1991;121(pt 1):25-32.

13. Paul JF, Mace L, Caussin C, et al: Multirow detector computed tomography assessment of intraseptal dissection and ventricular pseudoaneurysm in postinfarction ventricular septal defect. Circulation 2001;104:497-498.

14. Figueras J, Cortadellas J, Calvo F, Soler-Soler J: Relevance of delayed hospital admission on development of cardiac rupture during acute myocardial infarction: study in 225 patients with free wall, septal or papillary muscle rupture. J Am Coll Cardiol 1998;32:135-139.

15. Bethea CF, Peter RH, Behar VS, et al: The hemodynamic simulation of mitral regurgitation in ventricular septal defect after myocardial infarction. Cathet Cardiovasc Diagn 1976;2:97-104.

16. Meister SG, Helfant RH: Rapid bedside differentiation of ruptured interventricular septum from acute mitral insufficiency. N Engl J Med 1972;287:1024-1025.

17. Grant P, Patel P, Singh SP: Balloon catheter used in the treatment of a ventricular septal rupture following a myocardial infarction. N Engl J Med 1986;314:60-61.

18. Ryan TJ, Antman EM, Brooks NH, et al: 1999 update: ACC/AHA Guidelines for the Management of Patients With Acute Myocardial Infarction: Executive Summary and Recommendations: a report of the American College of Cardiology/American Heart Association Task Force on Practice Guidelines (Committee on Management of Acute Myocardial Infarction). Circulation 1999;100:1016-1030.

19. Beekman RH, Rocchini AP, Rosenthal A: Hemodynamic effects of hydralazine in infants with a large ventricular septal defect. Circulation 1982;65:523-528.

20. Deville C, Fontan F, Chevalier JM, et al: Surgery of post-infarction ventricular septal defect: risk factors for hospital death and long-term results. Eur J Cardiothorac Surg 1991;5:167-174.

21. Cummings RG, Califf R, Jones RN, et al: Correlates of survival in patients with postinfarction ventricular septal defect. Ann Thorac Surg 1989;47:824-830.

22. Thanopoulos BD, Tsaousis GS, Konstadopoulou GN, Zarayelyan AG: Transcatheter closure of muscular ventricular septal defects with the Amplatzer ventricular septal defect occluder: initial clinical applications in children. J Am Coll Cardiol 1999;33:1395-1399.

23. Lee EM, Roberts DH, Walsh KP: Transcatheter closure of a residual postmyocardial infarction ventricular septal defect with the Amplatzer septal occluder. Heart 1998;80:522-524.

24. Pesonen E, Thilen U, Sandstrom S, et al: Transcatheter closure of postinfarction ventricular septal defect with the Amplatzer Septal Occluder device. Scand Cardiovasc J 2000;34:446-448.

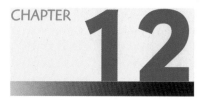

Papillary Muscle Rupture and Postinfarction Mitral Insufficiency

KEY POINTS

▸ In the context of an inferoposterior infarction and a new murmur, or an inferoposterior infarction with abrupt CHF or cardiogenic shock, maintain suspicion of PMR.

▸ The usual clinical syndrome is that of acute pulmonary edema and cardiogenic shock.

▸ The systolic murmur of mitral insufficiency is commonly atypical: shorter, softer, sometimes absent.

▸ V waves are usually present but may be absent.

▸ Echocardiography is the test of choice, but knowledge of detailed mitral imaging is required. TEE remains very useful to confirm the severity of mitral insufficiency and the basis of it.

▸ Vasodilators and IABP support and improve pulmonary congestion and forward output.

▸ Emergent or urgent surgery (mitral replacement) with aortocoronary artery bypass grafting is salvaging the majority of patients with the highest success rate of any form of myocardial rupture.

▸ Coronary angiography is indicated to address potential recurrent ischemia or reinfarction risks and to enable coronary artery bypass grafting at the time of valve surgery.

Papillary muscle rupture (PMR), one of the mechanical complications of infarction, has historically been identified as occurring in 1% of infarction cases, being responsible for 1% to 5% of deaths and 7% of cardiogenic shock cases. The current incidence is likely to be less. PMR results in acute left-sided heart failure and often in cardiogenic shock. In the SHOCK registry, 7% of shock cases were due to PMR. The 55% mortality of PMR cases in the SHOCK registry was nearly identical to the overall mortality (60%) and the mortality due to pump failure (59%).[1]

PMR is notable for the dual aspects of high early mortality (if untreated) and high surgical salvage rate, making it one of the most meaningful diagnoses in the CCU. PMR typically arises from the setting of a small underlying infarction, often a subendocardial infarction. Therefore, postoperative and long-term survival is generally characterized by freedom from heart failure. Although PMR is usually a solitary lesion, it may occur with other mechanical, electrical, or coronary complications of infarction. The concurrence of other mechanical complications of infarction, such as subacute rupture and tamponade, may delay recognition of PMR.[2]

Mitral insufficiency, due to adverse remodeling of the geometry of the ventricle and not due to rupture of a papillary muscle, occurs in about one sixth of patients after infarction (Table 12-1). The presence and the severity of postinfarction (non-PMR) mitral insufficiency are both predictive of worse 5-

year survival (38% ± 5% versus 61% ± 6%) (Figs. 12-1 and 12-2).[3] Effective regurgitant orifices of ≥20 mm², 1 to 19 mm², and 0 mm² are associated with 7-year survivals of 29 ± 9%, 47 ± 8%, and 61 ± 6%, respectively.[3]

HISTORICAL CONSIDERATIONS

The first postmortem diagnosis of postinfarction PMR was made by Merat in 1803, and the first antemortem diagnosis of postinfarction PMR was made by Davidson in 1948. In 1963, Burch described the first postinfarction papillary muscle dysfunction without rupture. Austen performed the first successful mitral valve repair for PMR in 1965, and Fluck performed the first successful mitral valve repair for papillary muscle dysfunction without rupture in 1966.

NATURAL HISTORY

The natural history of PMR involves 50% mortality within the first 24 hours and a further 30% mortality during the first 2 weeks. There are a few longer term survivors but very few long-term

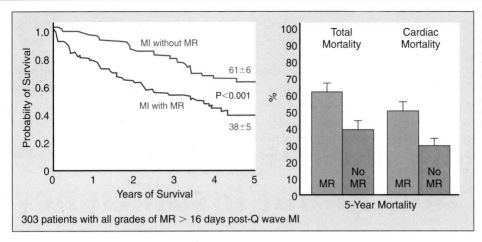

Figure 12-1. The presence of postinfarction mitral insufficiency is associated with increased total mortality and cardiac mortality. MI, myocardial infarction; MR, mitral regurgitation (From Grigioni F, Enriquez-Sarano M, Zehr KJ, et al: Ischemic mitral regurgitation: long-term outcome and prognostic implications with quantitative Doppler assessment. Circulation 2001;103:1759-1764.)

Table 12-1. Causes of Postinfarction Mitral Insufficiency

Non–papillary muscle rupture causes

  Global left ventricular distortion

    Dilation, "sphericalization"

  Regional left ventricular distortion

    Regional dilation

    Regional systolic dysfunction

Papillary muscle rupture

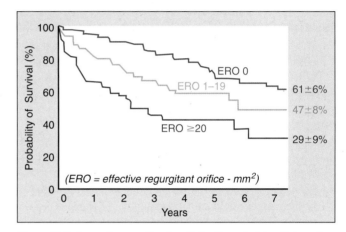

Figure 12-2. Increasing severity of postinfarction mitral insufficiency is associated with increasing mortality. ERO, effective regurgitant orifice. (From Grigioni F, Enriquez-Sarano M, Zehr KJ, et al: Ischemic mitral regurgitation: long-term outcome and prognostic implications with quantitative Doppler assessment. Circulation 2001;103:1759-1764.)

survivors because of the unsupportable combination of severe mitral insufficiency and left ventricular dysfunction within a background of underlying coronary artery disease.

Most PMRs occur within a 2- to 7-day period after acute infarction. There is some controversy as to whether ruptures of all forms occur more or less frequently after fibrinolytic treatment. Ruptures of all forms, whether or not there is an overall increase, appear to occur earlier in the era of reperfusion and fibrinolytics.

PATHOLOGY, PATHOGENESIS, AND PATHOPHYSIOLOGY

Almost invariably, there are two papillary muscle complexes in the left ventricle: the anterolateral papillary muscle (ALPM) complex and the posteromedial papillary muscle (PMPM) complex (Fig. 12-3). Papillary muscles subtend chordae tendineae that support the ipsilateral commissure of the mitral valve, preventing prolapse and retroversion of the mitral leaflets. The ALPM supports the anterolateral half of the mitral valve commissure, and the PMPM supports the posteromedial half of the mitral valve commissure. Contrary to belief, each papillary muscle apparatus does not support one leaflet. The ALPM, which is usually a single trunk, supports both leaflets of the anterolateral commissure. The PMPM, which is usually composed of dual heads or trunks, has each head or trunk supporting one leaflet of the posteromedial commissure. Therefore, rupture of the ALPM results in complete loss of support of the anterolateral commissure and

overwhelming mitral insufficiency. Rupture of one head or trunk of the PMPM usually results in loss of support or prolapse of one leaflet of the posteromedial commissure (symmetric prolapse) and overwhelming or severe mitral insufficiency. Similarly, partial rupture of a papillary muscle results in significant prolapse of a commissure and significant but less overwhelming mitral insufficiency. Papillary muscle anatomy is subject to variation.

Papillary muscle complexes involve a single trunk (or body), or a single body with two heads, or two trunks closely beside each other. Papillary muscle trunks attach directly to the underlying ventricular myocardium or indirectly through root-like connections. The attachment of papillary muscles occurs at the junction of the apical third and the middle third of the left ventricle. The papillary muscle basal attachment is widely used in cardiac imaging to segment the apical and the middle third of the left ventricular cavity. Most commonly, the ALPM complex comprises one trunk and head in 90% of cases and two trunks and heads in 10% of cases. Most commonly (75%), the PMPM complex comprises either two trunks or one trunk with two heads (Fig. 12-4). The two trunks or heads of the PMPM may be positioned to the side or beside each other, such that they can be well appreciated only in cross-sectional short-axis imaging, or they

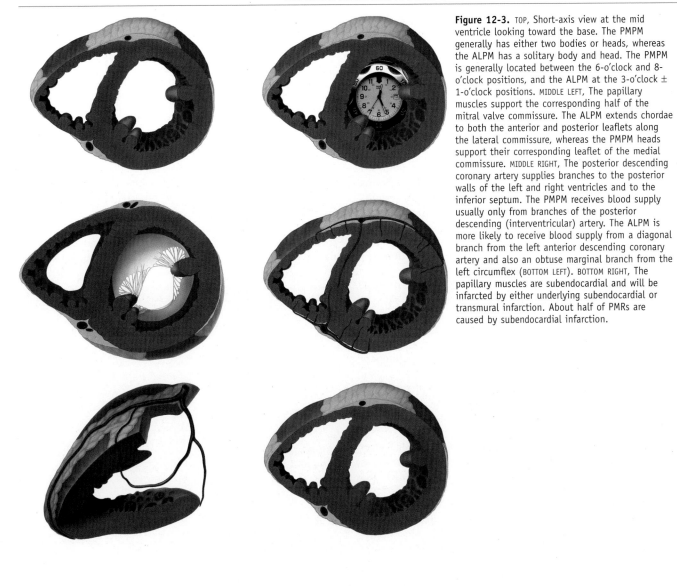

Figure 12-3. TOP, Short-axis view at the mid ventricle looking toward the base. The PMPM generally has either two bodies or heads, whereas the ALPM has a solitary body and head. The PMPM is generally located between the 6-o'clock and 8-o'clock positions, and the ALPM at the 3-o'clock ± 1-o'clock positions. MIDDLE LEFT, The papillary muscles support the corresponding half of the mitral valve commissure. The ALPM extends chordae to both the anterior and posterior leaflets along the lateral commissure, whereas the PMPM heads support their corresponding leaflet of the medial commissure. MIDDLE RIGHT, The posterior descending coronary artery supplies branches to the posterior walls of the left and right ventricles and to the inferior septum. The PMPM receives blood supply usually only from branches of the posterior descending (interventricular) artery. The ALPM is more likely to receive blood supply from a diagonal branch from the left anterior descending coronary artery and also an obtuse marginal branch from the left circumflex (BOTTOM LEFT). BOTTOM RIGHT, The papillary muscles are subendocardial and will be infarcted by either underlying subendocardial or transmural infarction. About half of PMRs are caused by subendocardial infarction.

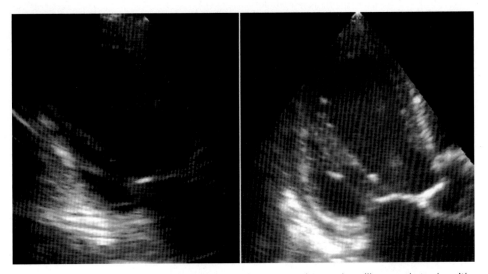

Figure 12-4. Usual variants of the posterior papillary muscle complex. LEFT, There are two (separate) papillary muscle trunks, with each supplying chordae to one leaflet—the more anterior trunk supports the anterior leaflet, and the more posterior trunk supplies the more posterior leaflet. Thereby, between the two, there is support for this posteromedial half of the commissure. RIGHT, There is one trunk with two heads, each of which supplies chordae, again the more posterior head supplying the posterior leaflet at this commissure and the more anterior head supporting the anterior leaflet. Note as well that some chordae supporting the anterior leaflet insert about 1 cm back from the free edge.

may be positioned over each other, such that their relation can be clearly appreciated on longitudinal plane imaging (long-axis views).

Papillary muscles contract in systole to maintain the correct length : tension relationship on the commissure as the left ventricle shortens along its longitudinal axis in systole, such that the mitral leaflets do not prolapse. Loss of papillary muscle contraction from infarction may confer prolapse to the less supported commissure, as left ventricular longitudinal shortening is not offset by papillary muscle shortening. However, what tends to oppose this occurrence is that the underlying infarction of the left ventricle wall reduces longitudinal shortening as well, preserving the balance (ratio) of left ventricular and papillary muscle shortening. Mitral valve coaptation normally occurs over a surface several millimeters long, rather than at a single point at the leaflet tips, affording a "coaptation reserve" to weather the load-dependent and systolic function–dependent variations of length : tension support to the valve.

Infarction is the usual but not the sole etiology of PMR (Table 12-2). The term papillary muscle *rupture* is preferable to *tear*, which is a term usually applied to *leaflet* disruption that occurs from different diseases. PMR may be complete, resulting in major loss of commissural support and severe or massive mitral insufficiency that clinically causes severe pulmonary edema, cardiogenic shock, or electromechanical dissociation (Fig. 12-5). Partial rupture of a papillary muscle complex may also occur, resulting in elongation of the papillary muscle, prolapse of a leaflet or commissure, and usually severe mitral insufficiency (see Fig. 12-5).

The papillary muscles are *entirely subendocardial* structures and may therefore infarct with subendocardial infarction alone. Hence, among the mechanical complications of infarction, PMRs are unique in occurring in about half of cases without ST elevation infarction—the requisite substrate for false aneurysms, ventricular septal rupture, and free wall rupture. Autopsy series of PMRs reveal that the responsible infarction is often subendocardial (12% to 55%)[4-6] and conspicuously small, averaging 3.8 cm × 2.8 cm (as small as 1 cm × 1.5 cm),[6] explaining why left ventricular function in surgical survivors tends to be very good and sometimes normal. The small size of infarction explains why residual mechanical forces within the left ventricle are capable of disrupt-

ing the papillary muscle. Because occlusion of a dominant right coronary artery (RCA) is responsible for most PMRs, concurrent right ventricular infarction is common (68%). In a small but elegantly assessed series of 9 cases of PMR, previous infarction was present in 2 cases; PMPM rupture accounted for 8 cases and ALPM rupture for 1 case. Rupture of one of two heads was the most common occurrence (4 cases); rupture of two heads occurred in 2 cases; rupture of an entire trunk occurred in 2 cases; and partial rupture occurred in 1 case. The time interval between PMR and death was less than 1 day in 3 cases, 1 day in 2 cases, 3 days in 2 cases, 30 days in 1 case, and 60 days in 1 case.[6]

The PMPM usually receives its blood supply solely from branches of the posterior descending (posterior interventricular) artery and is therefore highly susceptible to infarction from occlusion of this single vessel. In contradistinction, the ALPM usually receives blood supply from both an obtuse marginal branch of the left circumflex artery and a diagonal branch of the left anterior

Table 12-2. Causes of Papillary Muscle Rupture

Infarction
  Coronary artery disease
  Antiphospholipid antibody
  Prenatal hypoxia
Infections
  Infective endocarditis (abscess)
  Clostridial sepsis
Trauma (blunt)
  CPR
Iatrogenic
  CPR
  Mitral balloon valvuloplasty
  Aortic balloon valvuloplasty
  Subaortic membrane balloon dilation
Pacer electrode removal

CPR, cardiopulmonary resuscitation.

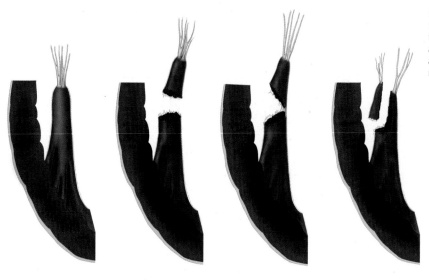

Figure 12-5. Illustration of a normal solitary papillary muscle apparatus (LEFT), an infarcted and completely ruptured papillary muscle (MIDDLE LEFT), an infarcted and partially ruptured papillary muscle (MIDDLE RIGHT), and an infarcted and partially ruptured papillary muscle with another type of tear (RIGHT).

descending coronary artery, and therefore it has a degree of resistance to ischemia and infarction. For anatomic reasons of coronary supply, the PMPM is far more commonly prone to infarction-related rupture (6 to 12 times[5]) than is the ALPM. On rarest of occasions, both the ALPM and the PMPM rupture concurrently.[7]

Complete rupture of the usually solitary ALPM trunk typically results in frank cardiogenic shock, electromechanical dissociation, or death. As the PMPM comprises two trunks or heads usually, and as rupture generally occurs of one of the two trunks or heads, its rupture generally results in severe pulmonary edema or cardiogenic shock.

Postinfarction Muscle Rupture Not Due to Papillary Muscle Rupture

Mild to moderate postinfarction mitral insufficiency not due to papillary muscle occurs in at least 10% to 20% of acute infarction cases. Postinfarction (non-PMR) mitral insufficiency may be due to several mechanisms, but the most common and most significant is that of left ventricular cavitary dilation, which may be

regional or global (sphericalization of the left ventricle). Dilation of the left ventricle regionally or globally may place the papillary muscles in incorrect spatial location to effectively support a commissure (Figs. 12-6 and 12-7). Lateral and apical displacement of the infarct zone and its overlying papillary muscle pulls the commissural coaptation line away from the annulus and into the left ventricle, reducing the surface available for coaptation. Dyskinesis outward of the infarction segment may compound the problem. Opposing the cavitary dilation effect on the commissures is papillary muscle noncontraction or even stretching, which adds length. The net result on mitral valve competence of regional and global dilation and remodeling, of infarct regional wall motion, and of papillary muscle akinesis or stretching, is highly unpredictable.

Of some note, postinfarction mitral insufficiency not due to rupture may be succeeded by papillary rupture—the two entities are not dichotomous.

Global left ventricular systolic dysfunction and radial cavitary dilation are the principal causes of postinfarction mitral insufficiency. Dog models of acute infarction demonstrate that the degree of mitral insufficiency is proportional to the degree of incomplete mitral leaflet closure ($r = 0.98$) and to the degree of left ventricular systolic dysfunction ($r = -0.92$ with dP/dt, and

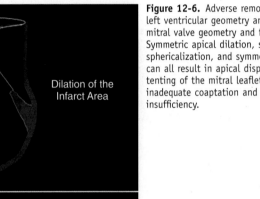

Figure 12-6. Adverse remodeling distorts left ventricular geometry and, secondarily, mitral valve geometry and function. Symmetric apical dilation, symmetric sphericalization, and symmetric dilation can all result in apical displacement or tenting of the mitral leaflets, causing inadequate coaptation and mitral insufficiency.

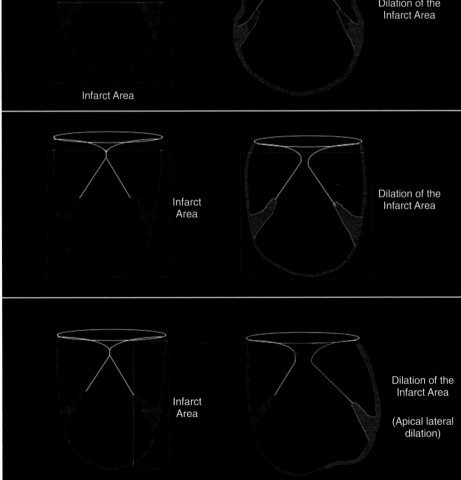

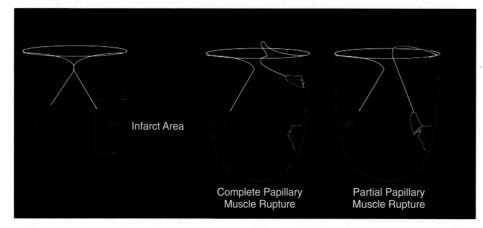

Figure 12-7. Complete PMR results in a flail papillary muscle and mitral leaflet. Partial PMR results in prolapse of a mitral leaflet or commissure from elongation of the papillary muscle.

Infarct Area

Complete Papillary
Muscle Rupture

Partial Papillary
Muscle Rupture

$r = 0.86$ with global left ventricular wall thickening) and not correlated with papillary muscle dysfunction ($r = -0.24$ ALPM, -0.38 PMPM) or regional left ventricular systolic dysfunction.[8] In a human study of 188 patients, of whom 13% had 3+ or 4+ mitral insufficiency, significant univariate predictors of mitral insufficiency were recurrent infarction, dilation of the left ventricle, sphericity index, inferoposterior asynergy, mitral annular dilation, and mitral leaflet restriction. Significant multivariate predictors of mitral insufficiency were recurrent infarction (odds ratio, 5.1), sphericity index (odds ratio, 1.1), and inferoposterior asynergy (odds ratio, 6.1).[9]

CLINICAL PRESENTATION

The most common clinical signs of PMR include the following:

- Post–myocardial infarction acute pulmonary edema
- Post–myocardial infarction cardiogenic shock
- Post–myocardial infarction electromechanical dissociation (pulseless electrical activity)
- Post–myocardial infarction systolic murmur

The diagnosis of PMR requires suspicion, and although it is often straightforward, it may require considerable persistence in some cases; but because of the availability of specific and often successful surgical repair, it is a critical diagnosis to make. PMR is revealing of limitations of diagnostic testing, clinical convention, and hemodynamics. A report of two cases of cardiogenic shock due to silent (no murmur) severe mitral insufficiency from PMR, without V waves on the pulmonary capillary wedge tracing, is evidence of this. One of these cases had only moderate mitral insufficiency on a poor-quality ventriculogram and had actually undergone urgent aortocoronary bypass the same day, in which the mitral valve was not inspected because there were no V waves on the pulmonary capillary wedge tracing. Transesophageal echocardiography had established the diagnosis of PMR, and the patient underwent emergent reoperation and mitral valve replacement and survived, despite renal acute tubular necrosis. The other patient, also in cardiogenic shock, without murmur but with low pulmonary artery pressures (40/20 mm Hg), pulmonary capillary wedge pressure of 18 mm Hg, and no V waves, had severe mitral regurgitation and at surgery was found to have rupture of both trunks of the PMPM. The patient survived.[10]

Most cases of PMR result in hypotension and tachycardia (due to the small or inadequate forward stroke volume) and marked pulmonary edema (due to markedly elevated left atrial pressure). PMR may result in different murmurs, which depend on the severity of the mitral insufficiency but mainly on the relative left ventricular and atrial systolic pressures. PMR without shock or severe heart failure may be associated with a holosystolic and loud murmur. However, most PMRs lower the left ventricular systolic pressure and raise the left atrial pressure dramatically, usually resulting in a short and softer murmur. The lesser left ventricular to left atrial gradient renders the murmur less loud, and the development of a high late systolic V wave may eliminate the left ventricle : left atrial gradient and the late systolic component of the murmur (Fig. 12-8). Massive mitral insufficiency with equilibration of left ventricular and left atrial pressure equalizes the left ventricular and left atrial systolic pressure, and hence in such cases, there is no systolic murmur. In a series of 19 cases of PMR, a murmur was detected in most (70%) partial PMRs but in very few (11%) complete PMRs. Overall, only about half (42%) of cases had a murmur.[5]

Other physical examination findings include hypotension, shock appearance, soft or absent S_1 (due to poor mitral closure, low left ventricle : left atrial gradient), loud P_2 (due to pulmonary hypertension), loud S_3 (due to elevated left atrial pressure), right-sided heart failure signs, and signs of pulmonary edema.

The differential diagnosis of a new systolic murmur after infarction includes "postinfarction" mitral insufficiency (non-PMR), PMR, ventricular septal rupture, ventricular false aneurysm, and a pericardial friction rub mistaken as a murmur or belated recognition of an antecedent murmur.

DIAGNOSTIC TESTING AND PAPILLARY MUSCLE RUPTURE

It is important to make a diagnosis of PMR for several reasons: (1) the lesion can be surgically repaired with good results (the best surgical outcomes of all the mechanical complications of infarction); (2) the mortality in untreated cases is enormous; and (3) the natural history of unrepaired postinfarction PMR is dramatically worse than that of postinfarction mitral insufficiency. PMR is a cardiac emergency and should entail an appropriately emergent response. Therefore, because of its high mortality if

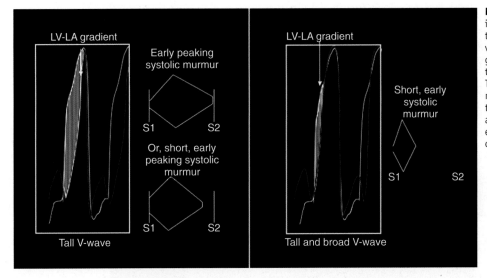

Figure 12-8. The murmur of mitral insufficiency is produced by vibration or turbulence of the jet driven by the left ventricle to left atrial (LV-LA) pressure gradient. The taller the V wave, the less the gradient and the softer the murmur. The broader the V wave, the shorter the murmur. When the V wave is massive and there is equalization of the left ventricular and left atrial pressures (common chamber effect), there is no murmur, despite the occurrence of massive mitral insufficiency.

untreated, yet good chance of salvage if treated, PMR is an important specific diagnosis to make.

Electrocardiography

There are no patterns specific to the rupture or due to the rupture. The electrocardiogram (ECG) usually demonstrates ST shifts or T-wave changes due to the underlying infarction. Q waves may not be present, as many PMRs may be due to only subendocardial infarction in about half of cases, unlike septal rupture, which nearly invariably is due to Q-wave or transmural infarction. ECG associations of PMR are less prominent than with other rupture because the responsible infarctions tend to be smaller and often subendocardial. Furthermore, posterior wall signs of infarction are less well represented on the ECG.

Chest Radiography

Acute (severe, often "bat-wing") signs of interstitial and airspace pulmonary edema are the norm. Pleural effusions, a sign of chronic and biventricular heart failure, tend to be absent. The size of the cardiopericardial silhouette is usually normal or only mildly increased, as there is seldom previous cardiac disease.

Transthoracic Echocardiography

Visualization of papillary muscles, which requires high spatial and temporal resolution, is generally most suitably performed by transthoracic echocardiography (TTE). In general, the PMPM is easier to image, and the ALPM is more difficult to image. In short-axis cross-sectional views, the PMPM is usually located at the 7-o'clock position (or 8-o'clock or 6-o'clock), and the ALPM is usually located at the 3-o'clock position (or 2-o'clock or 4-o'clock) (Fig. 12-9). To establish the integrity of a papillary muscle, long-axis visualization is far more useful than short-axis imaging (Figs. 12-10 and 12-11).

With PMR, severe mitral insufficiency is almost always present. The mitral valve appearance is abnormal in one of several ways. The velocity of the mitral insufficiency is less (<4 m/s) than usual (5 m/s) because of lower left ventricular systolic (driving) pressure and lower left ventricular systolic:left atrial systolic pressure gradient. Partial rupture that results in partial loss of commissural support results in prolapse of the commissure (Fig. 12-12). The leaflet thickness is normal, and the overall appearance is not usual for myxomatous disease. A partially ruptured papillary muscle can usually be appreciated to be wobbling or to have some form of excess or chaotic motion due to lesser attachment. Complete PMR results in a severed head or trunk that appears as an abnormal tangle of soft tissue (ruptured head) and chordae whipping from one side of the mitral valve to the other. In some cases, the severed muscle and chordae are tightly wound into a ball. An underlying wall motion abnormality is usually evident, generally small, and the remainder of the left ventricle is typically dynamic. TTE should be used to calculate the forward cardiac output and the right ventricular systolic pressure (RVSP) of CCU patients with mechanical and hemodynamic complications. In most cases, TTE can make the diagnosis of PMR.[11]

Transesophageal Echocardiography

Transesophageal echocardiography (TEE) is the best diagnostic imaging means by which to image and therefore to identify a complete or partial rupture of a papillary muscle (Figs. 12-13 and 12-14). Complete rupture is evident by the flailing motion of the severed component or a tangled mass of knotted chordae and muscle attached to leaflets (Fig. 12-15).

A partial rupture is evident by excessive motion of a papillary muscle with erratic sharp movement, and frank stretching is apparent. A series of 21 cases (20 left ventricular PMRs, 1 right ventricular PMR), surgically confirmed, established that in 35% of cases, the papillary muscle head did not appear in the left atrium as it was held by strands or knotted by its chords. Abnormal large-amplitude erratic motion of a large (1 cm) mass in the left ventricle was seen in 90% of cases.[12] The best echocardio-

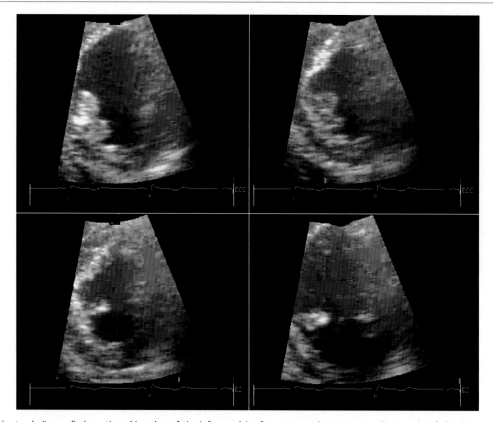

Figure 12-9. TTE short-axis "sweep" along the midportion of the left ventricle, from apex to base. TOP LEFT, Two trunks of the PMPM are seen (toward the apex). TOP RIGHT, Sweeping slightly more toward the base, both trunk bodies are still present. The frame is systolic, and the dyskinesis of the inferior wall and inferior septum is apparent by the angulation of the inferior septum. BOTTOM LEFT, Sweeping farther toward the base, there is only one papillary muscle body, the more anteromedial one. BOTTOM RIGHT, Sweeping nearly onto the mitral valve, again there is only the tip of a papillary muscle. This is a complete rupture of one trunk of the PMPM.

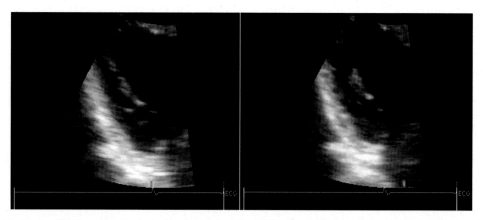

Figure 12-10. Apical 3-chamber TTE view along the long axis of a trunk of the PMPM. At end-diastole with no tension on the muscle (LEFT), the papillary muscle appearance is within normal. In systole (RIGHT) with tension on the muscle, there is separation of the trunk along its long axis—it is being held only by strands of tissue off the plane of imaging. This is a partial rupture of a trunk of the PMPM complex.

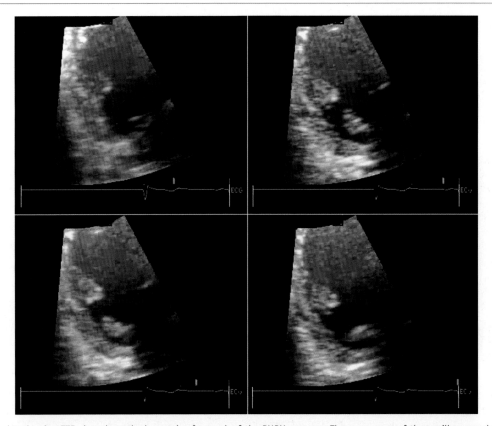

Figure 12-11. Apical 3-chamber TTE view along the long axis of a trunk of the PMPM. TOP LEFT, The appearance of the papillary muscle in this frame is not necessarily abnormal, although the muscle appears rather short. This may simply be due to imaging obliquely across the muscle rather than along its long axis. TOP RIGHT, In this frame, the appearance of the papillary muscle is distinctly abnormal as discontinuity is apparent. BOTTOM LEFT, Erratic motion and implausible alignment are seen, strongly suggesting rupture and loss of alignment and restraint. BOTTOM RIGHT, Further erratic alignment and motion signify a complete rupture of a trunk of the PMPM complex. In the top left image, the body of the ruptured papillary muscle trunk is actually faintly seen on the left atrial side of the mitral valve.

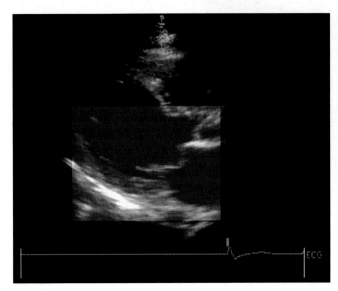

Figure 12-12. Parasternal long-axis TTE view. The central field has been brightness adjusted. There is prolapse of the body of the anterior leaflet, which does not have the myxomatous appearance of thickening and redundancy to explain the prolapse, nor is there drastic underfilling of the ventricle as an alternative explanation of the prolapse. The posterior wall is dilated outward, consistent with infarction. There is a paradox to the image—why, with dilation of the wall that supports the papillary muscle (not seen), is there prolapse rather than "tenting" or apical displacement? Further imaging identified a partially ruptured posterior papillary muscle head (the more anterior of two that supported the anterior leaflet at the medial commissure).

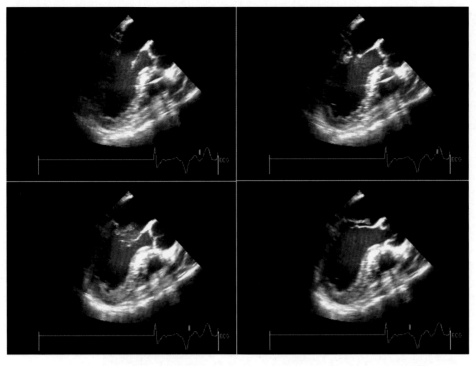

Figure 12-13. Lower esophageal 3-chamber TEE views reveal complete rupture of one of two trunks of the PMPM complex. During diastole (TOP LEFT), there is no definite abnormality of the mitral valve; but in all the other images at other times in the cardiac cycle, the body of the ruptured trunk of the PMPM that supported the posterior leaflet is seen windmilling about, attached by chordae to the posterior leaflet. The trunk of the PMPM complex to the anterior leaflet was intact, which is why the anterior leaflet is not prolapsing from lack of support.

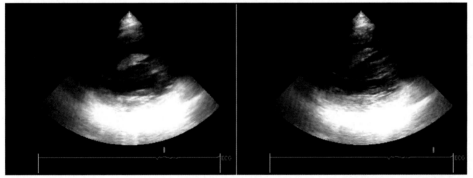

Figure 12-14. Transgastric vertical TEE views along the long axis of the PMPM show partial rupture of the PMPM complex. LEFT, The papillary muscle body is attached only by strands of tissue, probably endocardium. RIGHT, The erratic motion of the body is depicted by the angulation change, with illogical tip orientation toward the posterior wall.

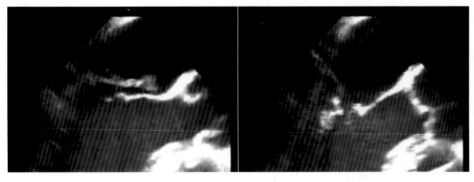

Figure 12-15. Shallow lower esophageal 3-chamber TEE views. One ruptured head of the PMPM is seen attached by chordae to the posterior leaflet and with free motion such that it moves back and forth from the atrium to the ventricle.

Table 12-3. Echocardiographic Views to Image the Papillary Muscle

	Posteromedial Papillary Muscle	Anterolateral Papillary Muscle
TTE	Parasternal long-axis view	Parasternal short-axis view
	Parasternal short-axis view	Apical 4-chamber view
	Apical 3-chamber view	
	Apical 2-chamber view	
TEE	Transgastric short-axis view	Transgastric short-axis view
	Transgastric long-axis view	Transgastric long-axis view
	Lower esophageal vertical 2-chamber view	Lower esophageal vertical 4-chamber view

TEE, transesophageal echocardiography; TTE, transthoracic echocardiography.

graphic views to image the papillary muscle are listed in Table 12-3 and illustrated in Figure 12-16.

Angiography and Catheterization Hemodynamics

Right-Sided Heart Balloon Catheterization

Right-sided heart balloon catheterization remains a useful technique to establish findings consistent with severe mitral insufficiency and to exclude septal rupture. When it first became available, in an era without echocardiography, right-sided heart catheterization revolutionized the assessment of acute infarction patients with hemodynamic deterioration and new systolic

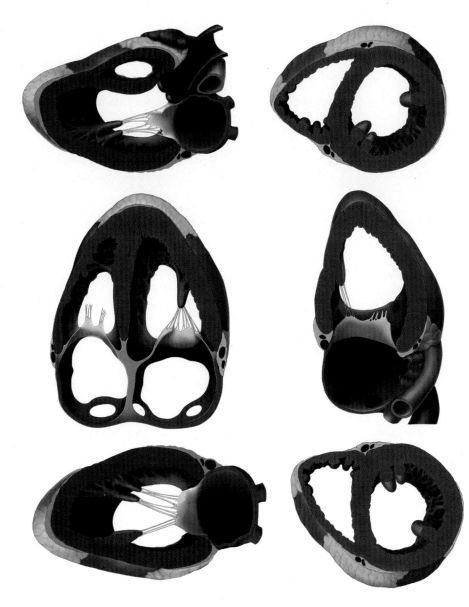

Figure 12-16. Echocardiographic views that depict papillary muscles. TOP LEFT, Parasternal long-axis view. In general, this plane falls along at least one component of the PMPM complex. TOP RIGHT, Parasternal short-axis view at the mid ventricular level. Both papillary muscle complexes can be imaged on this plane. MIDDLE LEFT, The apical 4-chamber (or 5-chamber) view generally depicts the ALPM. MIDDLE RIGHT, The apical 2-chamber (or 3-chamber) view generally images the PMPM. BOTTOM LEFT, Transgastric long-axis view along the plane of the papillary muscles. This view is very useful to identify disruption and partial or frank ruptures, and an imaging plane can often depict both the PMPM and ALPM complexes. BOTTOM RIGHT, Transgastric short-axis view is similar to the TTE short-axis image and enables the closest views of the posterior papillary muscles.

murmurs—who had either septal rupture or acute mitral insufficiency (often PMR)—and offered preoperative diagnosis. Echocardiography has assumed the primary diagnostic role for evaluation of acute infarction mechanical complications, but right-sided heart catheterization can build the case for severe mitral regurgitation (MR). Right-sided heart catheterization findings in PMR or non-PMR postinfarction MR include the following:

- Elevated pulmonary artery pressure
- Elevated pulmonary artery capillary wedge pressure
- V waves on pulmonary artery capillary wedge pressure (V wave more than 10 mm Hg greater than the mean pulmonary artery capillary wedge pressure) are commonly but not invariably seen with severe MR (Fig. 12-17). V waves reflect the pressure : volume relation (compliance curve) of the left atrium and are highly influenced by the degree of filling. V waves are neither sensitive (only 60%)[13] nor specific for severe mitral insufficiency[14] or even for mitral insufficiency[15]; they are also seen in states of left atrial overload such as congestive heart failure (CHF) from left ventricular dysfunction and aortic valve disease, mitral obstruction, and ventricular septal defects.[14,16,17] In the presence of large V waves, the trough of the *x* descent correlates best with the left ventricular end-diastolic pressure (LVEDP).
- Elevated right atrial pressure

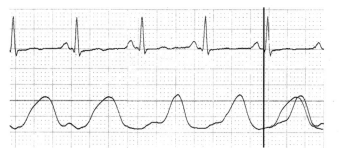

Figure 12-17. Right-sided heart balloon flotation catheter pressure recordings of severe acute mitral insufficiency. The balloon was said to be "not wedging." The left two systolic waveforms are pulmonary artery waveforms, with pressures of 66/25 mm Hg. The arterial blood pressure was 80/50 mm Hg. The next two systolic tracings are "wedge" pressure recordings, with massive V waves that are as tall as the pulmonary artery pressure tracings and in fact responsible for the magnitude of the pulmonary hypertension. The V wave is narrower than the pulmonary artery systolic waveform but may be as tall, as in this case. The right panel has the pulmonary artery systolic and pulmonary capillary wedge tracings superimposed. The wedge pressure is as tall and slightly temporally delayed compared with ventricular or, as in this case, arterial tracings.

- Reduced cardiac output and index
- Oximetry: an O_2 step-up is usually not present. On rare occasions, an O_2 step-up may be seen and is due to truly massive systolic regurgitation of oxygenated capillary blood.

A small series of predominantly *partial* PMRs tabulated the following average hemodynamic findings of PMR: LVEDP or pulmonary artery wedge pressure, 23 mm Hg; cardiac index, 2.4 L/min/m²; V wave, 55 mm Hg; and ejection fraction, 51%.[6] Figures 12-18 and 12-19 further illustrate the hemodynamics of PMR.

Coronary Angiography

Coronary angiography is indicated in PMR cases if clinical stability enables the additional time demand. Recurrent ischemia and infarction may occur without revascularization, and as the standard treatment is surgical repair, aortocoronary bypass grafting can be performed at the same setting. Angiographic findings in postinfarction rupture are summarized in Table 12-4.

Contrast Ventriculography

Contrast ventriculography will reveal severe mitral insufficiency when it is present and disclose this important finding is not already known at that point of case management. If it is confidently established by echocardiography that severe mitral insufficiency is present, the potential risk of contrast nephropathy among PMR cases seems to offset any yield. However, if the degree of mitral insufficiency is unclear and TEE is unavailable, contrast ventriculography is likely to be contributory to making a diagnosis, although establishing that severe mitral insufficiency is present does not explain its specific etiology. Assessment of the severity of mitral insufficiency by contrast ventriculography is summarized in Table 12-5.

PMR with severe mitral insufficiency is a class I ACC/AHA indication for each of the following[22]:

- Emergency or urgent surgical repair
- Emergency or urgent coronary artery bypass graft surgery
- Balloon flotation right-sided heart catheter monitoring
- Intra-aortic balloon counterpulsation (IABP)

MANAGEMENT

The definitive management of PMR is emergent or urgent surgical repair, and this perspective should be maintained during diag-

Table 12-4. Angiographic Findings in Postinfarction Rupture

Angiographic Disease	Septal Rupture			Papillary Muscle Rupture		Postinfarction MR, No Papillary Muscle Rupture	Free Wall Rupture
Reference	18	19	20	19	20	21	20
Single-vessel	50%	36%	57%	30%	46%	16%	58%
Two-vessel	40%	27%	33%	35%	29%	24%	38%
Three-vessel	11%	36%	10%	35%	25%	60%	4%

MR, mitral regurgitation.

12

nostic testing and stabilization so that undue time is not expended and renal insufficiency does not result in irreversible renal failure. Stabilization should be undertaken to keep the patient alive while arrangements are being made for surgery and to improve, when possible, pulmonary edema and peripheral perfusion, but stabilization should not delay surgery.

Provide airway protection and mechanical ventilation assistance as needed. If the patient has sufficient blood pressure and tissue perfusion, pure arterial vasodilators (such as hydralazine) may be used to facilitate forward ejection by the left ventricle (Figs. 12-20 to 12-22).[23] Inotropic support may be useful to maximize contractile function and to confer afterload reduction especially in hypotensive and congested patients. IABP improves

Table 12-5. Severity of Mitral Regurgitation by Contrast Ventriculography

MR Grade (Sellers)	Contrast Ventriculography Findings
1+	Contrast in LA < contrast in LV and clears from the LA in a single beat
2+	Contrast in LA > contrast in LV and clears from the LA in 3-5 beats
3+	Contrast in LA = contrast in LV
4+	Contrast in LA > contrast in LV
	± Opacification of the pulmonary veins
	± Opacification of the left atrial appendage

LA, left atrium; LV, left ventricle; MR, mitral regurgitation.

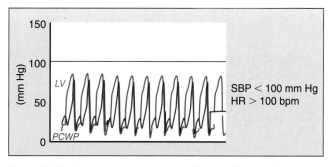

Figure 12-18. In acute severe or massive MR from PMR, the left ventricular systolic (arterial systolic) pressure is severely reduced, and the heart rate is elevated. The left atrial pulmonary capillary pressure is severely elevated, often with the pattern of a V wave.

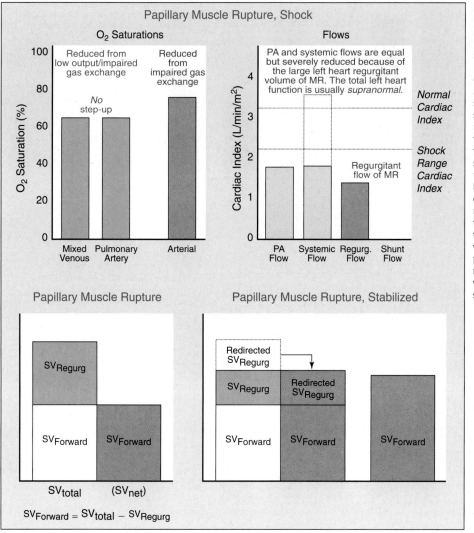

Figure 12-19. TOP, Hemodynamics of cardiogenic shock from severe MR due to PMR. There is no O_2 step-up detected on right-sided heart catheterization. Venous saturation is reduced because of reduced peripheral perfusion or increased peripheral extraction. Arterial saturation is decreased by impaired gas exchange. Right- and left-sided flows (Qp and Qs) are identical but severely reduced. There is a very large regurgitant volume-flow, more than 70% of the forward flow (i.e., more than half of the ejected blood is regurgitant). The summation of the net forward flow and the regurgitant flow is above normal, as the left ventricle is hyperdynamic. BOTTOM, The effect of afterload reduction on severe mitral insufficiency hemodynamics. In PMR, the total stroke volume (SV) is the sum of the regurgitant volume and the net forward volume. Afterload reduction, feasible in the presence of adequate blood pressure, redirects a proportion of the regurgitant volume forward, increasing the forward stroke volume.

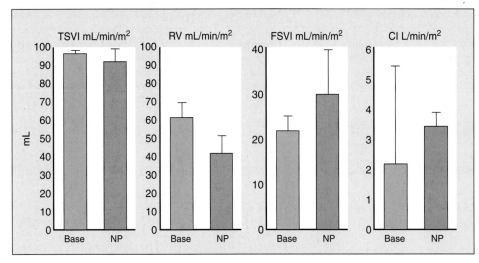

Figure 12-20. For patients with adequate blood pressure, arterial vasodilators (nitroprusside [NP]) reduce regurgitant volume (RV) and recover forward stroke volume index (FSVI) and cardiac index (CI). TSVI, total stroke volume index. (Data from Chatterjee K, Parmley WW, Swan HJ, et al: Beneficial effects of vasodilator agents in severe mitral regurgitation due to dysfunction of subvalvar apparatus. Circulation 1973;48:684-690.)

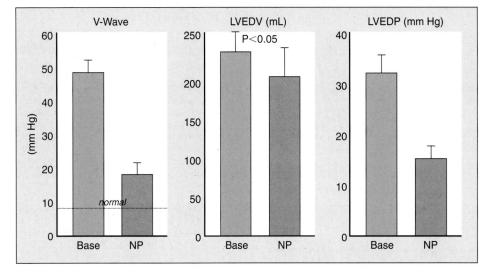

Figure 12-21. For patients with adequate blood pressure, arterial vasodilators (nitroprusside [NP]) reduce mitral regurgitation by enabling forward ejection: the magnitude of left atrial V waves reduces, as do the left ventricular end-diastolic volume (LVEDV) and pressure (LVEDP). (Data from Chatterjee K, Parmley WW, Swan HJ, et al: Beneficial effects of vasodilator agents in severe mitral regurgitation due to dysfunction of subvalvar apparatus. Circulation 1973;48:684-690.)

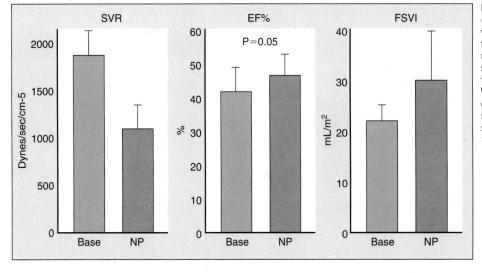

Figure 12-22. Arterial vasodilators (nitroprusside [NP]) reduce systemic vascular resistance (SVR), improve ejection fraction (EF), and increase forward regurgitant volume and recover forward stroke volume index (FSVI) and cardiac index. (Data from Chatterjee K, Parmley WW, Swan HJ, et al: Beneficial effects of vasodilator agents in severe mitral regurgitation due to dysfunction of subvalvar apparatus. Circulation 1973;48:684-690.)

acute mitral insufficiency hemodynamics.[24] IABP is the most effective means to improve systemic cardiac output and to alleviate pulmonary edema (Fig. 12-23).

Some cases of remarkable PMR salvages have occurred by extraordinary effort. A 59-year-old man in severe cardiogenic shock (blood pressure, 65/40 mm Hg; anuric) from postinfarction PMR who had been declined for surgery underwent percutaneous puncture of the left ventricular apex, then forceps introduction into the left ventricular cavity to grasp the ruptured papillary muscle and to provide traction onto the mitral apparatus. The degree of mitral insufficiency lessened, and the hemodynamics dramatically recovered (blood pressure, urine output). The patient was at that point accepted for surgery, survived, and was symptom free at follow-up.[25]

Mitral valve replacement is the usual intervention. Mitral valve repair may be effected in highly selected patients, when the ruptured papillary muscle head or trunk can be sewn to a viable adjacent papillary muscle (Fig. 12-24).[26] The likelihood of finding such a viable muscle in proximity to a ruptured one is small.

The surgical mortality of mitral valve replacement for PMR is approximately 25% for non–cardiogenic shock cases and at least 40% for cardiogenic shock cases (38% in the SHOCK registry). Although the surgical mortality is substantial, the focus should be on the dominant salvage from surgical intervention (60% to 70%). Factors that determine operative risk include the severity of heart failure, the presence or absence of cardiogenic shock, and the duration of shock. Urgent surgical intervention is important to lessen the risk accrued by low output (renal failure).

Ninety percent 1-year postoperative survival has been reported in several series. The straightforward nature of the surgical intervention is achieved because of good residual left ventricular function (smaller infarcts than with septal rupture) and less complex lesions and repairs than for false aneurysms and septal ruptures (Figs. 12-25 and 12-26).

Long-term survival is determined by the residual left ventricular systolic function, which is generally good.[26,27]

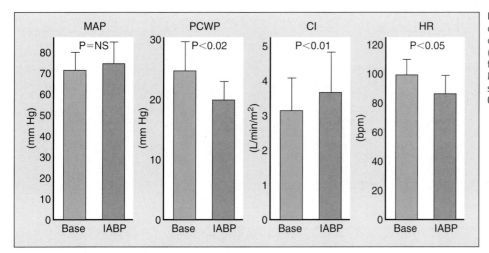

Figure 12-23. IABP lowers pulmonary capillary wedge pressure (PCWP), increases cardiac index (CI), and lowers heart rate (HR). MAP, mean arterial pressure. (Data from Kay GL, Kay JH, Zubiate P, et al: Mitral valve repair for mitral regurgitation secondary to coronary artery disease. Circulation 1986;74:I88-I89.)

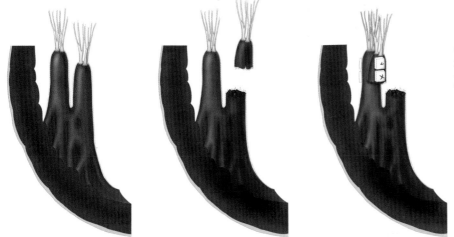

Figure 12-24. Illustration of a normal double-headed, single-trunk papillary muscle apparatus (LEFT IMAGE), an asymmetrically infarcted double-headed, single-trunk papillary muscle apparatus with complete rupture of one head (MIDDLE IMAGE), and a surgically repaired papillary apparatus with the ruptured head being sewn to the adjacent noninfarcted and intact papillary muscle head (RIGHT IMAGE).

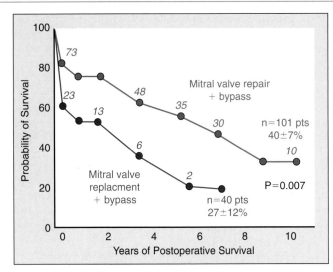

Figure 12-25. Among a population with severe mitral insufficiency, of which half of cases were PMR, performance of mitral valve repair and aortocoronary bypass surgery was associated with better postoperative survival than in patients undergoing mitral valve replacement (nonrandomized). (From Kay GL, Kay JH, Zubiate P, et al: Mitral valve repair for mitral regurgitation secondary to coronary artery disease. Circulation 1986;74:I88-I89.)

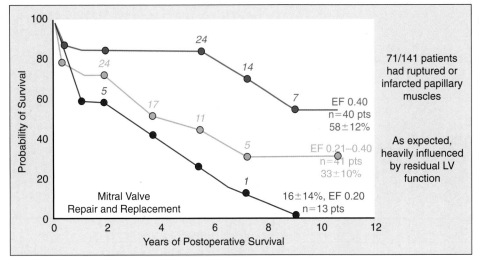

Figure 12-26. Among a population with severe mitral insufficiency, of which half of cases were PMR, postoperative survival was heavily influenced by systolic dysfunction. (From Kay GL, Kay JH, Zubiate P, et al: Mitral valve repair for mitral regurgitation secondary to coronary artery disease. Circulation 1986;74:I88-I89.)

CASE 1

History

▸ A 55-year-old man had presented to a community hospital with chest pains. He had been diagnosed with pleurisy (intermittent atypical, pleuritic chest pains; no rub, CK and troponins normal × 2).
▸ He returned to the emergency department several hours later in severe pulmonary edema and was transferred in cardiogenic shock.
▸ Intubated for respiratory support on arrival; IABP inserted for blood pressure support

Physical Examination

▸ BP 80/55 mm Hg, HR 115 bpm, ventilated
▸ Intubated, unresponsive; extremities cool—overt shock
▸ Venous distention, no edema
▸ S_1 soft or absent; S_2 loud
▸ 1/6 apical short and soft systolic murmur; no thrill
▸ Apex distinct, dynamic
▸ Urine output <10 mL/hr

Table 12-6. Hemodynamic Profile (with Inotropes)

	Physical Examination	Echocardiography	Catheterization
CVP	JVD (10 cm)	10 mm Hg	14 mm Hg
RVSP	Elevated (S_2 loud)	55 mm Hg	63 mm Hg
VSD	—	No evidence	No evidence
CI (systemic)	Shocky	1.4 L/min/m²	1.6 L/min/m²

CI, cardiac index; CVP, central venous pressure; JVD, jugular venous distention; RVSP, right ventricular systolic pressure; VSD, ventricular septal defect.

Clinical Impression

▸ Acute severe mitral insufficiency
▸ Rupture of the PMPM confirmed by TEE
▸ Small posterior infarction confirmed by TEE
▸ Cardiogenic shock and oliguria

Management and Evolution

▸ Surgery found ruptured PMPM and small inferoposterior infarction.
▸ Mitral valve replacement (mechanical) with aortocoronary bypass × 1 to the posterior descending coronary artery was performed.
▸ Ventilated for 5 days, discharged home in 12 days
▸ CCS class I, NYHA class I at follow-up
▸ Well for 3 months, then sudden development of shortness of breath and weakness
▸ Presented to community hospital hypotensive, in pulmonary edema, and transferred in cardiogenic shock

Subsequent Evolution and Outcome

▸ Emergent re-do mitral valve replacement for dehiscence
▸ Blood and tissue cultures negative. No clear evidence of endocarditis. Discharged 3 weeks later.
▸ The cycle of mitral valve replacement followed by dehiscence with heart failure or cardiogenic shock was repeated four times. The fourth mitral valve replacement was seated well enough to have only mild MR.
▸ On latest follow-up, although angina free, the patient has class II CHF and generalized debility after multiple surgeries aggravated by diaphragmatic paralysis.

Comments

▸ PMPM rupture (the most common) due to RCA disease
▸ Complete rupture and cardiogenic shock
▸ Treacherous presentation: non–Q wave myocardial infarction, presumably very late (possibly a week) presentation after biomarker normalization

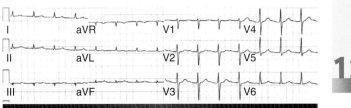

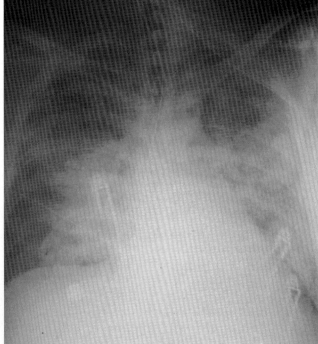

Figure 12-27. TOP, ECG shows sinus rhythm, no Q waves or ST deviations. This is a normal ECG with the exception of low voltages in the standard limb leads. BOTTOM, Chest radiograph shows normal cardiopericardial silhouette, severe bilateral airspace and interstitial (bat-wing) pulmonary edema, and IABP (tip low).

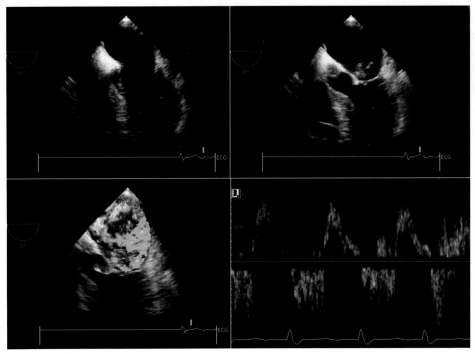

Figure 12-28. TEE. TOP LEFT, Lower esophageal 4-chamber view in diastole shows no apparent abnormality of the mitral valve. TOP RIGHT, Lower esophageal 4-chamber view in systole shows a complex mass on the atrial side of the mitral valve, probably a tangled complete rupture of the papillary muscle body and its chordae. The appearance of the closed mitral valve leaflets is abnormally angulated because of lack of tension support. BOTTOM LEFT, Severe mitral insufficiency. BOTTOM RIGHT, Pulmonary venous systolic flow reversal confirming severe mitral insufficiency.

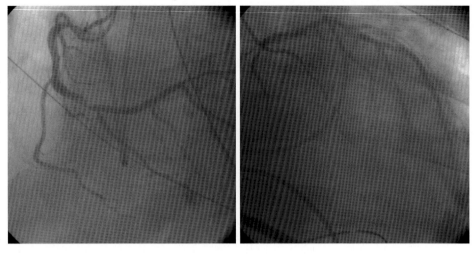

Figure 12-29. Selective coronary angiography. LEFT, RCA injection reveals dominance and a 70% proximal and a 90% distal stenosis. RIGHT, LCA injection does not reveal angiographically significant disease.

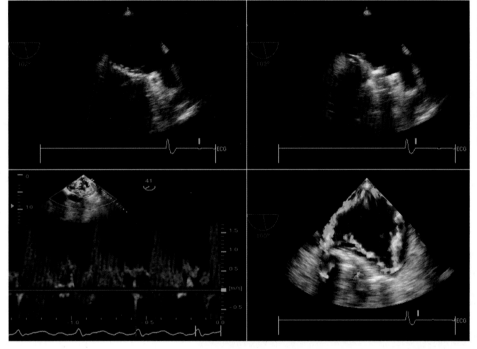

Figure 12-30. TEE. TOP IMAGES, The 2-chamber (vertical) views show frank rocking of the inferior portion of the mitral prosthesis. Mobile soft tissue elements on the atrial side are consistent with vegetations, or torn annular tissue. BOTTOM LEFT, Pulmonary venous flow. Systolic flow reversal confirms severe MR. BOTTOM RIGHT, The 2-chamber view with color Doppler flow mapping shows severe MR (large jet width and PISA) through the rocking portion of the mitral prosthesis.

▸ After initial surgery, the hemodynamics were normal, suggesting that the infarct was small and that the residual LV systolic function was normal.

▸ Operated on emergently before protracted oliguria; therefore, full renal function recovered postoperatively

▸ Murmur was soft and consistent with near-equilibration of LV and LA pressure. The S_1 was soft or absent because of low LV systolic pressure and noncoaptation of the mitral leaflets.

▸ Despite RCA occlusion with only one opacified acute marginal branch, no right ventricular infarction was apparent clinically, presumably because the RCA occlusion was chronic.

▸ Diagnosis by echocardiography to elucidate cardiac cause of shock

▸ Long and hard-fought course because of either septic or sterile annular necrosis

CASE 2

History

- 65-year-old woman presented to her family physician with 3 days of worsening shortness of breath
- Known COPD and long history of smoking. A chest pain episode had occurred 10 days before. The family physician identified a murmur and referred her for an echocardiogram.
- Severely distressed with respiratory fatigue in the echocardiography laboratory; transferred to the CCU for intubation

Physical Examination

- BP 110/55 mm Hg, HR 120 bpm (regular), ventilated
- Intubated, poorly responsive; extremities warm
- Venous distention, no edema
- S_1 soft, S_2 loud
- 3/6 short apical systolic murmur; no thrill
- Apex distant, dynamic
- Crepitations bilaterally
- Urine output < 20 mL/hr

Clinical Impression

- Rupture of the ALPM due to circumflex artery disease and lateral infarction
- Severe mitral insufficiency
- Cardiogenic shock and oliguria

Management and Evolution

- Surgery found rupture of the ALPM and small lateral wall infarction.
- Mitral valve replacement (mechanical) with aortocoronary bypass × 1 to the posterior descending coronary artery was performed.

- Excellent postoperative hemodynamics
- Slow (6 weeks) wean from ventilator

Subsequent Evolution and Outcome

- Developed gram-positive sepsis in the ICU
- Sudden development of a murmur and shock
- TEE revealed a dehisced mitral valve replacement
- Emergent repeated mitral valve replacement was performed.
- Although the hemodynamics were restored, respiratory failure was severe.
- The patient died in the ICU 3 months later.

Comments

- ALPM rupture (the uncommon PMR) due to nondominant circumflex disease and lateral STEMI; presumably, the pain 10 days before was the responsible infarction.
- Incomplete rupture and cardiogenic shock
- After initial surgery, the hemodynamics were normal, suggesting that the infarct was small and that the residual LV systolic function was normal.
- Emergency surgery avoided permanent renal dysfunction despite preoperative oliguria.
- The murmur was short, consistent with elevated left atrial pressure (V wave) and late systolic near-equilibration of LV and LA pressure.
- Long and hard-fought course initially because of underlying COPD and then from early prosthetic valve endocarditis, which is more commonly encountered with emergency valve surgery

12

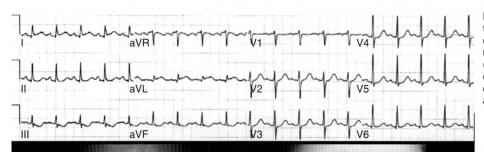

Figure 12-31. TOP, ECG shows sinus tachycardia, ST elevation in aVL, and down-sloping ST depression III, aVF. BOTTOM, Chest radiograph shows interstitial (acute) pulmonary edema, mild cardiomegaly, lung overinflation, and barrel chest (increased anteroposterior dimension and flat diaphragms).

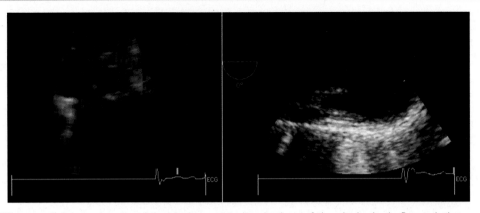

Figure 12-32. LEFT, TTE zoom apical 4-chamber view of the mitral apparatus shows prolapse of the mitral valve leaflets and what appears to be a partially torn papillary muscle head (round mass). RIGHT, TEE view of the descending aorta demonstrates protruding atheromatous material, which on real-time imaging included mobile elements.

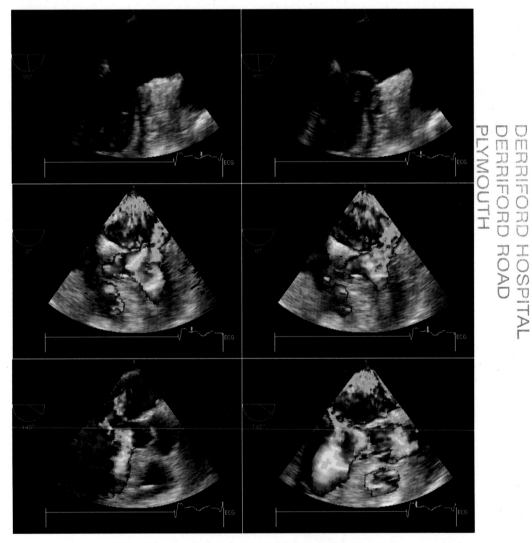

Figure 12-33. TEE view. TOP, Lower esophageal 2-chamber views in diastole (LEFT) and systole (RIGHT). There is prolapse of the mitral leaflets and a mobile round mass consistent with a partially ruptured papillary muscle body; by the location of the papillary muscle head (anteriorly), it is from the ALPM. MIDDLE, Color Doppler flow mapping shows a large PISA and a large regurgitation jet, consistent with severe mitral insufficiency. BOTTOM, The PISA from the mitral insufficiency is so large that it fills the LVOT.

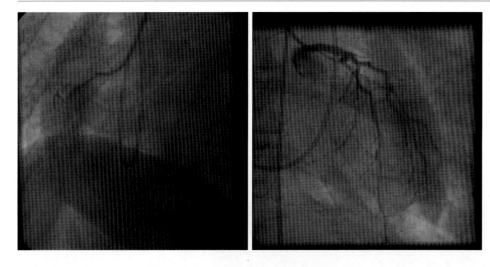

Figure 12-34. Selective coronary angiography. LEFT, RCA injection. The RCA is occluded proximally with only the conus branch or a first acute marginal branch filling. RIGHT, LCA injection reveals no angiographically significant disease to the left anterior descending coronary artery but mid circumflex disease and opacification of the distal RCA.

CASE 3

History

▸ 72-year-old man with no known past medical history had presented to a community hospital a week before with shortness of breath and chest pains due to an inferior myocardial infarction
▸ CHF developed and worsened, and a systolic murmur was heard.
▸ He was transferred for TEE because TTE image quality was poor.

Physical Examination

▸ BP 100/50 mm Hg, HR 100 bpm (regular), RR 24/min
▸ Alert, warm extremities
▸ Venous pressure and contour normal, no edema
▸ S_1, S_2 normal
▸ 3/6 short apical systolic murmur; no thrill
▸ Apex distant; crepitations bilaterally
▸ Urine output: 40 mL/hr

Clinical Impression

▸ Partial rupture of the PMPM
▸ Posterior infarction and associated right ventricular infarction
▸ Severe heart failure associated with the partial rupture

Management, Evolution, and Outcome

▸ Surgery found partially ruptured PMPM, posterior infarction, and right ventricular infarction.
▸ Mitral valve replacement (mechanical) with aortocoronary bypass × 1 to the posterior descending coronary artery was performed.
▸ Excellent postoperative hemodynamics
▸ Slow (2 weeks) wean from ventilator; discharged 2 weeks later
▸ CCS class I and NYHA class I at follow-up
▸ Died the following winter from pneumonia and COPD

Comments

▸ PMPM rupture (the more common PMR)
▸ Incomplete rupture caused mild cardiogenic shock.
▸ Associated right ventricular infarction
▸ After initial surgery, the hemodynamics were normal, suggesting that the infarct was small and that the residual LV systolic function was normal.
▸ Operated on emergently before protracted oliguria; therefore, renal function recovered postoperatively
▸ Initially prolonged admission because of underlying COPD

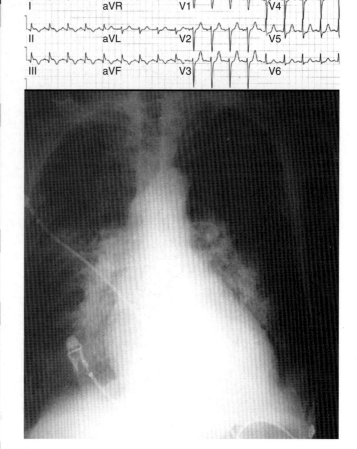

Figure 12-35. TOP, ECG shows sinus tachycardia, inferior ST elevation, and T-wave inversion, suggestive of a recent inferior myocardial infarction and no apparent posterior myocardial infarction. BOTTOM, Chest radiograph shows mild cardiomegaly and interstitial pulmonary edema (marked hyperinflation may be suggestive of emphysema).

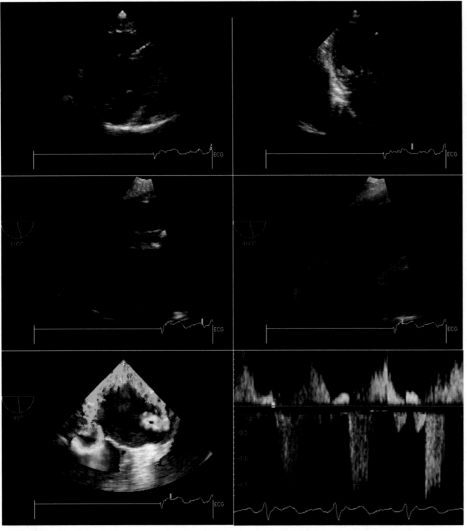

Figure 12-36. TOP LEFT, TTE parasternal short-axis view. Flipping soft tissue element at the medial mitral commissure. Inferior akinesis was present and normal septal contraction. TOP RIGHT, Apical 2-chamber view shows akinesis of the inferoposterior wall and possible disruption of a head of the PMPM. MIDDLE, TEE transgastric long-axis views of the mid left ventricle show discontinuity in the middle of the PMPM and marked wobbling of the body of the papillary muscle. The underlying LV wall is akinetic. BOTTOM LEFT, Vertical 2-chamber view with color Doppler mapping shows severe mitral insufficiency (large jet, large PISA). BOTTOM RIGHT, Spectral Doppler imaging of pulmonary venous flow shows flow reversal, indicative of severe mitral insufficiency.

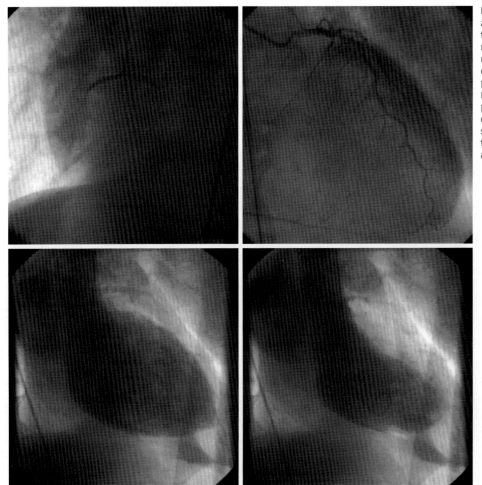

Figure 12-37. TOP ROW, Selective coronary angiography. RCA injection (LEFT) reveals total proximal occlusion (before the acute marginal branches). LCA injection (RIGHT) reveals only mild proximal disease and diagonal disease but collaterals to the posterior descending coronary artery. BOTTOM ROW, Contrast ventriculography (RAO projection) shows inferior akinesis but dynamic anterior wall contraction. There is severe mitral regurgitation (opacification of the pulmonary veins and atrial appendage) and left atrial dilation.

CASE 4

History

▸ 68-year-old woman transferred for coronary angiography; inferior STEMI 8 days before (received fibrinolytics at hour 1; CK 350)
▸ Postinfarction angina and mild heart failure. Reinfarction at day 5: CK peak 600, transient heart failure
▸ Past medical history is significant for hypertension, CCS class II angina for 2 years.

Physical Examination

▸ Venous pressure and contour normal, no edema
▸ S_1, S_2 normal
▸ No murmurs or rubs; apex distant; crepitations bilaterally
▸ Urine output: 80 mL/hr
▸ Angiography scheduled for the next morning
▸ New 3/6 pansystolic murmur noted and mild CHF; sudden pulseless electrical activity (PEA) arrest

Comments

▸ Acute rupture of the entire PMPM (the more common PMR)
▸ Complete rupture resulting in PEA cardiac arrest
▸ No murmur associated with the "wide-open" MR because there was equilibration of the left atrial and left ventricular pressures, with no tension on the mitral valve
▸ Infarction with reinfarction increases the risk of rupture.

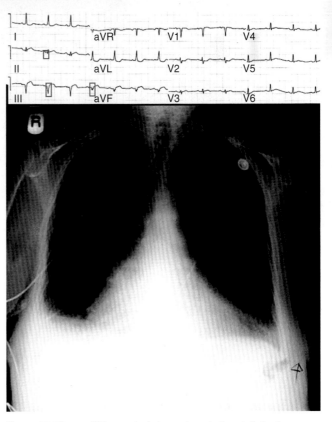

Figure 12-38. TOP, ECG on arrival shows sinus rhythm, inferior Q waves, and ST elevation, suggestive of a recent inferior myocardial infarction and no apparent posterior myocardial infarction. BOTTOM, Chest radiograph on arrival shows mild cardiomegaly and no pulmonary edema.

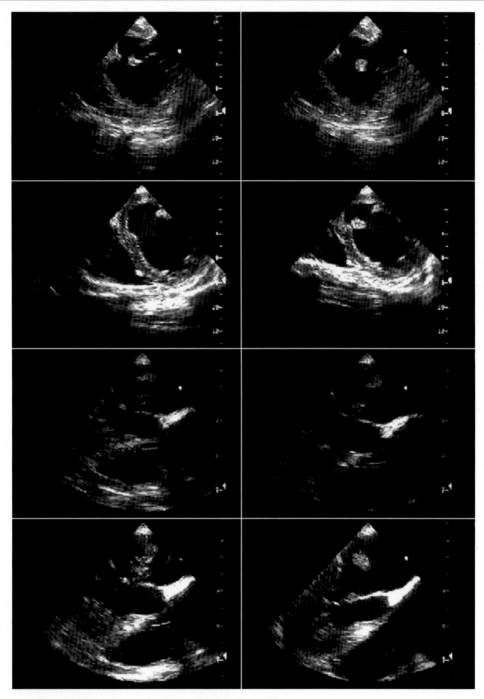

Figure 12-39. TEE images during cardiac arrest and resuscitation. TOP FOUR IMAGES, Transgastric short-axis views show a complete rupture of the PMPM, moving into and out of the plane of imaging. BOTTOM FOUR IMAGES, Basal transgastric views that also show the ruptured body of the papillary muscle in the left atrium, windmilling around erratically and tangled in chordae.

CASE 5

History

▸ 79-year-old woman 3 days after anterior STEMI (late presentation, no fibrinolytics)
▸ Initially no CHF, but CHF developed and progressed during 3 days.
▸ Past medical history is significant for hypertension.

Physical Examination

▸ Well appearing; BP 110/60 mm Hg (usual is 160/90), HR 90 bpm (on beta-blockers), RR 10/min
▸ Venous pressure and contour normal, no edema
▸ S_1, S_2 normal
▸ Apical 3/6 pansystolic murmur; no rubs
▸ Apex not dilated, displaced, or enlarged; no crepitations
▸ Urine output: 80 mL/hr

Clinical Impression

▸ Rupture of the ALPM was suspected but not proven by TTE.
▸ Lateral infarction
▸ Severe heart failure due to MR, not LV systolic dysfunction

Management, Evolution, and Outcome

▸ Surgery found ruptured ALPM and small lateral infarction.
▸ Mitral valve replacement (mechanical) with aortocoronary bypass × 2 (to OM2 and PDA) was obtained.

▸ In coming off cardiopulmonary bypass, the blood pressure was excellent; the lateral wall then ruptured through the infarct zone and underwent repair.
▸ Postoperative hemodynamics were excellent.
▸ Ventilated for 3 days, discharged home 8 days later
▸ CCS class I and NYHA class I at follow-up

Comments

▸ Non–Q wave myocardial infarction complicated by PMR, underscoring that papillary muscles are subendocardial and vulnerable to subendocardial infarction
▸ ALPM involved (accounts for only 10% of all PMRs)
▸ Hypertension may have contributed to the papillary and free wall ruptures.
▸ Mitral valve replacement normalized hemodynamics, which is the usual case because PMR is usually associated with small infarctions of previously normal ventricles.
▸ Although the diagnosis was suspected clinically, it was not made by TTE and was made definitively only at surgery.

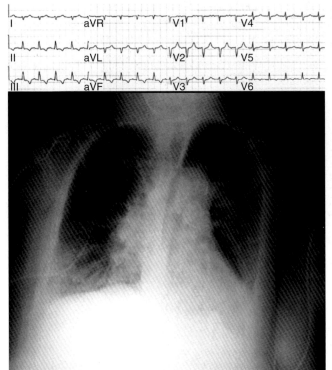

Figure 12-40. TOP, ECG shows sinus tachycardia, small R waves and voltages in leads I and aVL. Widespread ST-T abnormalities suggest a lateral infarction. BOTTOM, Chest radiograph shows severe interstitial pulmonary edema, enlarged and calcified aortic arch, and normal cardiopericardial silhouette.

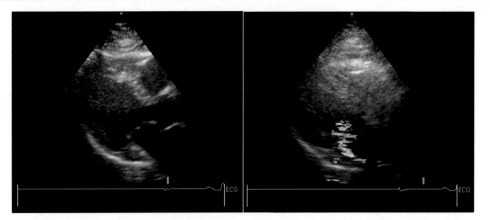

Figure 12-41. TTE parasternal long-axis views showing dynamic anterior septal and posterior walls and normal-size RV(OT). There is anterior mitral prolapse. The papillary muscle body is not visualized. Color Doppler flow mapping achieves only poor visualization of mitral insufficiency. Eccentric jet suggests severe MR, the mechanism of which is unclear.

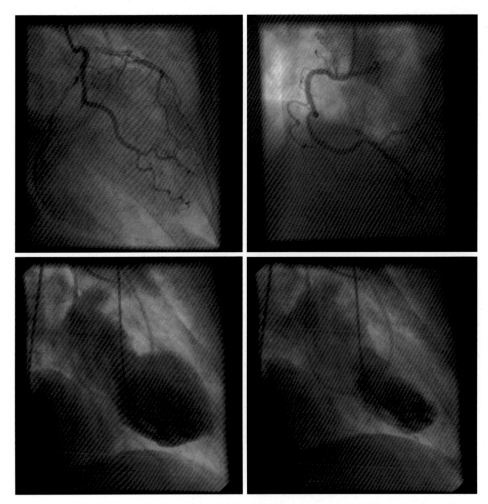

Figure 12-42. TOP ROW, Selective coronary angiography. LCA injection (LEFT) reveals minor disease in the left anterior descending coronary artery and occlusion of the left circumflex artery after a large marginal branch. RCA injection (RIGHT) reveals dominance of the artery and a mild lesion in the midportion after an acute marginal branch. BOTTOM ROW, Contrast ventriculography (RAO projection) shows akinetic inferior wall and dynamic anterior wall. There is left atrial dilation. Opacification of the pulmonary veins and left atrial appendage is indicative of severe MR.

CASE 6

History

▸ 51-year-old man after lateral non-STEMI
▸ Aortic valve replacement (mechanical) 5 years previously for aortic insufficiency from endocarditis of a bicuspid valve
▸ Three subtherapeutic INRs were recorded, then a small lateral wall myocardial infarction. At catheterization 5 years before, there was no angiographic coronary artery disease. Presumed embolic myocardial infarction
▸ Uneventful post–myocardial infarction course other than mild CHF and a new murmur of MR

Physical Examination

▸ Normal appearance, blood pressure, heart rate, and R-R interval
▸ Normal venous pressure and contour

▸ Normal opening and closing clicks, S₃ gallops
▸ 2/6 early peaking systolic ejection murmur at base; no murmur of aortic insufficiency
▸ 4/6 pansystolic murmur with axillary radiation; no thrill; no anterograde flow rumble
▸ Normal apex, no crepitations

Management and Outcome

▸ Surgery found partial rupture of the ALPM and small anterolateral infarction.
▸ Mitral valve replacement (mechanical) was obtained.
▸ Excellent postoperative hemodynamics
▸ Discharged home in 5 days
▸ CCS class I and NYHA class I at follow-up

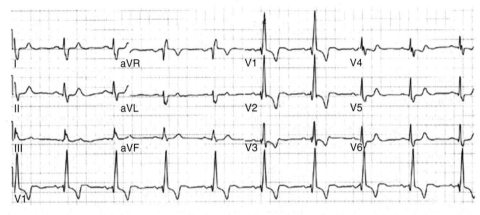

Figure 12-43. ECG shows sinus rhythm, right bundle branch block (old), and nonspecific lateral repolarization abnormalities.

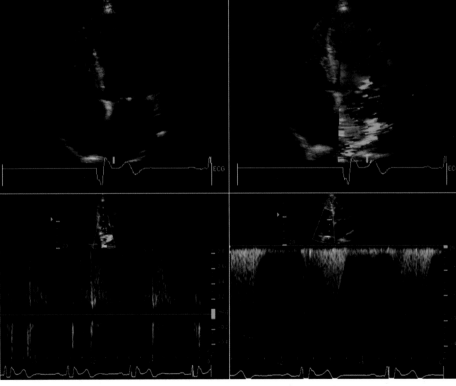

Figure 12-44. TTE apical 4-chamber views show poor endocardial definition, no obvious wall motion abnormalities, and no major abnormalities of the mitral apparatus, but there is severe MR. There is systolic flow reversal in the pulmonary vein (BOTTOM LEFT), consistent with severe MR. There is high-velocity TR, consistent with pulmonary hypertension (RVSP, 65 mm Hg).

Comments

▸ MR was unexpectedly due to papillary muscle infarction after myocardial infarction.
▸ The papillary muscles were never well visualized, hence the lack of anticipation of rupture.

▸ The ALPM is the more difficult to image.
▸ PMR due to subendocardial infarction
▸ Infarction due to embolization from the nontherapeutically anticoagulated aortic valve replacement
▸ Partial PMR and associated severe MR with heart failure

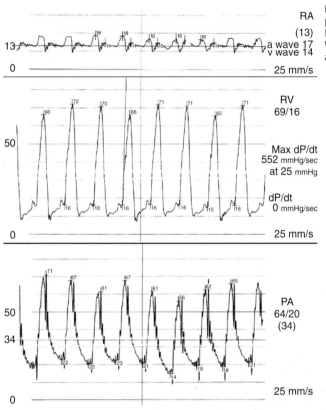

Figure 12-45. Cardiac catheterization tracings reveal moderate to severe pulmonary hypertension. TOP, Right atrium. MIDDLE, Right ventricle. BOTTOM, Pulmonary artery. There is elevation of the mean RA pressure and significant V waves. There is moderate to severe right ventricular systolic hypertension and elevation of the RV diastolic pressure.

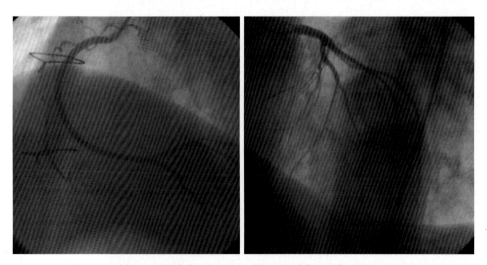

Figure 12-46. Selective coronary angiography shows no significant disease in either the right or left coronary artery.

CASE 7

History

▸ Frail and elderly 85-year-old woman admitted with a late-presentation non-STEMI
▸ Past medical history is significant for hypertension, chronic renal insufficiency.
▸ CK 1000. CHF worsened progressively during the next 3 days, requiring mechanical ventilation.
▸ A murmur of MR was heard on the second day; echocardiography that day showed MR with intact papillary muscles.

Physical Examination

▸ BP 90/60 mm Hg, HR 110 bpm (regular), ventilated
▸ Venous distention, no edema
▸ S₁ soft, S₂ loud
▸ 3/6 apical pansystolic murmur; no thrill
▸ Apex distant, dynamic
▸ Crepitations throughout lung fields
▸ Urine output: 25 mL/hr

Clinical Impression

▸ Inferoposterior infarction
▸ Borderline cardiogenic shock

▸ Severe MR, papillary muscles intact. The PMPM is clearly sitting in the middle of the infarct territory and, by virtue of its stretching, appears infarcted but intact.

Evolution and Outcome

▸ Refractory shock led to progression of renal failure, followed by death.

Comments

▸ PMPM rupture (the more common PMR)
▸ Incomplete rupture caused mild but eventually lethal cardiogenic shock.
▸ Q-wave myocardial infarction was the culprit in this case (as it is in 50% of all cases).
▸ Initially had severe MR from infarction of the papillary muscle, then developed worsened MR from frank rupture of the papillary muscle
▸ Murmur was short, consistent with elevated LA pressure (V wave) and late systolic near-equilibration of LV and LA pressure.

12

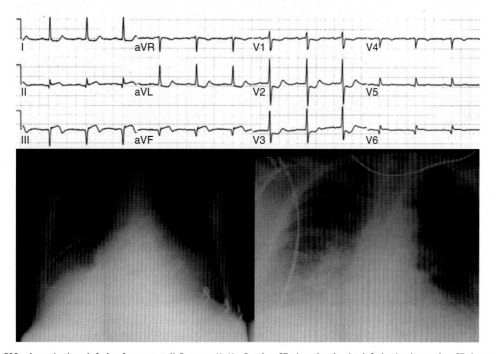

Figure 12-47. TOP, ECG: sinus rhythm; inferior Q waves, tall R waves V₁-V₃. Resting ST elevation in the inferior leads, resting ST depression V₂, V₃. V₄R not elevated. Inferoposterior infarction. BOTTOM LEFT, Chest radiograph on day 1 shows no heart failure. BOTTOM RIGHT, Chest radiograph on day 4 shows interstitial (acute) pulmonary edema.

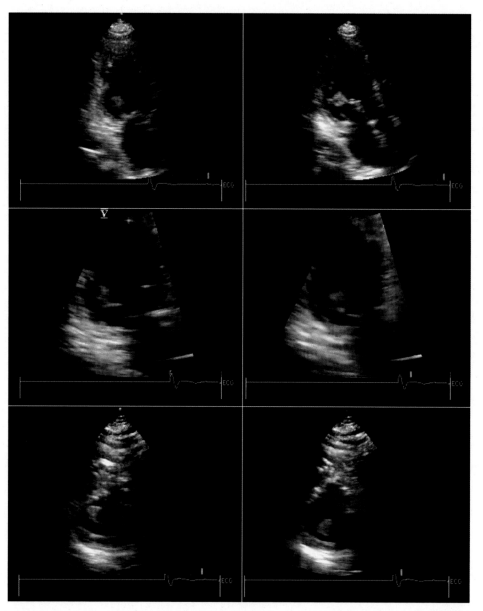

Figure 12-48. TTE apical and parasternal short-axis views demonstrating erratic motion and unclear attachment of the head of the PMPM.

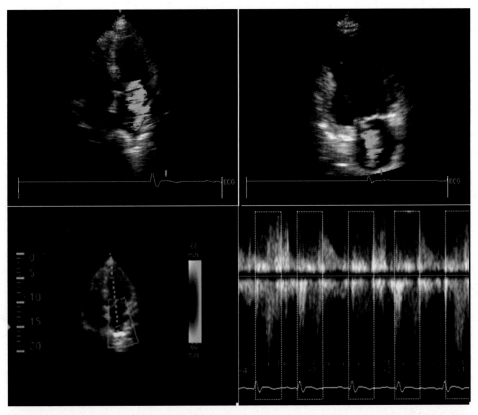

Figure 12-49. Color Doppler flow mapping reveals a large jet of MR consistent with severe MR. Pulmonary venous pulsed wave spectral recording detects systolic flow reversal diagnostic of severe MR. Other Doppler-derived findings included an RVSP of 70 mm Hg and a cardiac output of 1.6 L/min/m².

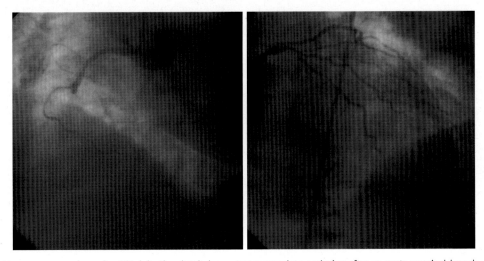

Figure 12-50. Selective coronary angiography. RCA injection (LEFT) demonstrates complete occlusion after an acute marginal branch. LCA injection (RIGHT) reveals small-caliber vessels and moderate disease of the proximal left anterior descending coronary artery and first diagonal. The distal RCA fills from the left injection.

CASE 8

History

▸ Very fit and active 80-year-old man presented to a community hospital with an inferior STEMI (received fibrinolytics at hour 4; CK 900).
▸ Uncomplicated course until day 3, when he developed sudden-onset severe shortness of breath without chest pain.

Physical Examination

▸ BP 90/60 mm Hg, HR 110 bpm (regular)
▸ Alert, cool extremities
▸ Marked venous distention, no edema
▸ S_1 soft, S_2 loud
▸ 1/6 short and soft apical systolic murmur; no thrill
▸ Apex distant, dynamic
▸ Crepitations throughout lung fields
▸ Urine output: 35 mL/hr

Clinical Impression

▸ Partial rupture of the PMPM
▸ Posterior infarction
▸ Borderline cardiogenic shock

Management, Evolution, and Outcome

▸ Surgery found ruptured PMPM, inferoposterior infarction, and RV infarction
▸ Mechanical mitral valve replacement with aortocoronary bypass × 2 to the left anterior descending coronary artery and to the posterior descending coronary artery was obtained.
▸ Excellent postoperative hemodynamics
▸ 1 week on the ventilator, discharged 5 weeks later
▸ Died of a pulmonary embolism while convalescing

Comments

▸ PMPM rupture (the more common PMR)
▸ Incomplete rupture caused mild cardiogenic shock.
▸ Q-wave myocardial infarction responsible in this case, as it is in 50% of cases.
▸ After initial surgery, the hemodynamics were normal, suggesting that the infarct was small and that the residual LV systolic function was normal.
▸ Operated on emergently before protracted oliguria; thus, renal function recovered postoperatively.
▸ Murmur was short, consistent with elevated LA pressure (V wave) and late systolic near-equilibration of LV and LA pressure, diagnosed by echocardiography.
▸ Although postoperative hemodynamics were excellent, his age-related slow convalescence unfortunately did not elude medical complications.

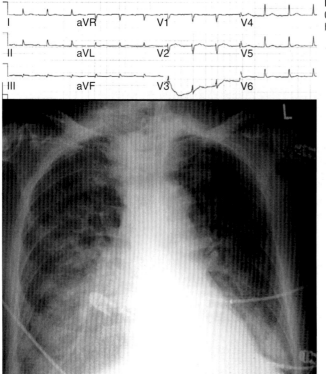

Figure 12-51. TOP, ECG shows sinus rhythm and inferior Q waves. BOTTOM, Chest radiograph shows interstitial (acute) pulmonary edema and normal heart size.

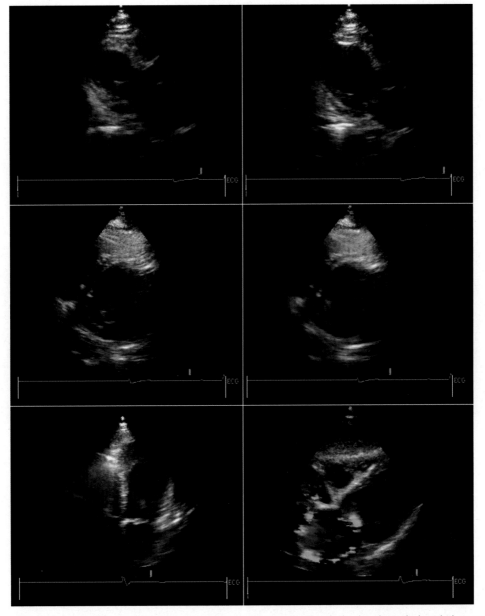

Figure 12-52. TTE. TOP, Parasternal long-axis views. MIDDLE, Parasternal short-axis views in diastole (LEFT) and systole (RIGHT) show erratic motion of the trunk of the PMPM and prolapse of the mitral valve. BOTTOM LEFT, Apical 4-chamber view also demonstrating prolapse of the mitral valve. BOTTOM RIGHT, Subcostal image demonstrating severe MR that extends all the way around the left atrium. Other Doppler-derived findings included an RVSP of 60 mm Hg and a cardiac output of 2.3 L/min/m².

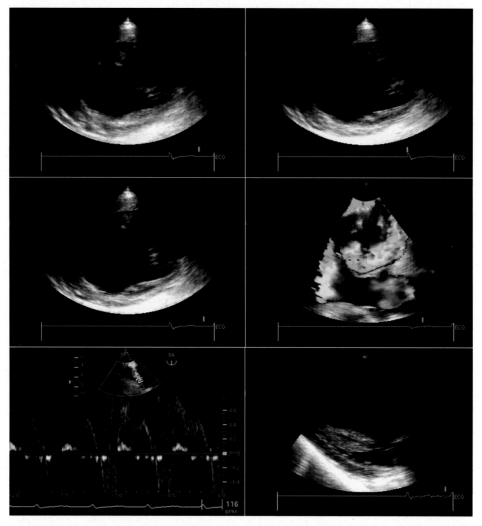

Figure 12-53. TEE. TOP, Transgastric long-axis views of the mid left ventricle show excess mobility of the PMPM. MIDDLE, Severe MR by color Doppler flow mapping and a large PISA. BOTTOM LEFT, Pulmonary venous flow reversal detected by pulsed wave Doppler sampling. BOTTOM RIGHT, Intactness of the ALPM is seen in its long axis.

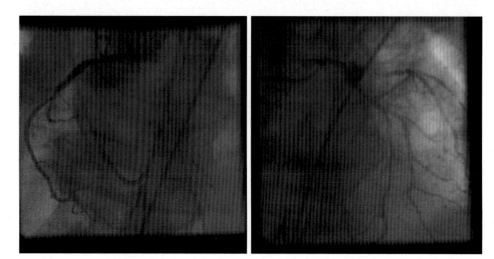

Figure 12-54. Selective coronary angiography. RCA injection (LEFT) shows a dominant RCA with subtotal occlusion in the midportion. LCA injection (RIGHT) reveals aneurysm of the left main coronary artery and a 60% mid left anterior descending coronary artery stenosis.

CASE 9

History

▸ 78-year-old woman admitted with an inferior STEMI
▸ Past medical history is significant for hypertension.
▸ Killip I at presentation; received fibrinolytic at hour 4
▸ Initial post–myocardial infarction evolution unremarkable: CK 800; no CHF
▸ At day 4, suddenly developed shock and severe pulmonary edema and was intubated emergently

Physical Examination

▸ BP 75/40 mm Hg, HR 120 bpm (regular), ventilated
▸ Unresponsive, cool extremities
▸ Venous distention, no edema
▸ S_1 soft, S_2 loud
▸ 2/6 short and soft apical systolic murmur; no thrill
▸ Apex distant, dynamic
▸ Crepitations throughout lung fields
▸ Urine output < 20 mL/hr

Clinical Impression

▸ Partial rupture of the PMPM
▸ Inferoposterior lateral infarction
▸ Cardiogenic shock and oliguria

Management, Evolution, and Outcome

▸ Mechanical mitral valve replacement with aortocoronary bypass × 3 (PDA, OM, left anterior descending coronary artery) was obtained.
▸ Surgery found ruptured PMPM and small posterolateral infarction.
▸ Excellent postoperative hemodynamics
▸ Ventilated for 6 days, discharged home in 2 weeks
▸ CCS class I and NYHA class I at follow-up

Comments

▸ Abrupt near-complete rupture of the PMPM (the more common PMR)
▸ Sudden development of cardiogenic shock
▸ Q-wave myocardial infarction responsible in this case
▸ After initial surgery, the hemodynamics were normal, suggesting that the infarct was small and that the residual LV systolic function was normal.
▸ Operated on emergently before protracted oliguria; therefore, renal function recovered postoperatively.
▸ Murmur was short, consistent with elevated left atrial pressure (V wave) and late systolic near-equilibration of left ventricular and left atrial pressure.
▸ Good outcome despite age and three-vessel coronary artery disease

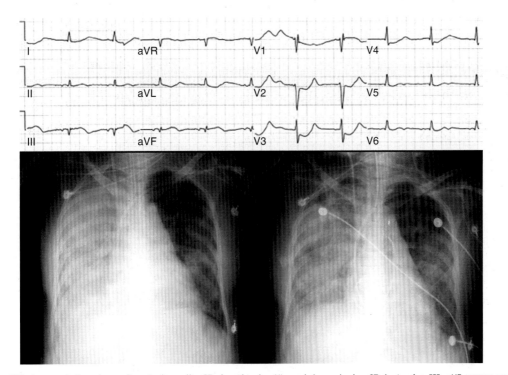

Figure 12-55. TOP, ECG at presentation shows sinus tachycardia, ST elevation in aVL, and down-sloping ST depression III, aVF. BOTTOM LEFT, Chest radiograph shows severe interstitial (acute) pulmonary edema, borderline cardiomegaly, ET tube in correct position. BOTTOM RIGHT, Chest radiograph showing IABP in correct position and PA catheter "looped" in right side of the heart.

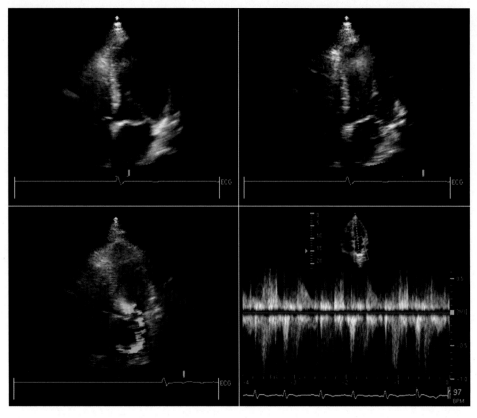

Figure 12-56. TTE. The plane of imaging falls along the PMPM complex. The body of the PMPM has an abnormal appearance (round) and motion (wobbling) and inconsistent continuity with the underlying myocardium.

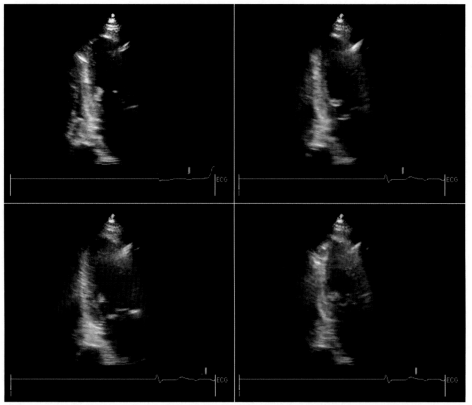

Figure 12-57. TTE apical 4-chamber views. Dynamic left ventricle on this plane of imaging. The ALPM comes into view (TOP RIGHT) and is intact. The plane of mitral coaptation is normal, but there is severe mitral insufficiency with an eccentric jet. BOTTOM RIGHT, Spectral display of pulsed wave Doppler recording of pulmonary venous flow. There is systolic flow reversal and aliasing consistent with severe mitral insufficiency.

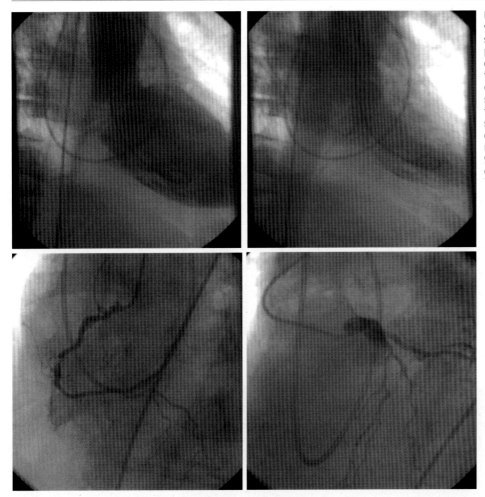

Figure 12-58. TOP, Contrast ventriculography in the RAO projection shows severe MR (opacification of the pulmonary veins and left anterior descending coronary artery appendage) and inferior hypokinesis. BOTTOM, Selective coronary angiography. RCA injection (LEFT) shows a dominant RCA with a 95% stenosis in the midportion. LCA injection (RIGHT) shows a 50% mid left anterior descending coronary artery stenosis and also a 50% mid left circumflex artery stenosis, but 90% stenosis of the first and second obtuse marginal branches.

12

CASE 10

History

▸ Frail 83-year-old demented man from a nursing home initially admitted with an upper GI bleed, requiring transfusions. He then developed dyspnea. Chest radiograph showed pulmonary edema. ECG changes were noted. There had been no chest pains.
▸ Mechanical ventilation was required when he experienced a respiratory arrest.

Physical Examination

▸ BP 95/55 mm Hg, HR 115 bpm (regular), RR 16/min
▸ Venous distention, no edema
▸ S_1 soft, S_2 loud, S_3 present; no rubs
▸ 3/6 apical pansystolic murmur; no thrill
▸ Apex distant, dynamic
▸ Crepitations throughout lung fields
▸ Urine output < 20 mL/hr

Clinical Impression

▸ Partial rupture of the PMPM
▸ Posterior infarction
▸ Severe heart failure from the severe MR

Evolution and Outcome

▸ His neurologic function had deteriorated because of the hypoxia before respiratory arrest.
▸ Given the age of the patient, underlying dementia, and recent severe hypoxic brain damage, surgical repair was not attempted.
▸ The patient never woke up and died a week later.

Comments

▸ Abrupt partial (nearly complete) rupture of the PMPM (the more common PMR)
▸ Localized posterior, non–Q wave myocardial infarction was responsible in this case.
▸ Several challenging aspects to the case: no chest pains, ECG changes appeared subendocardial but were not.
▸ The utility of establishing the cause of the murmur in a patient with an acute myocardial infarction was well demonstrated in this case.
▸ Medical comorbidities determined the outcome.

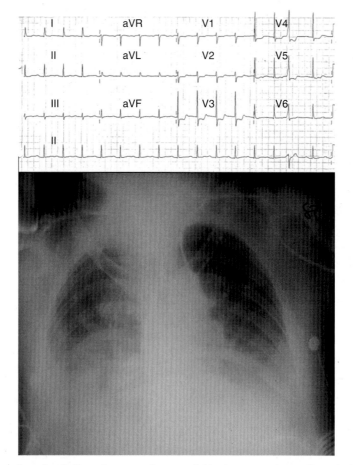

Figure 12-59. TOP, ECG shows sinus tachycardia, ST depression across the precordial leads. BOTTOM, Chest radiograph shows severe interstitial (acute) pulmonary edema and borderline cardiomegaly.

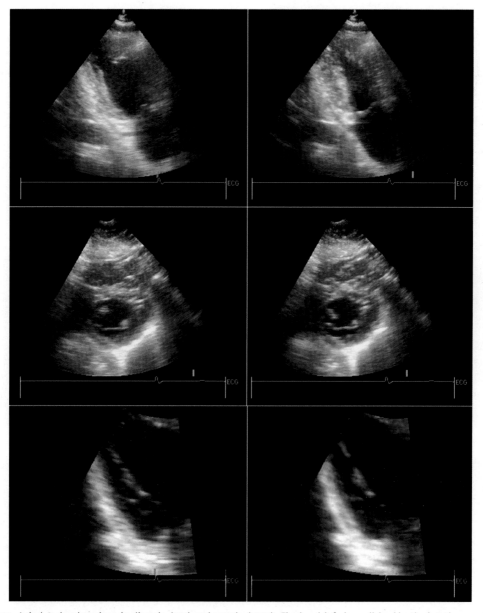

Figure 12-60. TTE. TOP, Apical 2-chamber views in diastole (LEFT) and systole (RIGHT). The basal inferior wall is akinetic, but the overall systolic function is good. MIDDLE, Parasternal short-axis views at the basal level of the LV show basal inferior akinesis. BOTTOM, Apical 2-chamber views in diastole (LEFT) and systole (RIGHT). The PMPM appears almost normal in diastole, other than a questionable interruption. In systole, the papillary muscle is stretched and more obviously partially disrupted in the middle portion.

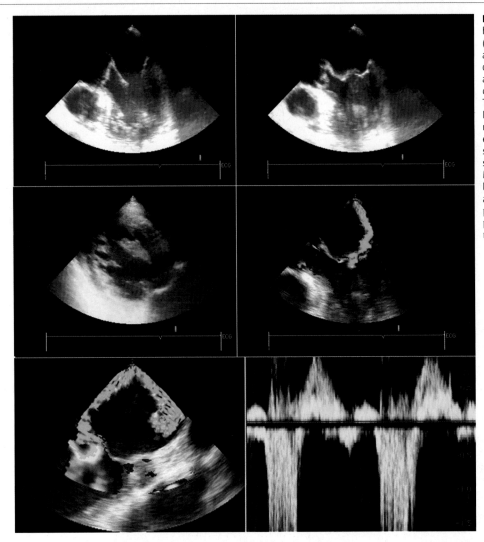

Figure 12-61. TEE. TOP, Lower esophageal horizontal 4-chamber views in diastole (LEFT) and systole (RIGHT). The mitral appearance in diastole is unremarkable. In diastole, there is prolapse of the anterior and the posterior leaflets due to loss of commissural support. MIDDLE LEFT, Transgastric long-axis view through the PMPM shows disruption of the papillary muscle body that is retained only by thin endocardial strands. MIDDLE RIGHT, From the site of commissural prolapse, there is severe, eccentric MR. BOTTOM LEFT, Severe MR is evident by large PISA and large and long jet to and around the posterior left atrium. BOTTOM RIGHT, Spectral display of pulsed wave Doppler sampling of pulmonary venous flow shows systolic flow reversal and aliasing.

CASE 11

History

▸ A 77-year-old man was transferred for angiography after an inferior infarction. On arrival, he was initially normotensive and comfortable. Shortly before undergoing angiography, he became distressed and restless and his blood pressure fell below 100 mm Hg systolic.
▸ While undergoing angiography, he became so distressed and hypotensive that he was intubated and sedated, and a dopamine infusion and IABP were started.
▸ Echocardiography was obtained to establish the cause of the deterioration.

Clinical Impression

▸ Near-complete rupture of the PMPM and severe MR complicating the infarction

Management, Evolution, and Outcome

▸ Emergent surgical mitral valve repair was obtained, with three-vessel aortocoronary bypass grafting.
▸ Surgery found partial, nearly complete rupture of the PMPM and small inferior infarction.

Outcome

▸ The patient survived.

Comments

▸ Inferior infarction: abrupt postinfarction shock from PMR and severe MR
▸ PMR from a small infarction

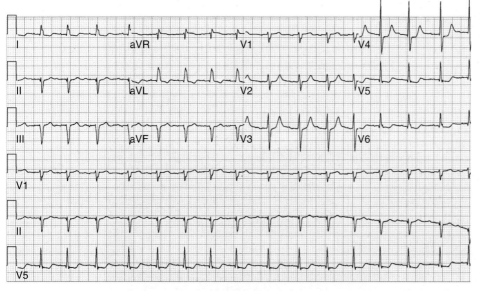

Figure 12-62. ECG shows sinus tachycardia with ST depression V₄-V₆.

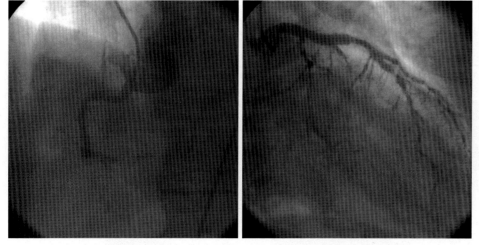

Figure 12-63. Selective coronary angiography. LEFT, RCA injection shows a subtotal occlusion in the midportion with a large volume of distal thrombus. RIGHT, LCA injection reveals angiographically significant disease of the left circumflex and left anterior descending arteries.

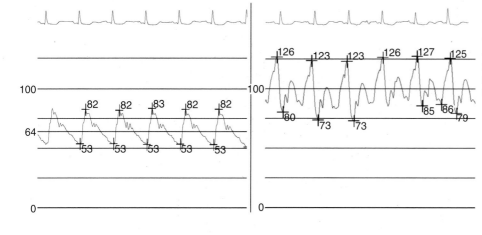

Figure 12-64. LEFT, Native-state hemodynamic study shows severe hypotension and a small pulse pressure. The patient is beta-blocked, reducing the tachycardic response to the hypotension. RIGHT, After IABP insertion (1:1 assistance) and dopamine infusion. Augmented pressures are prominently increased.

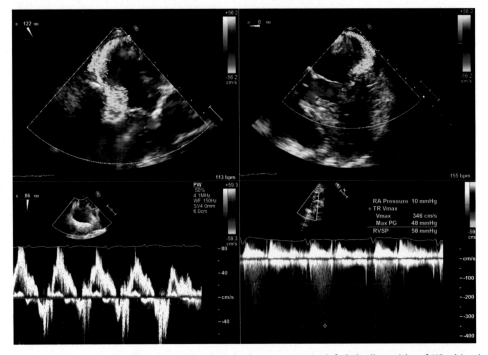

Figure 12-65. LEFT IMAGES, Transesophageal views. RIGHT IMAGES, Transthoracic views. TOP LEFT, An inferiorly directed jet of MR with a large PISA identifies severe MR and indirectly establishes that an anterior leaflet suspension problem is responsible. TOP RIGHT, By transthoracic imaging, the jet is clearly also laterally directed, also consistent with an anterior leaflet suspension problem. BOTTOM LEFT, TEE pulmonary venous sampling documents pulmonary venous systolic flow reversal and confirms that the MR is hemodynamically severe. BOTTOM RIGHT, Transthoracic parasternal Doppler sampling reveals high-velocity TR and a calculated RVSP of 58 mm Hg, consistent with hemodynamic severity.

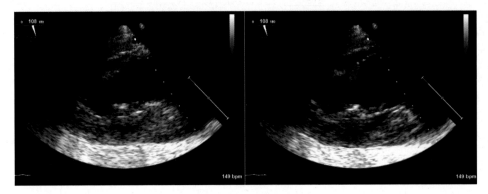

Figure 12-66. TEE transgastric views along the long axis of the PMPM. LEFT, The PMPM has a peculiar posterior angulation. RIGHT, The head of the trunk of the PMPM is severely, abnormally angulated, strongly suggestive of tissue discontinuity.

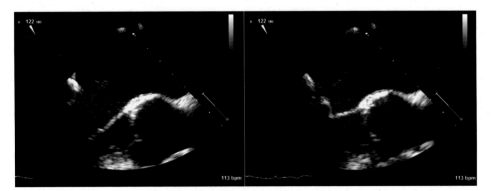

Figure 12-67. TEE lower esophageal images. LEFT, Diastolic image shows a normal-looking mitral valve. RIGHT, Systolic image shows a distinct prolapse of the anterior mitral leaflet, but the leaflets do not appear myxomatous.

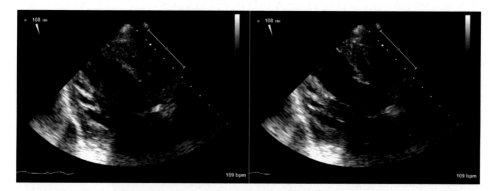

Figure 12-68. TEE transgastric views along the long axis of the PMPM. LEFT, The PMPM in diastole, without tension on it, appears normal. RIGHT, The abrupt "slice" across the body of the papillary muscle suggests disruption and rupture.

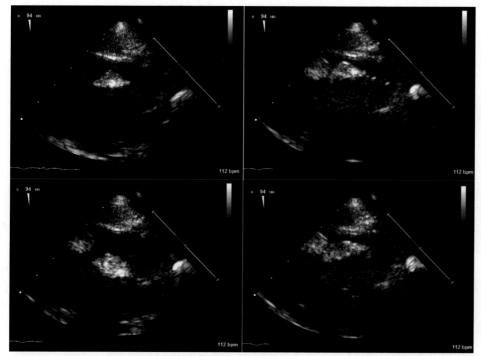

Figure 12-69. TEE transgastric views along the long axis of the PMPM. TOP LEFT, The head of the posteromedial trunk does not appear connected to a base. TOP RIGHT, A cleft is present in the trunk of the PMPM. BOTTOM LEFT, The cleft stretches to a wide gap in systole as tension is applied along it. BOTTOM RIGHT, There is a peculiar angulation of the long axis of the PMPM as it falls back into place in diastole.

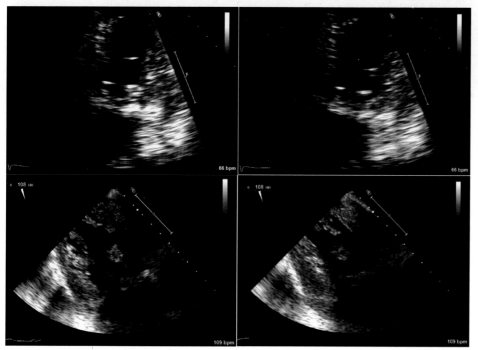

Figure 12-70. TOP ROW, TTE views of the LV cavity. Real-time images slightly but not definitely suggested a papillary muscle problem. BOTTOM ROW, TEE transgastric views along the long axis of the PMPM. Its variable separation from its base establishes that it has ruptured.

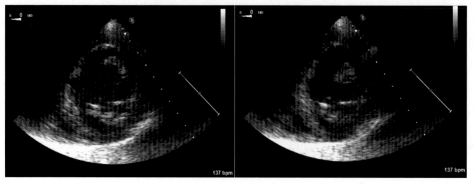

Figure 12-71. TEE transgastric short-axis views at the mid ventricle. The PMPM (at the 2-o'clock position) has excessive and erratic motion.

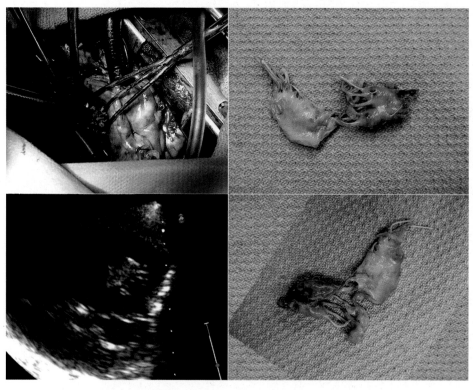

Figure 12-72. TOP LEFT, The chest is opened, the heart is stopped, and the left atrium is opened. The free end of the ruptured papillary muscle is being grasped by forceps. TOP RIGHT, Excised leaflets attached to ruptured papillary muscle. BOTTOM LEFT, TEE image of the partially ruptured papillary muscle in the left ventricle, askew at an odd angle, with chordal attachments to the mitral leaflets. BOTTOM RIGHT, Corresponding surgical specimen photograph.

References

1. Thompson CR, Buller CE, Sleeper LA, et al: Cardiogenic shock due to acute severe mitral regurgitation complicating acute myocardial infarction: a report from the SHOCK Trial Registry. SHould we emergently revascularize Occluded Coronaries in cardiogenic shocK? J Am Coll Cardiol 2000;36(Suppl A):1104-1109.
2. Srichai MB, Casserly IP, Lever HM: Cardiac tamponade masking clinical presentation and hemodynamic effects of papillary muscle rupture after acute myocardial infarction. J Am Soc Echocardiogr 2002;15:1000-1003.
3. Grigioni F, Enriquez-Sarano M, Zehr KJ, et al: Ischemic mitral regurgitation: long-term outcome and prognostic implications with quantitative Doppler assessment. Circulation 2001;103:1759-1764.
4. Coma-Canella I, Gamallo C, Onsurbe PM, Jadraque LM: Anatomic findings in acute papillary muscle necrosis. Am Heart J 1989;118:1188-1192.
5. Vlodaver Z, Edwards JE: Rupture of ventricular septum or papillary muscle complicating myocardial infarction. Circulation 1977;55:815-822.
6. Nishimura RA, Schaff HV, Shub C, et al: Papillary muscle rupture complicating acute myocardial infarction: analysis of 17 patients. Am J Cardiol 1983;51:373-377.
7. Lobo FV, El King D, Heggtveit HA: Rupture of both left ventricular papillary muscles following acute myocardial infarction. Can J Cardiol 1990;6:66-70.
8. Kaul S, Spotnitz WD, Glasheen WP, Touchstone DA: Mechanism of ischemic mitral regurgitation. An experimental evaluation. Circulation 1991;84:2167-2180.
9. Van Dantzig JM, Delemarre BJ, Koster RW, et al: Pathogenesis of mitral regurgitation in acute myocardial infarction: importance of changes in left ventricular shape and regional function. Am Heart J 1996;131:865-871.
10. Goldman AP, Glover MU, Mick W, et al: Role of echocardiography/Doppler in cardiogenic shock: silent mitral regurgitation. Ann Thorac Surg 1991;52:296-299.
11. Joseph MX, Disney PJ, Da Costa R, Hutchison SJ: Transthoracic echocardiography to identify or exclude cardiac cause of shock. Chest 2004;126:1592-1597.
12. Moursi MH, Bhatnagar SK, Vilacosta I, et al: Transesophageal echocardiographic assessment of papillary muscle rupture. Circulation 1996;94:1003-1009.
13. Haskell RJ, French WJ: Accuracy of left atrial and pulmonary artery wedge pressure in pure mitral regurgitation in predicting left ventricular end-diastolic pressure. Am J Cardiol 1988;61:136-141.
14. Fuchs RM, Heuser RR, Yin FC, Brinker JA: Limitations of pulmonary wedge V waves in diagnosing mitral regurgitation. Am J Cardiol 1982;49:849-854.
15. Pichard AD, Kay R, Smith H, et al: Large V waves in the pulmonary wedge pressure tracing in the absence of mitral regurgitation. Am J Cardiol 1982;50:1044-1050.
16. Hawley JG, Little RC, Feil H: Further studies on the cardiodynamics of experimental intraventricular communications. Circulation 1950;1:321-328.
17. Drobac M, Schwartz L, Scully HE, Utley-Taylor MM: Giant left atrial V-waves in post–myocardial infarction ventricular septal defect. Ann Thorac Surg 1979;27:347-349.
18. Crenshaw BS, Granger CB, Birnbaum Y, et al: Risk factors, angiographic patterns, and outcomes in patients with ventricular septal defect complicating acute myocardial infarction. GUSTO-I (Global Utilization of Streptokinase and TPA for Occluded Coronary Arteries) Trial Investigators. Circulation 2000;101:27-32.
19. Kishon Y, Iqbal A, Oh JK, et al: Evolution of echocardiographic modalities in detection of postmyocardial infarction ventricular septal defect and papillary muscle rupture: study of 62 patients. Am Heart J 1993;126 (pt 1):667-675.
20. Figueras J, Cortadellas J, Calvo F, Soler-Soler J: Relevance of delayed hospital admission on development of cardiac rupture during acute myocardial infarction: study in 225 patients with free wall, septal or papillary muscle rupture. J Am Coll Cardiol 1998;32:135-139.
21. Edwards BS, Edwards WD, Edwards JE: Ventricular septal rupture complicating acute myocardial infarction: identification of simple and complex types in 53 autopsied hearts. Am J Cardiol 1984;54:1201-1205.
22. Ryan TJ, Antman EM, Brooks NH, et al: 1999 update: ACC/AHA Guidelines for the Management of Patients With Acute Myocardial Infarction: Executive Summary and Recommendations: a report of the American College of Cardiology/American Heart Association Task Force on Practice Guidelines (Committee on Management of Acute Myocardial Infarction). Circulation 1999;100:1016-1030.
23. Chatterjee K, Parmley WW, Swan HJ, et al: Beneficial effects of vasodilator agents in severe mitral regurgitation due to dysfunction of subvalvar apparatus. Circulation 1973;48:684-690.
24. Gold HK, Leinbach RC, Sanders CA, et al: Intraaortic balloon pumping for ventricular septal defect or mitral regurgitation complicating acute myocardial infarction. Circulation 1973;47:1191-1196.
25. Sochman J, Vrbska J, Fridl P, et al: Catheter-based fixation of the mitral valve after acute papillary muscle rupture: a new technique for temporary hemodynamic stabilization. Catheter Cardiovasc Interv 1999;46:446-449.
26. Kay GL, Kay JH, Zubiate P, et al: Mitral valve repair for mitral regurgitation secondary to coronary artery disease. Circulation 1986;74:I88-I89.
27. Fasol R, Lakew F, Wetter S: Mitral repair in patients with a ruptured papillary muscle. Am Heart J 2000;139:549-554.

12

Index

Note: Page numbers followed by f indicate figures; those followed by t indicate tables.